Textbook for
DIPLOMA IN OPTOMETRY
II Year

Textbook for
DIPLOMA IN OPTOMETRY
II Year

As per the Syllabus and Curriculum of DO

Ajay Kumar Bhootra
B Optom DOS FAO FOAI FCLI
ICLEP FIACLE (Australia)
Diploma in Sportvision (UK)

Ex-CEO and Dean
Krishnalaya School of Optometry
Kolkata, West Bengal, India

Sumitra Agarwal
BHMS DMBS MD (Bio) M Optom B Optom DOS
Diploma in Sportvision (UK)

Optometrist and Ocularist
Private Practitioner

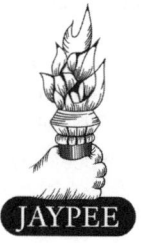

JAYPEE BROTHERS MEDICAL PUBLISHERS
The Health Sciences Publisher
New Delhi | London

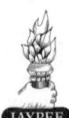 **Jaypee Brothers Medical Publishers (P) Ltd**

Headquarters

Jaypee Brothers Medical Publishers (P) Ltd
EMCA House, 23/23-B
Ansari Road, Daryaganj
New Delhi 110 002, India
Landline: +91-11-23272143, +91-11-23272703
+91-11-23282021, +91-11-23245672
Email: jaypee@jaypeebrothers.com

Corporate Office

Jaypee Brothers Medical Publishers (P) Ltd
4838/24, Ansari Road, Daryaganj
New Delhi 110 002, India
Phone: +91-11-43574357
Fax: +91-11-43574314
Email: jaypee@jaypeebrothers.com

Overseas Office

J.P. Medical Ltd
83 Victoria Street, London
SW1H 0HW (UK)
Phone: +44 20 3170 8910
Fax: +44 (0)20 3008 6180
Email: info@jpmedpub.com

Website: www.jaypeebrothers.com
Website: www.jaypeedigital.com

© 2024, Jaypee Brothers Medical Publishers

The views and opinions expressed in this book are solely those of the original contributor(s)/author(s) and do not necessarily represent those of editor(s) and publisher of the book.

All rights reserved. No part of this publication may be reproduced, stored or transmitted in any form or by any means, electronic, mechanical, photocopying, recording or otherwise, without the prior permission in writing of the publishers.

All brand names and product names used in this book are trade names, service marks, trademarks or registered trademarks of their respective owners. The publisher is not associated with any product or vendor mentioned in this book.

Medical knowledge and practice change constantly. This book is designed to provide accurate, authoritative information about the subject matter in question. However, readers are advised to check the most current information available on procedures included and check information from the manufacturer of each product to be administered, to verify the recommended dose, formula, method and duration of administration, adverse effects and contraindications. It is the responsibility of the practitioner to take all appropriate safety precautions. Neither the publisher nor the author(s)/editor(s) assume any liability for any injury and/or damage to persons or property arising from or related to use of material in this book.

This book is sold on the understanding that the publisher is not engaged in providing professional medical services. If such advice or services are required, the services of a competent medical professional should be sought.

Every effort has been made where necessary to contact holders of copyright to obtain permission to reproduce copyright material. If any have been inadvertently overlooked, the publisher will be pleased to make the necessary arrangements at the first opportunity.

Inquiries for bulk sales may be solicited at: jaypee@jaypeebrothers.com

Textbook for Diploma in Optometry—II Year

First Edition: **2024**

ISBN: 978-93-5696-482-2

Printed at: Sterling Graphics Pvt. Ltd.

Preface

Discover the intricate world of optometry, where scientific expertise merges seamlessly with compassionate care, all in pursuit of enhancing and safeguarding one of our most invaluable senses—vision. This comprehensive guide is your gateway into the multifaceted realm of optometry, covering a spectrum of topics ranging from ocular diseases to the intricacies of mechanical optics, lenses and precise prescription techniques, right through to the nuances of nursing care procedures.

Whether you are a seasoned optometrist seeking to deepen your knowledge or a budding student venturing into this captivating field, this book is your indispensable companion. It serves as a beacon of insight and practical wisdom, illuminating every aspect of optometry with clarity and depth. In a discipline where innovation and research continually redefine the landscape, this guide is meticulously crafted to not only provide a robust foundation in optometric principles but also to offer a tantalizing glimpse into the future of vision care.

From the fundamental principles of refraction to the nuanced management of ocular diseases, each chapter is meticulously curated to offer a blend of theoretical comprehension and real-world application. As your journey through these pages, you will gain not only a deeper understanding of the core tenets of optometry but also a profound appreciation for its transformative potential in shaping the future of vision health.

Ajay Kumar Bhootra
Sumitra Agarwal

Acknowledgments

Writing a book is not a solitary endeavor; it is a collaborative journey enriched by the support, encouragement, and contributions of many individuals. As we pen down these words of acknowledgment, we extend our deepest gratitude to those whose presence and efforts have shaped this work.

First and foremost, we express our heartfelt thanks to our family members for their unwavering support and understanding during the countless hours spent immersed in research and writing.

To our mentors and advisors, their guidance have been invaluable. Their wisdom, constructive feedback, and expert insights have played a pivotal role in shaping the content of this book.

We extend our special thanks to Dr Madhu Chaudhary (Director—Educational Publishing) and Dr Upma Tomar (Development Editor) of Jaypee Brothers Medical Publishers who have believed in us and motivated us to take the initiative.

We are also indebted to Shri Jitendar P Vij (Group Chairman), Mr Ankit Vij (Managing Director), Mr MS Mani (Group President), Ms Pooja Bhandari [Director-Production (Books and Journals)], Ms Sunita Katla (EA to Group Chairman and Publishing Manager), Mr Ajay Kumar Sharma [DGM (Books and Journals)], Ms Samina Khan (EA to Director-Educational Publishing), Mr Rajesh Sharma (Production Coordinator), Ms Seema Dogra (Cover Visualizer) and Neha Verma (Graphic Designer) of Jaypee Brothers Medical Publishers (P) Ltd., New Delhi for production process. Their dedication to excellence and attention to detail have transformed the manuscript into a polished and professional work.

Last but not least, we extend our gratitude to the readers. We hope the pages ahead offer insights, inspiration, and a meaningful contribution to the subject matter.

Contents

1. **Details of Diseases of Eye** 1
   - Common Symptoms in Ophthalmology and Examination of Eye *1*
     » Common Symptoms *1*
   - Error of Refraction *6*
     » Myopia *7*
     » Hypermetropia *9*
     » Astigmatism *9*
     » Presbyopia *11*
   - Diseases of Lacrimal Apparatus *12*
     » Dry Eyes *12*
     » Watering of Eyes *14*
     » Lacrimal Tumors *15*
     » Dacryocystitis *17*
   - Diseases of Eyelids *18*
     » Stye *18*
     » Chalazion *20*
     » Blepharitis *21*
     » Ptosis *23*
     » Lagophthalmos *25*
     » Trichiasis *26*
     » Blepharospasm *28*
     » Entropion *29*
     » Ectropion *30*
   - Diseases of Conjunctiva *31*
     » Conjunctivitis *31*
     » Pterygium *34*
     » Pinguecula *35*
     » Red Eyes *36*
   - Diseases of Cornea *37*
     » Keratitis *37*
     » Corneal Ulcer *39*
     » Corneal Opacity *40*
     » Keratoconus *41*
     » Keratoplasty *43*
   - Diseases of Sclera *44*
     » Episcleritis *44*
     » Scleritis *45*
     » Staphyloma *46*
   - Diseases of Uvea *47*
     » Uveitis *47*
     » Endophthalmitis *48*
     » Panophthalmitis *48*
   - Diseases of Lens *48*
     » Cataract *48*
     » Latest Techniques in Surgery of Cataract *50*
     » Subluxation/Dislocation of Lens *51*
   - Diseases of the Angle of Anterior Chamber *52*
     » Glaucoma *52*
   - Diseases of Vitreous *54*
     » Vitreous Hemorrhage *54*
     » Vitreous Opacities *56*
     » Vitrectomy *57*
   - Diseases of Retina *58*
     » Diabetic and Hypertensive Retinopathy *58*
     » Retinal Detachment *59*
     » Central Serous Retinopathy *61*
     » Cystoid Macular Edema *62*
     » Retinoblastoma *62*
     » Central Retinal Artery Occlusion *62*
     » Central Retinal Vein Occlusion *63*
     » Branch Retinal Artery Occlusion *63*
     » Branch Retinal Vein Occlusion *63*
     » Eale's Disease *63*
   - Diseases of Optic Nerve *63*
     » Optic Neuritis *63*
     » Papilledema *64*
     » Optic Atrophy *64*
   - Destructive Surgeries of Eyeball *64*
     » Enucleation *64*
     » Evisceration *65*
     » Orbital Exenteration *65*
   - Strabismus *65*
     » Paralytic Squint *65*
     » Non-paralytic Squint *66*

- Diseases of Orbit *68*
  - » Proptosis *68*
  - » Orbital Fracture *68*
  - » Orbital Cellulitis *68*
- Community Ophthalmology *68*
  - » Blindness—Various Programs Related of Blindness *68*
- Miscellaneous *70*
  - » Vitamin A Deficiency *70*
  - » Impaired Tear Production *71*
  - » Low Vision Aids *71*
  - » First-aid in Ocular Injuries *73*
- Amblyopia *74*
- Color Blindness *74*

2. **Nursing Procedures like Vital Recording, IM/IV/SC Injection, Oxygen Therapy, Nebulization and IV Infusion**.................**76**
- Temperature Monitoring and Fever *76*
  - » Methods of Measurement *76*
  - » Normal Body Temperature *76*
- Pulse Monitoring *78*
  - » Normal Resting Heart Rate *78*
  - » Methods of Pulse Monitoring *78*
- Blood Pressure Monitoring *78*
  - » Normal Blood Pressure Range *79*
  - » Monitoring Blood Pressure at Home *79*
  - » Lifestyle Factors Affecting Blood Pressure *79*
- Respiration Monitoring *79*
  - » Respiratory Rate *80*
  - » Respiratory Depth *80*
  - » Respiratory Rhythm *80*
- Types of Injection Routes *81*
  - » Intramuscular *81*
  - » Subcutaneous *81*
  - » Intradermal *81*
  - » Intravenous *81*
  - » Intraosseous *81*
  - » Intraperitoneal *81*
  - » Intrathecal *82*
  - » Epidural *82*
  - » Intravenous Push *82*
- IM Injection *82*
  - » Location of Injection *82*
  - » Needle Size *82*
  - » Common Medications *82*
- IV Injection *83*
  - » Location of Injection *83*
  - » Needle and Catheter *83*
  - » Types of IV Injections *83*
- SC Injection *84*
  - » Location of Injection *84*
  - » Needle Size *84*
- Oxygen Therapy *84*
  - » Indications *85*
  - » Delivery Systems *85*
- Nebulization *86*
  - » Indications *86*
  - » Nebulizer Device *86*
- IV Infusion (also with Infusion Pump) *87*
  - » Indications for IV Infusion *87*
  - » IV Infusion Set-up *87*
- Care of Unconscious Patient *88*
  - » Common Reasons for Unconsciousness *88*

3. **Mechanical Optics, Lenses and Lens Prescription**..........................**91**
- A Brief History of Ophthalmic Lenses and Spectacles *91*
  - » History of Ophthalmic Lenses *91*
  - » History of Spectacles *95*
- Terms used in Lens Workshop *97*
  - » Lens Blank *97*
  - » Lens Surfacing *97*
  - » Lens Prescription *97*
  - » Lens Diameter *97*
  - » Effective Diameter *97*
  - » Refraction Index *98*
  - » Abbe Number *98*
  - » Crown *98*
  - » CR-39 *98*
  - » Spherical *98*
  - » Cylinder *98*
  - » Axis *99*
  - » Meridian *99*
  - » Optical Cross *99*
  - » Near Add *100*
  - » Prism *100*
  - » Decentration *100*
  - » Base Curve *100*
  - » Ocular Curve *100*
  - » Cross Curve *100*
  - » Surface Power *101*
  - » Surface Curvature *101*

- » Corridor Length *101*
- » Free-Form Technology *101*
- » Lacquer *101*
- » Etching *101*
- » Generator *102*
- » Lens Surfacing *102*
- » Lens Polishing *102*
- » Chiller *102*
- » Varnish *102*
- » Edging *102*
- » Glazing *102*
- » Bevel *102*
- » Lens Grooving *103*
- » Emery *103*
- » Abrasives *103*
- » Chuck *103*
- » Newton's Ring *103*
- » Test Plate *103*
- » Button *103*
- » Depression Curve *103*
- » Cribbing *103*
- » Shanking *104*
- » Trepanning Tool *104*
- » Lens Form *104*
- » Lens Marking *104*
- » Surface Power *104*
- » Transverse Test *104*
- » Vertex *104*
- » C-Sizer *104*
- » Caliper *104*
- » Colmascope *104*
- » Crazing *105*
- » Edger Vomit *105*
- » Equithin *105*
- » Groover *105*
- » Hide-A-Bevel *105*
- » Hydro-Phobic *105*
- » Image Jump *105*
- » Impact Resistance *105*
- » Segment Inset *105*
- » Laminated *105*
- » Lap *105*
- » Lens Clock *105*
- » Lens Washer *106*
- » Safety Bevel *106*
- » Swarf *106*
- Ophthalmic Lens Material *106*
  - » Glass Lens *106*
  - » Resin Lens *106*
  - » Curve Variation Factor *111*
- Lens Standards *113*
  - » ISO 8980 *113*
  - » ISO 12870 *113*
  - » ISO 14889 *113*
  - » ISO 16034 *113*
  - » ISO 21987 *114*
  - » ANSI Z80.1 *114*
  - » EN 1836 *114*
  - » AS/NZS 1067 *114*
- Ophthalmic Lens Blank Manufacture—Glass and Plastic *116*
  - » Glass Lens Blank Manufacturing *116*
  - » Plastic Lens Blank Manufacturing *122*
- Ophthalmic Prescription Lens Making *124*
- Lens Defects *126*
  - » Optical Aberrations *126*
- Ophthalmic Lens Designs *130*
- Types of Ophthalmic Lenses *133*
  - » Aspheric Lens *133*
  - » High Index *133*
  - » Multifocal Lenses *134*
  - » Bifocal and Trifocal Lenses *134*
  - » Photochromatic Lenses *136*
  - » Polarized Lenses *136*
  - » Tinted Lenses *138*
  - » Protective Lenses *139*
- Spectacles Frames: History, Nomenclature, Terminology and Classification *141*
  - » History of Spectacle Frames *141*
  - » Nomenclature and Terminology *146*
  - » Classification *151*
- Types of Frame Material *154*
  - » Plastic Frames *155*
  - » Metal Frames *157*
- Types of Human Faces and Choice of Frames *159*
  - » Types of Human Faces *159*
- Cosmetic and Functional Dispensing of Spectacles *161*
  - » Dispensing of Spectacles *161*
  - » Functional Aspect Spectacle Dispensing *163*
  - » Cosmetic Aspect Spectacle Dispensing *166*

- Measurement for Ordering Spectacles: IPD and VD *171*
  - » Interpupillary Distance *171*
  - » Vertex Distance Measurement *173*
  - » Special Measurement for Fitting Special Types of Lenses *174*
  - » Special Dispensing Measurements *174*
- Fitting of Lenses in Various Types of Frames *181*
  - » Lens Insertion into Zyl Frames *181*
  - » Lens Insertion into Supra Frames *182*
  - » Lens Insertion into Rimless Frames *183*
  - » Lens Insertion into Full-rim Metal Frames *183*
- Spectacles Intolerance *184*
  - » Reasons for Intolerance *184*
- Special Types of Spectacles *186*
  - » Task Specific Spectacles *186*
- Dispensing of Prisms and Prismatic Effect of Lens *189*
  - » Prismatic Effect of Lens *189*
  - » Dispensing of Prisms *193*
- Contact Lenses *195*
- Low Vision Aids *205*
- Magnifications of Lenses *208*

4. **Instruments and Equipment used in Eye** **213**
   - Refractometer *213*
   - Tonometer *215*
   - Lensmetry *218*
   - Ophthalmoscope *222*
   - Operating Microscope *224*
   - Slit Lamp Biomicroscope *225*
   - Gonioscope *249*
   - Pachymeter *250*
   - Ishihara Chart *251*
   - Perimeter *253*
   - Exophthalmometer *254*
   - A and B Scan *255*
     - » A-Scan (Amplitude Scan) *255*
     - » B-Scan (Brightness Scan) *256*
   - ERG, EOG and VER *257*
     - » ERG (Electroretinogram) *257*
     - » EOG (Electrooculogram) *257*
     - » VER (Visual Evoked Response or Visual Evoked Potential) *257*
   - Synoptophore *258*
   - Other Orthoptic Instruments *259*
     - » Amblyoscopes *259*
     - » Haploscopes *259*
     - » Bagolini Striated Glasses *260*
     - » Maddox Rod *260*
     - » Worth 4-Dot Test *260*
   - Keratometer *260*
     - » General Principle of Keratometer *260*

5. **Community Ophthalmology** **263**
   - National Programme for Control of Blindness *265*
     - » Objectives of National Programme for Control of Blindness *265*
     - » Plan of Action *267*
     - » Activities *269*
   - Blindness: Causes and its Prevention *276*
     - » Causes of Blindness *276*
     - » Strategies to Address Eye Conditions to Avoid Vision Impairment *278*
   - National Immunization Programme *279*
     - » Immunization *280*

6. **Drugs used in Optometry** **283**
   - Vascular Endothelial Growth Factor *283*

Index *285*

CHAPTER 1

Details of Diseases of Eye

Ajay Kumar Bhootra, Sumitra Agarwal

COMMON SYMPTOMS IN OPHTHALMOLOGY AND EXAMINATION OF EYE

COMMON SYMPTOMS

Vision and refractive-related symptoms in ophthalmology are often associated with issues affecting the clarity and focusing of vision and are indicative of refractive errors such as myopia, hyperopia, astigmatism, or presbyopia. The following is the list of common vision and refractive-related symptoms:

Blurred Vision

Blurry vision is the loss of sharpness of eyesight, making the objects appear out of focus and hazy. The loss of sharpness occurs because of defocused image. It can also be because of degraded and deshaped image. While the defocused image is brought to focus by spherical correction, degraded and deshaped image is corrected by cylinder correction with its axis placed at appropriate direction. Numerous possible combinations of sphere powers, cylinder powers, and cylinder axes can be used to correct. Blurred vision can manifest in various ways, and different types of blurriness may indicate different underlying eye conditions, for example:
❖ Blur vision can be permanent or transient.
❖ Blur vision can be intermittent and fluctuating.
❖ Blur vision can be episodic or sudden with the condition worsening over time.

Permanent blur vision can be because of defocused, degrade and deshape image. It can be caused by ocular condition or refractive error or presbyopia. Transient blur vision can occur due to local and systemic causes. Pressure from a tumor or swelling of lids may involve transient astigmatic changes. Certain eye drops and medications can also cause blurring of vision. Intermittent blur vision in near viewing distance may be because of dry eyes. Insufficient tear production or poor quality tears can cause blurred vision, particularly when reading, using a computer, or watching TV for extended periods. Intermittent blur vision at distance may be because of accommodative spasm. Intermittent blur vision may simply mean tiredness, eye strain or over-exposure to sunlight. Fluctuating vision refers to frequent changes in the clarity of vision. A patient may have blurred vision that comes and goes. Fluctuating vision may be a sign of diabetes or hypertension which are chronic conditions that can damage the blood vessels in the retina. Any damage to the retina can cause permanent vision loss, and so a patient with fluctuating vision should seek immediate medical attention. Episodic visual blurring is an important clinical indicator of vascular insufficiency in the occipital cortex of the brain. Sudden blur vision can be a medical emergency and include stroke, steep increase in blood pressure, hyphema, retinal detachment, concussion, infection of the eye and its tissues, migraine, eye injury. In addition to above blurred vision may be for distance vision, near vision, night vision, monocular, binocular, and peripheral blurred vision.

Asthenopia

Asthenopia refers to eye strain or discomfort that can result from prolonged or intense use of the eyes. It is a common condition that may occur in individuals of all ages, and it is often associated with activities that involve visual concentration. Asthenopia can be temporary and relieved with rest, but in some cases, it may be a symptom of an underlying vision problem or other eye-related issues. The symptoms of asthenopia may include eye fatigue, headaches, pain, sensation of burning or irritation in the eyes, light sensitivity, focusing difficulties, etc.

Dry Eyes

Dry eyes are a common visual symptom that occurs when the eyes do not produce enough tears or when the quality of the tears is compromised. Tears are essential for maintaining the health of the front surface of the eye and for clear vision. When the eyes are dry, it can lead to discomfort and various visual symptoms. Dry eyes can cause fluctuations in vision, making objects appear intermittently blurry. The eyes may feel itchy and irritated. It may also cause a burning or stinging sensation, leading to discomfort. Paradoxically, dry eyes can sometimes trigger an overproduction of reflex tears, resulting in watering of eyes.

Double Vision

Double vision, also known as diplopia, can sometimes be related to refractive errors, but it can also be associated with other underlying eye conditions. It is important to note that double vision can also be a symptom of more serious eye conditions or health issues that may include muscle imbalance, cataracts, neurological issues or trauma. Head injuries or trauma to the eye area can damage the muscles or nerves involved in eye movement, leading to double vision.

Glare, Flare and Halos around the Light

Glare, flare, and halos around lights are visual symptoms that individuals may experience, and they can be associated with various eye conditions. These symptoms are often related to issues with how the eye handles light, and they can impact visual comfort and clarity. Glare refers to excessive brightness or dazzling light that can be discomforting and may interfere with vision. Flare is the scattering of light within the eye, leading to the perception of scattered light or veiling glare. Halos are circular rings of light that surround a light source, often seen at night. Glare may be caused by oncoming headlights while driving at night, sunlight reflecting off surfaces and bright lights in an indoor environment. Presence of bright light sources in the visual field and light scattering in the eye due to certain eye conditions or abnormalities may cause flare. Cataracts and corneal abnormalities or irregularities may cause glare and halos.

Distorted Vision

Distorted vision refers to a condition where objects appear misshapen, blurred, or distorted. This visual symptom can be caused by various eye conditions or abnormalities in the visual system. Astigmatism may lead to distorted vision at all distances, keratoconus may cause distorted vision, and macular degeneration can lead to distorted central vision. Retinal detachment, diabetic retinopathy and glaucoma can cause distorted vision. Some individuals may experience visual distortions during a migraine headache. Certain medications may have visual side effects, leading to distorted vision in some cases. Physical trauma to the eye or head can cause changes in the structure of the eye or affect the visual pathways, resulting in distorted vision. Dislocation or displacement of the eye's natural lens can lead to distorted vision.

Red Eyes

Red eyes are caused by the dilation of blood vessels on the eye's surface, and it can be associated with various factors, conditions, or external irritants. Conjunctivitis, dry eye syndrome, environmental irritants, subconjunctival hemorrhage, corneal ulcer, uveitis, blepharitis, glaucoma are several reasons that may lead to red eyes. If red eyes persist, cause discomfort, or are accompanied by other concerning symptoms.

Stringy Mucus in or around the Eyes

The presence of stringy mucus in or around the eyes can be a visual symptom associated with various eye conditions or factors affecting the tear film. This symptom is often indicative of issues with tear production, tear quality, or the overall health of the ocular surface. Some common causes of stringy mucus in or around the eyes are Dry eye syndrome, allergic conjunctivitis, blepharitis, conjunctivitis, meibomian gland dysfunction (MGD), subconjunctival hemorrhage, etc. Certain systemic conditions, such as autoimmune diseases or rheumatoid arthritis, can affect the health of the ocular surface and contribute to stringy mucus.

Increased Blinking

Blinking is a normal and necessary function of the eyes, helping to spread tears evenly over the ocular surface, protect the eyes from foreign objects, and maintain overall eye health. However, an increase in blinking frequency or duration may be associated with certain conditions or factors, the common among them are dry eye syndrome, eye irritation or allergies, corneal abrasions or foreign bodies, conjunctivitis, nervous system disorders, and medication side effects. Uncorrected or under-corrected refractive errors can lead to eye strain, discomfort, and increased blinking. Prolonged periods of intense visual concentration, such as staring at a screen for extended periods and blepharospasm may lead to increased blinking.

Eye Squeezing

Eye squeezing can be a behavior exhibited for various reasons, and it may be associated with different visual symptoms. Squeezing the eyes can be a natural response to shield the eyes from excessive light. Prolonged periods of visual concentration, such as reading or using digital devices, can lead to eye strain and fatigue. Squeezing the eyes may provide a brief relief from strain. Individuals experiencing headaches or migraines may find relief by squeezing their eyes shut, especially if light sensitivity is associated with the headache. Stress or tension can manifest in various ways, including tightness or discomfort around the eyes. Squeezing the eyes may be a response to stress. During intense concentration or focus, individuals may squeeze their eyes shut momentarily. This behavior can be observed in various activities, such as problem-solving or deep thinking. Allergic reactions, especially those affecting the eyes, can cause itching and discomfort. Squeezing the eyes may be an attempt to relieve the itching. Some individuals may habitually squeeze eyes.

Foreign Body Sensation

The sensation of a foreign body in the eye, despite the absence of an actual object, is known as a "foreign body sensation" or "feeling of something in the eye." This symptom can be quite uncomfortable and may be associated with various underlying causes that may include dry eye syndrome, conjunctivitis, corneal abrasions or scratches, allergic conjunctivitis, blepharitis, conjunctival papillae. Exposure to smoke, dust, wind, or other irritants may also lead to foreign body sensation, redness, tearing.

Flashes of Light

Flashes of light are visual symptoms characterized by the perception of brief, flickering, or flashing lights in the visual field. These flashes can appear as sparks, streaks, or arcs of light and may be described by individuals as seeing "stars" or "lightning." Flashes of light can be associated with various underlying causes that may include retinal detachment, posterior vitreous detachment, and vitreous floaters. A blow to the head or eye can stimulate the retina and cause flashes of light.

Floaters

Floaters are visual symptoms characterized by the perception of small, dark spots, specks, or cobweb-like shapes that seem to "float" in the field of vision. These floaters move with the eye's movements and are most noticeable against a bright background, such as a clear sky or a white wall. Floaters are typically caused by the presence of tiny particles or clumps of gel-like substance in the vitreous, the gel that fills the inside of the eye. The common causes of floaters include age-related changes, posterior vitreous detachment (PVD), retinal tears or detachment. Blood in the vitreous, often due to a retinal blood vessel hemorrhage, can cause floaters. Conditions like diabetic retinopathy or vascular disorders may contribute to bleeding. Inflammatory conditions within the eye, such as uveitis, can result in the presence of floaters. Individuals with high myopia may be more prone to developing floaters due to the elongation of the eyeball and changes in the vitreous.

Loss of Peripheral Vision

The loss of peripheral vision, also known as peripheral visual field loss or tunnel vision, refers to a reduction or absence of vision in the outer areas of the visual field. This can affect an individual's ability to see objects or movement to the side or around the edges of their visual field. Peripheral vision loss can be associated with various eye conditions or neurological disorders. Some of the common among them are glaucoma, retinitis pigmentosa, optic nerve disorders, stroke or brain injury, retinal detachment, chronic retinal diseases, hypertensive retinopathy.

Difficulty Focusing

Problems adjusting focus between near and distant objects are often related to difficulties with accommodation, a process by which the eyes change their focus to see objects at different distances. This issue is commonly associated with accommodative insufficiency, accommodative excess, convergence insufficiency, and refractive errors.

Examination of Eye

The examination of the eyes refers to various tests and procedures applied to eye examination conducted by eye care professionals to assess the health and visual function of the eyes. Eye examinations can detect a variety of eye conditions, vision problems, and systemic health issues. The overview of the different tests and procedure is as follows:

Visual Acuity Test

The patient is asked to read letters or symbols from an eye chart to assess how well they see at various distances. This test helps determine the clarity of vision and the presence of refractive errors.

Contrast Sensitivity Test

Contrast sensitivity testing is a visual assessment that measures a person's ability to distinguish between subtle differences in light and dark or in the contrast between different objects. Unlike traditional visual acuity tests that focus on the ability to see fine details, contrast sensitivity tests assess the visual system's sensitivity to differences in contrast. Contrast sensitivity testing is often part of a comprehensive eye examination, especially when evaluating visual function beyond standard visual acuity. The results can provide valuable information for understanding an individual's overall visual capabilities and addressing specific visual challenges. The interpretation of contrast sensitivity results is typically done by eye care professionals who consider various factors, including age, lighting conditions, and the individual's visual needs.

Color Vision Testing

Color vision is a component of overall visual function. Testing color vision provides insights into the integrity of the visual system and its ability to perceive and interpret visual stimuli accurately. The primary diagnostic purpose of color vision tests is to identify color vision deficiencies. Certain medical conditions, such as retinal diseases, optic nerve disorders, or systemic diseases, can lead to acquired color vision problems. Color vision testing can be part of a comprehensive eye examination to detect and monitor these conditions.

Clinical Refraction

Clinical refraction includes multiple tests in the eye examination process aim to measure refractive error that includes spherical, cylinder and near addition for the purpose of correction either by surgical or non-surgical method. The procedure is not only about achieving clear vision but also about optimizing visual comfort and reducing eye strain. Eye care professionals consider factors such as working distance, reading habits, and individual visual needs when prescribing corrective lenses. It is a collaborative process between the practitioner and the patient and the collaboration ensures that the prescribed lenses meet the patient's visual requirements and contribute to overall eye health and well-being.

Retinoscopy

Retinoscopy is an objective method to determine the refractive status of the eye with respect to the point of fixation. The test is not dependent upon the subject's response. Often the test is the first test used to peep inside the patient's eyes.

Slit Lamp Examination

Slit lamp examination provides a detailed view of the anterior segment of the eye, including the cornea, iris, and lens.

Tonometry

Tonometry measures intraocular pressure to assess for conditions like glaucoma.

Dilated Fundus Examination

Dilated fundus examination involves dilating the pupil to examine the retina, optic nerve, and blood vessels at the back of the eye.

Visual Field Test

Visual field test assesses peripheral vision and can detect abnormalities indicative of certain eye conditions.

Ophthalmoscopy

Direct examination of the interior of the eye, including the retina and optic nerve, using an ophthalmoscope is a common procedure of comprehensive eye examination.

Corneal Topography

Corneal topography maps the shape of the cornea which is useful for evaluating conditions like keratoconus.

Ultrasound Imaging

Ultrasound imaging uses sound waves to create images of the eye's internal structures, helpful for assessing conditions in opaque media.

Optical Coherence Tomography

Optical coherence tomography (OCT) provides high-resolution cross-sectional images of the retina and optic nerve.

Fluorescein Angiography

Fluorescein angiography involves injecting a dye to evaluate blood flow in the retina and identify abnormalities.

Visual Evoked Potential

Visual evoked potential (VEP) records electrical activity in the visual cortex of the brain to assess visual function.

ERROR OF REFRACTION

The term "error of refraction" refers to a condition in which the eye has difficulty focusing light onto the retina, leading to blurred vision. The most common types of errors of refraction are shown in **Flowchart 1.1**.

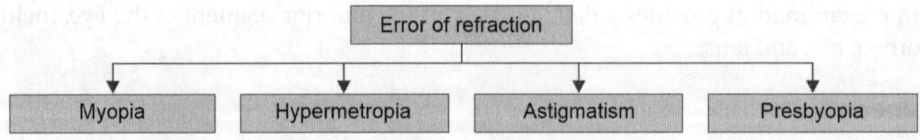

Flowchart 1.1: Error of refraction.

MYOPIA

Myopia, commonly known as nearsightedness, is a refractive error of the eye where close objects can be seen clearly, but objects at a distance appear blurry. This occurs when the eyeball is too long or the cornea has too much curvature. As a result, light entering the eye is focused in front of the retina instead of directly on it.

Myopia is a common refractive error affecting the eye's ability to focus on distant objects, leading to blurred vision. Beyond its impact on visual clarity, myopia can exert far-reaching consequences, influencing career choices and heightening the risk of serious vision-threatening disorders. The hallmark indication of myopia is difficulty seeing objects at a distance, a condition typically correctable with appropriate minus-power lenses.

However, the prevalence of myopia is a cause for concern due to its widespread occurrence and the potential to contribute to visual impairment. Managing myopia is of paramount importance, not only to enhance visual acuity but also to mitigate the associated risks of vision-threatening conditions such as glaucoma, retinal fractures, and detachment. The myopic eye presents a significant challenge due to its propensity to contribute to visual morbidity.

Efforts in myopia management involve tailored interventions, ranging from corrective lenses to advanced treatments aimed at controlling the progression of myopia, particularly in younger individuals. Regular eye examinations are crucial for early detection and appropriate management, ensuring that individuals with myopia receive the necessary care to safeguard their long-term eye health. As ongoing research explores the multifaceted aspects of myopia, comprehensive strategies for its effective management continue to evolve, underscoring the importance of proactive measures in preserving vision and minimizing associated risks.

Signs and Symptoms

The signs and symptoms of myopia may vary in severity, and they can include:
- Difficulty seeing objects clearly at a distance is a primary symptom of myopia. This is particularly noticeable when trying to read road signs or see the board in a classroom.
- People with myopia often unconsciously squint in an attempt to bring distant objects into focus. Squinting temporarily changes the shape of the eye's lens, helping to improve vision.
- Strain or discomfort in the eyes, especially after prolonged periods of reading, driving, or other activities that require focusing on distant objects, can be a symptom of myopia.
- Eyestrain and the effort to see clearly at a distance can lead to tension headaches, particularly during activities that involve looking at distant objects for extended periods.
- Myopia can make it challenging to see clearly in low-light conditions, such as at night or in dimly lit environments. This is known as night myopia.
- Individuals with myopia may notice that their prescription for glasses or contact lenses needs to be updated regularly as their nearsightedness progresses.
- The eyes may feel tired or fatigued, especially after engaging in tasks that require sustained focus on nearby objects.

Investigations

Comprehensive Eye Examination

A thorough eye examination by an optometrist or ophthalmologist is essential. This includes assessing visual acuity, determining the refractive error (degree of myopia), and examining the health of the eyes.

Refraction Test

A refraction test helps determine the specific prescription needed for corrective lenses (glasses or contact lenses).

Dilated Eye Exam

Dilating the pupils allows the eye care professional to examine the health of the retina and optic nerve, which is crucial, especially in cases of high myopia.

Corneal Topography

Corneal topography is a mapping of the cornea's surface and can be useful in assessing corneal irregularities, which may impact myopia management.

Management

Corrective Lenses

Prescription glasses with concave lenses are commonly prescribed to correct myopia and provide clear distance vision. Contact lenses offer an alternative for vision correction and may be preferred, especially in certain lifestyle situations.

Orthokeratology (Ortho-K)

Ortho-K involves using specially designed rigid gas permeable contact lenses worn overnight to reshape the cornea temporarily. This can provide clear vision during the day without the need for glasses or lenses.

Atropine Eye Drops

Low-dose atropine eye drops have been studied for their ability to slow the progression of myopia in children. However, their use requires careful monitoring and consultation with an eye care professional.

Environmental and Lifestyle Interventions

Encouraging outdoor activities and minimizing screen time can be beneficial in managing myopia, particularly in children.

Myopia Control Lenses

Specialized lenses, such as multifocal or dual-focus contact lenses, have been developed to slow the progression of myopia in some individuals.

Surgical Interventions

In cases of severe myopia, refractive surgeries like LASIK or implantable collamer lenses may be considered. However, these are typically reserved for adults with stable prescriptions.

The management of myopia is often individualized based on factors such as age, the degree of myopia, lifestyle, and overall eye health. Regular follow-up visits with an eye care professional are crucial to monitor changes in prescription and address any potential issues promptly. Early intervention and a comprehensive approach to myopia management can help reduce the risk of associated complications and maintain good eye health.

HYPERMETROPIA

Hypermetropia, also known as farsightedness, is a common refractive error of the eye. People with hypermetropia can see distant objects more clearly than nearby objects. This condition occurs when the eyeball is too short or the cornea has too little curvature, causing light entering the eye to focus behind the retina instead of directly on it.

Signs and Symptoms

Hypermetropia can be present from birth and may change over time. The symptoms of hypermetropia can include:
- People with hypermetropia often have difficulty with tasks that require seeing objects up close, such as reading or using a computer.
- Extended periods of close work may lead to headaches.
- The near objects are not clear, the subject may feel eye straining while performing close-up tasks.

Investigations

The investigation of hypermetropia involves a comprehensive eye examination which may include:
- **Refraction:** The clinical refraction measures the degree of refractive error and helps determine the prescription needed for corrective lenses.
- **Visual acuity test:** Visual acuity test assesses the clarity of vision, both at a distance and up close.
- **Retinal examination:** An examination of the back of the eye, including the retina is critical to ensure there are no underlying eye conditions.

Management

Prescription of Corrective Lenses

Convex lenses are prescribed to help focus light directly on the retina, improving close-up vision which may either used as spectacle lenses or contact lenses.

Refractive Surgery

In some cases refractive surgery may be an option. LASIK involves reshaping the cornea using a laser to improve the focus of light on the retina.

Vision Therapy

In some cases vision therapy may be recommended for certain individuals, especially children, to improve eye coordination and focusing abilities.

ASTIGMATISM

Astigmatism is a common refractive error. 1 in 3 people across the world have some degree of astigmatism. It can be comfortably corrected by cylindrical lens power both in contact lenses as well as in spectacle lenses. Astigmatism is caused by an irregularity in the shape of the cornea and/or the eye's crystalline lens. The shape of the eye is more like a rugby ball than a football, which can cause distorted or blurry vision. Astigmatic error exists independent of spherical error and can only be effectively corrected using cylinder lens power. The irregular shape can cause light to focus on more than one point on the retina, leading to blurred or distorted vision. The cylinder lens corrects vision in one dimension without affecting the perpendicular dimension.

Signs and Symptoms

Astigmatism can cause a variety of signs and symptoms related to vision, the common among them are:
- **Blurred or distorted vision:** Objects at any distance may appear blurry or distorted.
- **Eyestrain:** Prolonged or intense use of the eyes, especially for tasks such as reading or using a computer, may result in eyestrain.
- **Headaches:** Astigmatism can contribute to frequent headaches, particularly after activities that require visual focus.
- **Difficulty seeing at night:** Poor night vision or difficulty seeing in low-light conditions may be a symptom of astigmatism.
- **Eye discomfort:** Some individuals with astigmatism may experience general discomfort or irritation in the eyes.

Investigations

The investigation of astigmatism involves a comprehensive eye examination which may include:
- **Refraction:** The clinical refraction measures the degree of refractive error and helps determine the prescription needed for corrective lenses.
- **Visual acuity test:** Visual acuity test assesses the clarity of vision, both at a distance and up close.
- **Retinal examination:** An examination of the back of the eye, including the retina is critical to ensure there are no underlying eye conditions.

Management

The management of astigmatism typically involves corrective measures to improve visual acuity. The most common methods include:

Eyeglasses

Prescription eyeglasses with lenses that have a specific curvature to compensate for the irregular shape of the cornea or lens are a common and effective way to correct astigmatism. The prescription is determined based on the individual's degree of astigmatism.

Contact Lenses

Toric contact lenses are designed specifically for astigmatism. These lenses have different powers in different meridians to correct the irregularities in the cornea or lens. They are available in both soft and rigid gas-permeable materials.

Refractive Surgery

In some cases, individuals may opt for refractive surgery to reshape the cornea and correct astigmatism. LASIK (laser-assisted in situ keratomileusis) is a common surgical procedure for this purpose. Other surgical options include PRK (photorefractive keratectomy) and astigmatic keratotomy.

PRESBYOPIA

Presbyopia is a prevalent age-related vision condition that typically becomes noticeable around the age of 40. This occurs when the natural lens of the eye loses its flexibility, diminishing its ability to focus on close objects effectively. Consequently, individuals with presbyopia experience a range of visual changes accompanied by specific traits and symptoms.

The onset of presbyopia is often sudden, leading to a perplexing realization for many individuals who suddenly struggle with tasks like reading. This abrupt change can evoke frustration and annoyance as they grapple with difficulties in performing close-up activities. The initial impact of presbyopia is particularly pronounced, causing individuals to question why their near vision has suddenly become challenging.

For some, the need for reading glasses, bifocals, or other vision aids can trigger self-consciousness and potentially lead to social withdrawal. The reluctance to engage in social situations or activities requiring close-up tasks in public may arise as individuals navigate the adjustment to their changing vision.

Despite these challenges, many presbyopic individuals develop coping strategies, fostering increased resilience. They learn to accept the necessity of reading glasses or other visual aids, adapting to accommodate their evolving vision. This adaptive process is crucial for maintaining a sense of normalcy and functionality in daily activities.

Presbyopic myopes or hyperopes may struggle to focus on near objects even when wearing their distance prescription. This difficulty arises from the aging process making accommodation more challenging, preventing the crystalline lens from providing the necessary increase in power, resulting in a blurry image with the focus formed behind the retina.

Signs and Symptoms

It is important to note that presbyopia is a normal part of the aging process and affects nearly everyone to some degree as they get older. Common signs and symptoms of presbyopia include:

- **Difficulty reading small print:** One of the earliest signs of presbyopia is difficulty reading small print or doing close-up tasks like threading a needle.
- **Blurred vision at close range:** Objects held at a close distance may appear blurry, requiring you to hold them at arm's length to see them clearly.
- **Eye strain:** Extended periods of reading or performing close-up work may cause eyestrain, headaches, or fatigue.
- **Needing more light:** The patient may find needing more light to see clearly up close.
- **Difficulty seeing in low light:** Presbyopia can make it challenging to see clearly in low-light conditions, especially when trying to read or perform tasks up close.
- **Changes in the ability to focus quickly between near and far objects:** It may take longer for your eyes to adjust when shifting focus between near and far objects.
- **Need for reading glasses:** Many people with presbyopia find that they need reading glasses to help compensate for the difficulty in focusing on close objects.

Management

The management of presbyopia involves various options to help individuals cope with the difficulty of focusing on close objects. The common approaches to managing presbyopia are:

- **Reading glasses:** This is one of the simplest and most common solutions. Reading glasses are designed to provide clear vision for close-up tasks. They come in various strengths, typically labelled in diopters, and can be purchased over-the-counter or prescribed by an eye care professional.

- **Bifocal or multifocal glasses:** These glasses have different prescriptions in different parts of the lens. The upper part is usually set for distance vision, while the lower part is for close-up tasks. Multifocal lenses may have additional segments for intermediate distances.
- **Progressive lenses:** Similar to bifocals, progressive lenses provide a gradual transition between different prescriptions, eliminating the visible line found in bifocals. They offer a more natural and seamless adjustment for various distances.
- **Contact lenses:** Multifocal contact lenses are available for those who prefer not to wear glasses. These lenses have different prescriptions within the lens to address both distance and near vision.
- **Monovision:** In monovision, one eye is corrected for distance vision, while the other eye is corrected for close-up tasks. This can be achieved with contact lenses or through refractive surgery.
- **Refractive surgery:** Surgical options for presbyopia include procedures like monovision LASIK or conductive keratoplasty. These surgeries aim to reshape the cornea to improve near vision.
- **Implantable lenses:** In some cases, an intraocular lens can be surgically implanted to replace the natural lens of the eye. This procedure is less common and typically considered for individuals undergoing cataract surgery.

DISEASES OF LACRIMAL APPARATUS

Lacrimal apparatus consists of lacrimal gland which is a secretary portion and the lacrimal passage which is excretory portion. Lacrimal glands are main organs that release tears. There are two types of lacrimal glands—main lacrimal glands and accessory lacrimal gland. The main lacrimal gland is located in the upper and outer part of the eye socket in a fossa. It is divided into two portions—a large superior or orbital portion and a small inferior or palpebral portion. The superior or orbital portion lies in the lacrimal fossa whereas palpebral portion is just above the lacrimal aspect of superior fornix. The main gland secrets tears only when it receives a nerve impulse like in cases of eye irritation, crying etc, i.e., it is responsible for reflex secretion. The accessory lacrimal glands known as Krause's glands and Wolfring's glands are situated within the conjunctiva. They secret throughout the day and form basal secretion and maintain normal amount of tears on the surface of conjunctiva. This helps overcome the effect of tear evaporation. Lacrimal passage also known as drainage system consists of following parts:
- Lacrimal puncta
- Lacrimal canaliculi
- Lacrimal sac
- Nasolacrimal duct

DRY EYES

Condition

Dry eyes, also known as keratoconjunctivitis sicca, are a common eye condition characterized by a lack of sufficient lubrication and moisture on the surface of the eye. Broadly, dry eyes may be classified into two categories—aqueous deficient dry eyes and evaporative dry eyes. **Table 1.1** shows the difference between the two types of dry eyes.

It is important to note that some individuals may have a combination of both aqueous-deficient and evaporative factors contributing to their dry eye symptoms. Effective treatment often requires a personalized approach tailored to the specific underlying causes and symptoms experienced by each patient.

Table 1.1: Differences between aqueous deficient and evaporative dry eyes.

Aqueous deficient dry eyes	Evaporative dry eyes
Insufficient tear production, often due to issues with the lacrimal glands	Normal tear production, but tears evaporate too quickly due to issues with meibomian glands
Decreased tear production, resulting in reduced tear volume	Normal or increased tear production; however, tears lack proper composition
Schirmer's test and tear osmolarity are often used to diagnose aqueous-deficient dry eyes	Meibomian gland evaluation and lipid layer assessment are common in diagnosing evaporative dry eyes
Artificial tears, prescription medications to stimulate tear production (e.g., cyclosporine), and punctal plugs to retain tears may be recommended	Warm compresses, lid hygiene, omega-3 supplements, and in some cases, meibomian gland expression may be recommended

Causes

Several factors can contribute to the development of dry eyes, including:
- As people get older, tear production often decreases.
- Women are more likely than men to experience dry eyes, especially after menopause.
- Exposure to wind, smoke, dry air, or pollution can exacerbate the symptoms of dry eyes.
- Conditions such as diabetes, rheumatoid arthritis, and thyroid disorders can increase the risk of dry eye syndrome.
- Certain medications, such as antihistamines, decongestants, and antidepressants, can reduce tear production.
- Spending extended periods looking at screens (computers, smartphones) can reduce the frequency of blinking, which helps distribute tears over the eye's surface.

Signs and Symptoms

Dry eyes can lead to various symptoms and discomfort, including:
- Dry eyes can cause a scratchy, burning, or stinging sensation in the eyes.
- The eyes may appear bloodshot.
- Paradoxically, dry eyes can sometimes trigger excessive tearing as a reflex response to the irritation.
- A lack of tears can disrupt the smoothness of the eye's surface, leading to fluctuating visual acuity.
- Dry eyes can make the eyes more sensitive to light.
- Stringy mucus in or around the eyes.
- Foreign body sensation and tired eyes
- Rapid tear break up time and low tear meniscus
- Conjunctival staining

Investigations

Diagnosing and investigating dry eyes typically involves a thorough evaluation. The following are some common diagnostic procedures and tests used to assess and investigate dry eyes:
- The first step in the evaluation process is discussing the patient's symptoms, their duration, and any underlying medical conditions or medications that may contribute to dry eye syndrome. A detailed medical history can provide valuable insights.

- The doctor will ask about the specific symptoms you are experiencing, such as eye discomfort, redness, burning, or blurred vision.
- The eye care specialist will perform an external examination of your eyes to check for signs of inflammation, infection, or other conditions that could be contributing to dry eye symptoms.

Tear Film Evaluation

- Schirmer's test to measures tears production.
- Tear break-up time measures how long it takes for the tear film to break-up
- Tear osmolarity test to measure the salt concentration in your tears, which can help in diagnosing dry eye syndrome. High tear osmolarity indicates that the tears are more concentrated and salty, which can be a sign of dry eye disease. Tear osmolarity values above a certain threshold are associated with dry eye syndrome.
- The eye care practitioner may examine the meibomian glands located on the eyelids. Dysfunction of these glands can lead to evaporative dry eye. Meibomian gland expression may be performed to assess their function.
- A slit lamp biomicroscope is used to closely examine the eyes, including the eyelids, cornea, conjunctiva, and tear film. This allows the eye care practitioner to identify abnormalities or signs of dry eye.
- Special dyes are applied to the surface of the eye to check for damage to the cornea or irregularities in the tear film.
- In some situations, more specialized tests and imaging techniques, such as meibography (imaging of meibomian glands) or tear film interferometry (evaluating the lipid layer of the tear film), may be used to provide additional information.
- The eye care practitioner will review your current medications and assess for any underlying medical conditions that might be contributing to dry eyes.

Management

The treatment options for dry eyes may include:
- Over-the-counter artificial tear drops or ointments can provide temporary relief by adding moisture to the eyes.
- In some cases, your doctor may prescribe medications like cyclosporine (Restasis) or lifitegrast (Xiidra) to help increase tear production.
- Punctal plugs are tiny plugs inserted into the tear ducts to block drainage and keep the tears on the eye's surface longer.
- Taking steps to improve environmental conditions (e.g., using a humidifier, avoiding smoke) and practicing good eye hygiene can alleviate symptoms.
- Omega-3 fatty acids found in fish oil can help improve tear quality and reduce dry eye symptoms.
- In cases where meibomian gland dysfunction is the cause, your eye doctor may perform a procedure to clear blocked glands, improving the quality of the tears.

WATERING OF EYES

Condition

Excessive tearing or watering of the eyes, known as epiphora, can be caused by various factors, including eye irritation, environmental conditions, underlying medical issues, or blocked tear ducts.

Causes

The common causes of epiphora are:
- Foreign objects, such as dust, pollen, or small debris, can irritate the eyes and trigger excessive tearing. Allergies to airborne irritants or allergens can also cause watery eyes.
- Dry eyes can lead to excessive tearing. When the eyes are too dry, they can become irritated, causing a reflex response in which they produce more tears to compensate for the dryness.
- Conjunctivitis is an inflammation of the conjunctiva, the clear tissue that covers the front of the eye. It can lead to watery eyes, along with redness and discharge.
- Blepharitis which involves inflammation of the eyelids can lead to irritated, watery eyes. It is often associated with crusty eyelids and a burning sensation.
- Exposure to windy, smoky, or dusty conditions can cause excessive tearing.
- Allergic reactions to substances like pollen, pet dander, or certain foods can trigger watery eyes along with itching and other allergy symptoms.
- When the tear drainage system is partially or completely blocked, tears cannot drain properly from the eye, leading to excessive tearing. This can be due to a variety of factors, including congenital issues, infections, or aging.
- Abnormalities in the eyelids, such as ectropion (where the lower eyelid turns outward) or entropion (where the lower eyelid turns inward), can cause tears to pool in the eye and lead to watering.
- Trichiasis, can cause irritation and lead to tearing.
- Certain medical conditions, such as sinusitis or Sjögren's syndrome, can lead to watery eyes.

Investigations

Investigating the cause of epiphora typically involves a comprehensive evaluation by an eye care specialist which may include:
- Medical history and discussing symptoms are very critical.
- A thorough examination of the eyes and surrounding structures is conducted. The eye care specialist will inspect for signs of irritation, inflammation, infections, or other abnormalities.
- Fluorescein dye is used to assess the integrity of the tear film and check for abnormalities on the surface of the eye. It can reveal irregularities that may be contributing to epiphora.
- A slit lamp biomicroscope is used to closely examine the eyes, eyelids, cornea, conjunctiva, and tear film.
- If the practitioner suspects an obstruction in the tear drainage system, he may perform a procedure where a saline solution is flushed through the tear ducts. This can help identify and sometimes clear blockages.
- In cases of suspected tear duct blockage, imaging studies like dacryocystography or dacryoscintigraphy may be used to visualize and assess the tear drainage system.

Management

Treatment for watering eyes depends on the underlying cause. Treatment may involve addressing eye irritation, managing allergies, treating infections, or addressing structural issues in the eye or tear drainage system. In some cases, surgical interventions may be necessary to correct tear duct obstructions or eyelid abnormalities.

LACRIMAL TUMORS

Condition

Lacrimal tumors are rare growths that can develop in or around the lacrimal system, which is responsible for producing and draining tears **(Fig. 1.1)**. The lacrimal system includes the

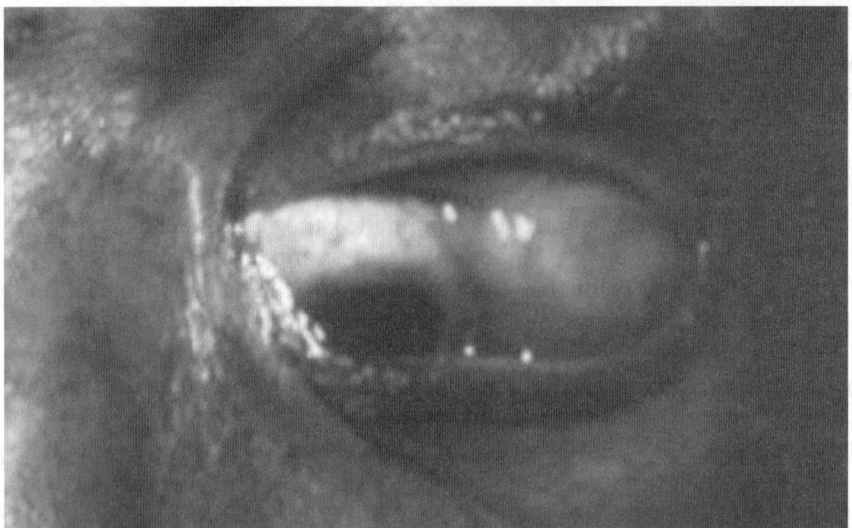

Fig. 1.1: Lacrimal tumor.

lacrimal glands, located above the eye, and the tear ducts and canaliculi that help drain tears from the eye to the nose. Lacrimal tumors can be benign (non-cancerous) or malignant (cancerous) and can lead to various symptoms and complications.

Signs and Symptoms

- Watery eyes or epiphora
- Mass or swelling around the eye
- Pain, redness, or irritation of the eye
- Decreased vision
- Double vision
- Changes in the appearance of the eye
- Eyelid abnormalities

Investigations

Lacrimal tumors are diagnosed through a combination of a physical examination, imaging studies (such as CT or MRI scans), biopsy, and evaluation by an ophthalmologist or oculoplastic surgeon. Biopsy is essential to determine the type and nature of the tumor, whether it's benign or malignant.

Management

Lacrimal tumors are relatively rare, and the management of these tumors often involves a multidisciplinary approach with specialists in ophthalmology and oncolog. Early diagnosis and prompt treatment are critical for achieving the best outcomes for patients with lacrimal tumors. Treatment depends on the type, location, size, and stage of the lacrimal tumor.

Benign tumors may be surgically removed, often with the goal of preserving as much lacrimal function as possible. Malignant tumors may require more extensive surgery, such as orbital exenteration (removal of the eye and surrounding tissues), radiation therapy, and in some cases, chemotherapy.

DACRYOCYSTITIS (FIG. 1.2)

Condition

Dacryocystitis is the inflammation or infection of the lacrimal sac, which is a small, tear-collecting pouch located at the inner corner of the eye. The lacrimal sac is part of the lacrimal drainage system and serves as a reservoir for tears before they are drained into the nasal passages. Dacryocystitis typically occurs when the drainage system is blocked or obstructed, leading to the build-up of tears and creating a favorable environment for infection.

Causes

The most common cause of dacryocystitis is a blockage in the nasolacrimal duct, which is the tube that carries tears from the eye to the nasal cavity. The obstruction can be caused by various factors, such as congenital issues, age-related changes, injuries, or the presence of foreign bodies. When the tear drainage system is blocked, tears can stagnate in the lacrimal sac, providing a breeding ground for bacteria to multiply and cause an infection.

Signs and Symptoms

- Tearing (epiphora)
- Redness and swelling at the inner corner of the eye
- Pain, tenderness, or a feeling of pressure in the area
- Mucopurulent discharge (yellow or greenish discharge) from the eye
- Blurred vision
- Fever in cases of severe infection

Investigations

An ophthalmologist or an oculoplastic surgeon can diagnose dacryocystitis through a physical examination of the eye and lacrimal sac. Sometimes, diagnostic tests, such as dye disappearance tests may be used to assess the level of tear flow and any underlying blockages.

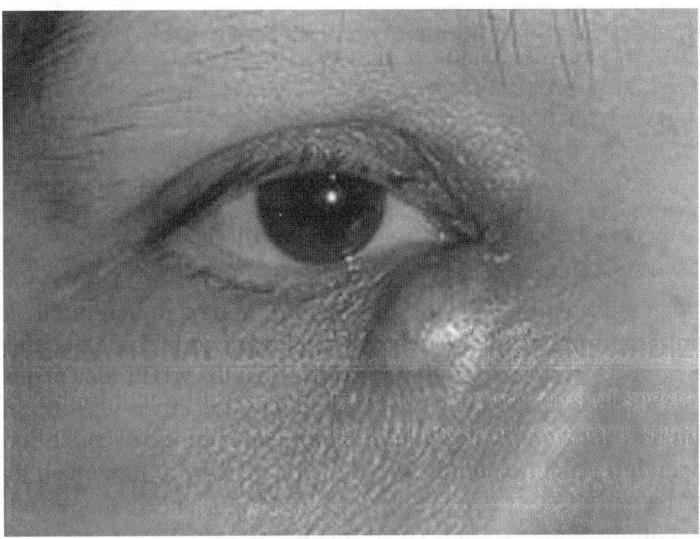

Fig. 1.2: Dacryocystitis.

Management

Mild cases of dacryocystitis may respond to warm compresses, massage of the tear sac, and the use of antibiotic eye drops or ointment. However, in cases of persistent or recurrent dacryocystitis, a surgical procedure called DCR or dacryocystorhinostomy may be recommended. DCR creates a new drainage pathway for tears to bypass the obstruction and drain into the nasal passages. This can be done either externally (external DCR) or endoscopically (endoscopic DCR).

DISEASES OF EYELIDS

The eyelids are two movable folds of skin covering the orbital cavity and the anterior eyeball. The upper eyelid moves over the eyeball and the lower eyelid sits below the eye. The upper eyelid extends up to the eyebrow and lower eyelid merges with the skin of cheeks. The edges of either eyelid are called eyelid margins. The margins of the upper and lower lids meet at the medial and lateral angles called the canthi. The lid margin is about 2 mm broad. Its anterior border is rounded, while posterior border is sharp. The free border of the lid carries the eyelashes. The eyelashes are short and stout hair arranged in two or three rows. The upper eyelid lashes are 100 to 150 in number and are directed upwards and lower eyelid lashes approximately 20% less and they turn downwards, so that when the lids are closed, the lashes do not interlace. Eyelashes are absent near medial canthus as lacrimal punctum is present. Eyelashes do not grey with aging and they regenerate within a span of 10 weeks. Hairs of eyelashes are replaced after every 3–5 months. The follicles of eyelashes pass into the lid obliquely and attached with Gland of Zeis. The meibomian glands open just in front of the posterior border of the lid margin. Eyelid diseases encompass a variety of conditions that affect the structures surrounding the eye. These can range from minor annoyances to more serious conditions that require medical intervention. Some common eyelid diseases include ptosis, lagophthalmos, blepharitis, stye, chalazion, internal hordeolom, trichiasis, entropion, ectropion, blepharospasm.

STYE

Condition

Stye, also known as hordeolum is an infection of the eyelid's oil glands **(Fig. 1.3)**. It appears as a painful, red bump on the eyelid, usually near the base of the eyelashes. Styes can be uncomfortable and cause localized swelling and tenderness. There are two main types of styes as described in **Table 1.2**.

Causes

Styes are primarily caused by an infection, often by the bacterium Staphylococcus aureus bacteria. This bacteria can enter the oil glands (sebaceous glands) located along the eyelid margins, leading to inflammation and blockage of the gland's opening and results in the formation of a painful bump.

Signs and Symptoms

- ❖ Painful, red bump on the eyelid, resembling a pimple or small boil
- ❖ Swelling and tenderness around the bump
- ❖ Discomfort or pain, especially when blinking or touching the affected area
- ❖ Crusting and matting of the eyelashes near the bump
- ❖ Watering of the eye due to irritation

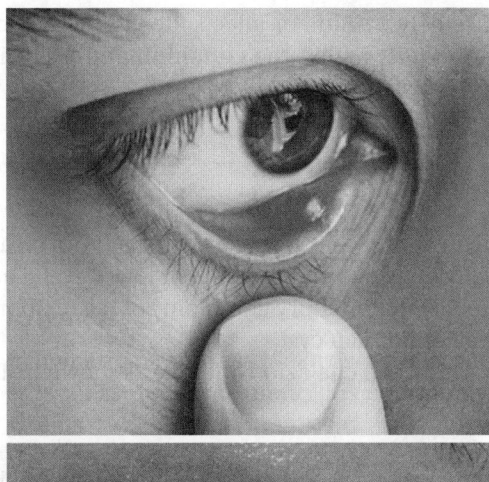
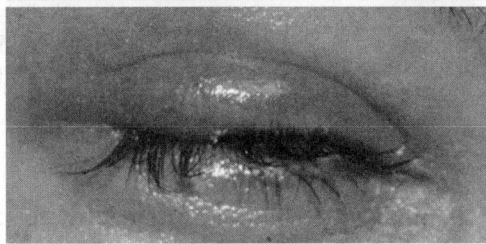

Fig. 1.3: Stye.

Table 1.2: Types of stye.	
Types	Description
External stye	External stye develops at the base of an eyelash follicle, usually on the outer surface of the eyelid
Internal stye	Also called an internal hordeolum, it forms on the underside of the eyelid due to an infection in a Meibomian gland

Investigations

The diagnosis of a stye (hordeolum) is primarily based on clinical examination by a healthcare professional. The appearance, location, and symptoms of the stye usually provide enough information for diagnosis. The healthcare provider will visually inspect the affected eyelid and surrounding area to assess the size, location, and appearance of the stye. They will also ask symptoms and medical history. They might gently palpate the stye to assess its tenderness and firmness. If there is a suspicion of an internal stye, the eyelid might need to be everted to examine the inside of the lid and the affected gland.

Management

Most styes resolve on their own within a week or so, as the body's immune system fights off the infection. However, the following management may be recommended to alleviate symptoms and promote healing:
- Warm compresses
- Good hygiene
- Avoid squeezing

If the stye persists, becomes extremely painful, or affects the vision, medical consultation is advisable. The medical practitioner can assess the condition and prescribe appropriate treatment, including oral antibiotics if necessary.

CHALAZION

Condition

A chalazion is a localized swelling or bump that forms on the eyelid, typically caused by a blocked oil gland **(Fig. 1.4)**. It usually develops on the upper or lower eyelid and appears as a painless, firm lump. It is a non-specific inflammatory granuloma of the meibomian gland. It is sometimes called an eyelid cyst or a meibomian cyst.

It is nice to gather the differences between chalazion and stye as shown in **Table 1.3**.

Causes

Chalazion is typically caused by a blockage of one of the small oil glands (meibomian glands) located within the eyelid. This blockage leads to the accumulation of oil and inflammation. Excess rubbing of eyes to gain clear vision may also cause chalazion.

Signs and Symptoms

- Chalazion appears as small pea size nodular swelling away from lid margin.
- It is firm and non-tender. Patient also does not report pain.
- Skin over swelling is normal and free from it.
- On lid eversion the tarsal conjunctiva underneath the nodule is velvety red or purple.

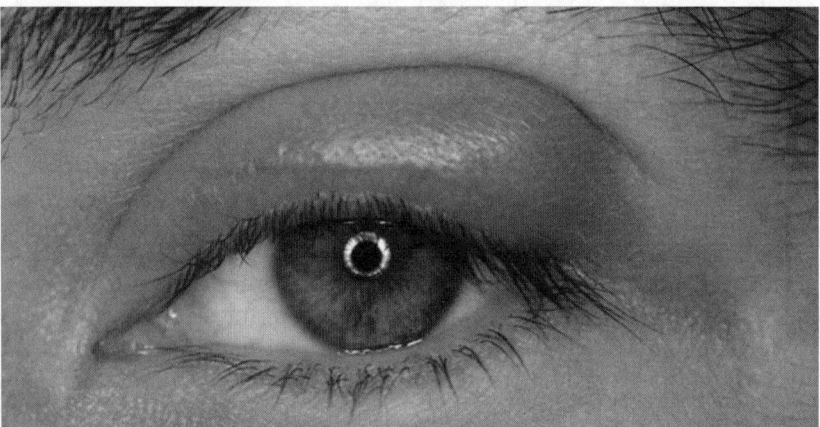

Fig. 1.4: Chalazion.

Table 1.3: Differences between chalazion and stye.

Chalazion	Stye
Chalazion is a non-infectious blockage of an oil gland	Stye is an infected eyelid gland or follicle
Chalazion usually occur on the upper eyelid, closer to margin. It may also develop on the lower eyelid	Stye can occur on either upper or lower eyelid found closer to the eyelash line
Chalazion tends to be firmer and more gradual in development	Style causes pain and tenderness

Investigations

The diagnosis of a chalazion is usually straightforward and can often be made through a physical examination by an eye care professional. He assesses the size, location, and characteristics of the lump that helps distinguish between a chalazion and other similar conditions, such as a stye or an eyelid infection.

Management

The management of a chalazion involves a combination of at-home care and, in some cases, medical interventions. The goal is to reduce inflammation, promote drainage, and relieve discomfort.

- Applying warm compresses to soften the blockage, promote drainage, and relieve discomfort.
- Gently massage the eyelid to help encourage drainage. Wash your hands thoroughly before doing this.
- Keep the eyelid areas clean using baby shampoo to prevent further irritation and infection.
- It is important not to try to squeeze or "pop" the chalazion like you might with a pimple. This can lead to further irritation and potential infection.
- If the chalazion does not respond to home treatments or becomes very large and uncomfortable, medical interventions may be considered. These might include injection of corticosteroids to reduce inflammation and promote resolution. In some cases, especially if the chalazion is very large and persistent, a minor surgical procedure may be performed to drain the contents of the lump.
- If there is evidence of infection or if a stye is present alongside the chalazion, antibiotic ointments or oral antibiotics might be prescribed to treat the infection.

BLEPHARITIS

Condition

Blepharitis is an inflammation of the eyelids (**Fig. 1.5**). Eyelid becomes red, irritated and itchy. Dandruff-like scales form on the eyelashes. It is usually caused by either bacteria or a skin

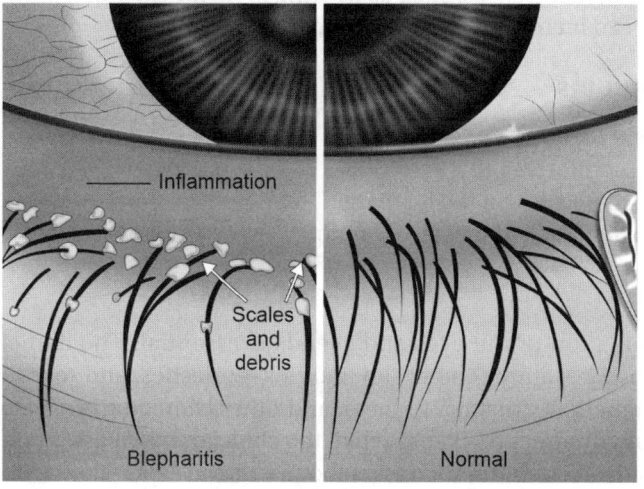

Fig. 1.5: Blepharitis.

Table 1.4: Types of blepharitis.

Types of blepharitis	Description
Anterior blepharitis	It occurs at the outside front edge of the eyelid where the eyelashes attach
Posterior blepharitis	It affects the inner edge of the eyelid that touches the eyeball

condition, such as dandruff of the scalp or rosacea. It primarily affects the eyelid margins where the eyelashes are attached. The condition can be either acute (short-term) or chronic (long-term) and may cause discomfort and irritation.

Blepharitis is classified into two types as shown in **Table 1.4**.

Causes

Blepharitis can have various causes, and in many cases, it is caused by a combination of factors. The condition typically arises from a combination of inflammation, bacteria, and issues with the oil glands in the eyelids.

- Anterior blepharitis is commonly caused by bacteria staphylococcal blepharitis or dandruff of the scalp.
- Seborrheic dermatitis is a skin condition characterized by oily, flaky skin. When it affects the eyelids, it can contribute to the development of blepharitis.
- Demodex mites are tiny organisms that naturally reside on the skin, including the eyelids. An overgrowth of these mites can lead to anterior blepharitis.
- Posterior blepharitis can occur when the meibomian glands of the eyelids irregularly produce oil.
- Posterior blepharitis can also develop as a result of other skin conditions, such as rosacea and scalp dandruff.
- Poor hygiene of the eyelids can lead to the accumulation of debris, oil, and bacteria, contributing to blepharitis.
- Environmental factors such as pollution, dry air, and wind can contribute to the development or exacerbation of blepharitis symptoms.
- Improper use of contact lenses, such as wearing them for extended periods or not cleaning them properly, can increase the risk of blepharitis.

Signs and Symptoms

- Redness of eyelid margins
- Burning and discomfort
- White dandruff like scales on the lid margin
- Itching, lacrimation and soreness of lid margin

Investigations

A thorough examination of the eyes and eyelids is essential. The clinician uses slit lamp microscope to closely examine the eyelid margins, eyelashes, and tear film. They will look for signs of inflammation, crusting, redness, and other characteristic features of blepharitis. If meibomian gland dysfunction is suspected, the clinician might assess the function of these oil-producing glands. Techniques such as meibomian gland expression or imaging may be used to evaluate the glands' condition and flow of oil.

Management

The management of blepharitis involves a combination of at-home care, lifestyle adjustments, and, in some cases, medical interventions. The specific approach will depend on the type and severity of blepharitis.
- Eyelid hygiene that includes regular and proper eyelid hygiene is a cornerstone of blepharitis management. Use a mild, non-irritating cleanser or baby shampoo diluted with water.
- Gently massage the eyelid margins to help remove debris and unclog oil glands. Rinse thoroughly and pat dry.
- Apply a warm compress to your closed eyelids for about 5–10 minutes. Warmth helps soften crusts, open blocked oil glands, and improve circulation. It can be done several times a day, especially before eyelid hygiene.
- Depending on the type of blepharitis, the clinician might prescribe antibiotic or corticosteroid eye drops or ointments to reduce inflammation and control bacterial overgrowth.
- Avoid makeup, especially eye makeup, during flare-ups, as it can exacerbate symptoms.
- A break from wearing contacts during a blepharitis flare-up.
- Regular visits to your eye care professional are important to monitor your condition and adjust your treatment plan.

PTOSIS (FIG. 1.6)

Condition

Ptosis, also known as "drooping eyelid," is a condition characterized by the sagging or drooping of the upper eyelid. It can affect one or both eyelids and may vary in severity, ranging from a mild droop that only slightly covers the eye to a more significant droop that impairs vision.

Causes

Ptosis can be caused by various factors, including:
- Ptosis is often associated with aging, as the muscles responsible for lifting the eyelid can weaken over time.
- Some individuals are born with ptosis due to underdeveloped or weak eyelid muscles. This condition is present from birth and may require surgical correction if it affects vision.
- Certain neurological disorders or injuries to the nerves or muscles that control eyelid movement can lead to ptosis.

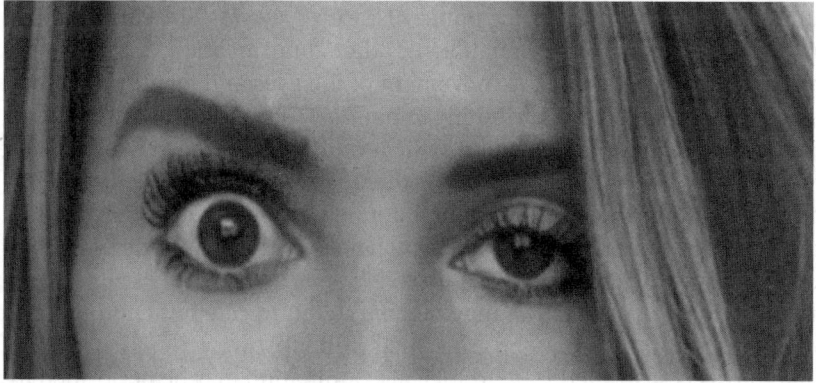

Fig. 1.6: Ptosis.

- Injuries to the eye area or eyelid muscles can cause temporary or permanent ptosis.
- Medical conditions like myasthenia gravis, a neuromuscular disorder, and Horner's syndrome, a neurological disorder, can result in ptosis.
- Some medications, such as those used to treat glaucoma or as side effects of other drugs, can cause ptosis.

Signs and Symptoms

Ptosis, or drooping eyelid, can manifest with various signs and symptoms, which may include:
- The most noticeable sign of ptosis is the drooping of one or both upper eyelids. The degree of droopiness can vary from mild drooping to more pronounced that partially or completely covers the eye.
- In more severe cases, ptosis can obstruct the field of vision. The drooping eyelid may interfere with the person's ability to see objects clearly, especially when looking upward or straight ahead.
- To compensate for the drooping eyelid and improve vision, individuals with ptosis may raise their eyebrows excessively. This can lead to wrinkles on the forehead and a constantly raised eyebrow on the affected side.
- Trying to keep the drooping eyelid open can lead to eye fatigue and strain.
- Ptosis can cause asymmetry between the two eyes, with one eye appearing smaller or less open than the other.
- Some people with ptosis may tilt their head backward or to the side to improve their field of vision. This compensatory head posture can be a sign of ptosis.

Investigations

The evaluation of ptosis typically involves a series of investigations and examinations by an eye specialist. The goal is to determine the underlying cause of ptosis and its severity to guide appropriate treatment.
- The eyecare practitioner will begin by taking a detailed medical history, including information about when the ptosis started, any recent injuries or surgeries, family history of eye conditions, and any associated symptoms or medical conditions.
- A thorough physical examination of the eyes and eyelids will be conducted. This includes assessing the degree of ptosis, the presence of any other eyelid abnormalities, and the overall health of the eye and surrounding structures.
- Visual acuity test
- The examination of the external appearance of the eyes, eyelids, and surrounding structures, looking for signs of trauma, inflammation, or other abnormalities.
- Ocular motility test to evaluate the movement of the eyes and identify any issues with eye muscle function that may be contributing to ptosis.
- Assessment of the strength and function of the levator muscle, which is responsible for lifting the eyelid. It helps determine if the ptosis is due to muscle weakness.
- A slit lamp examination is a detailed examination of the eye's anterior structures, including the cornea, lens, and anterior chamber. This can help identify any underlying eye conditions that may be causing or contributing to ptosis.
- A test to measure tear production may be conducted to rule out conditions like dry eye syndrome, which can sometimes be associated with ptosis.
- If acquired ptosis is suspected, a neurological examination may be performed to assess the function of the nerves that control eyelid movement and to rule out neurological disorders.

Management

The treatment for ptosis depends on its underlying cause and severity. Mild ptosis may not require treatment, while more severe cases that affect vision or aesthetics may be corrected through surgery.
- Ptosis surgery involves tightening the muscles responsible for lifting the eyelid or repositioning the eyelid to a higher position.
- If ptosis is secondary to an underlying medical condition, such as myasthenia gravis, Horner's syndrome, or a neurological disorder, the primary focus of treatment may be managing the underlying condition. This can involve medications, physical therapy, or other specialized treatments.
- In cases where surgery is not immediately possible or appropriate, especially in individuals who are not surgical candidates, temporary solutions like eyelid crutches or ptosis props may be used to help lift the eyelid and improve vision.

LAGOPHTHALMOS (FIG. 1.7)

Condition

Lagophthalmos is a medical condition characterized by the inability to fully close the eyelids, leaving a gap between the upper and lower eyelids when the eyes are closed. This condition can affect one or both eyes and may result from various underlying causes.

Causes

Lagophthalmos can be caused by several factors, including:
- One of the most common causes is facial nerve paralysis, often resulting from Bell's palsy, trauma, or other neurological conditions. When the facial nerve is affected, it can lead to weakness or paralysis of the muscles responsible for closing the eyelids.
- In some cases, lagophthalmos can occur as a complication of eyelid surgery, particularly if too much skin or muscle is removed during a blepharoplasty.
- Trauma or fractures involving the bones of the orbit can disrupt the normal function of the eyelids, leading to lagophthalmos.
- Some thyroid conditions, such as Graves' disease, can cause eye-related symptoms, including lagophthalmos.
- Rarely, congenital factors can contribute to lagophthalmos, such as abnormalities in the eyelid structure.

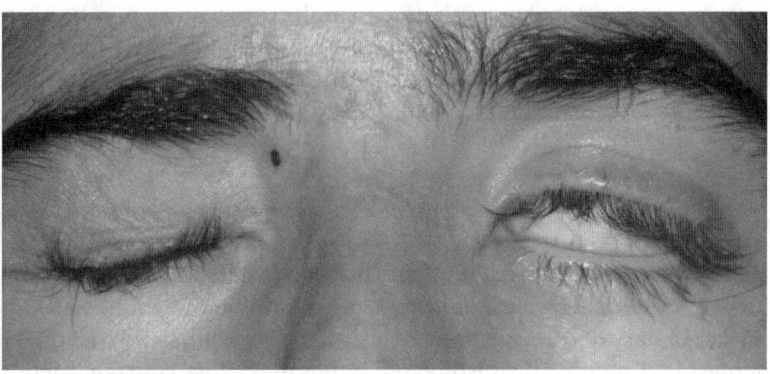

Fig. 1.7: Lagophthalmos.

Signs and Symptoms

The primary symptom of lagophthalmos is the inability to fully close the eyelids. This can result in several issues, including:
* Exposure of the cornea and other parts of the eye, which can lead to dryness, irritation, and damage to the cornea.
* Increased sensitivity to light.
* Foreign body sensation in the eye.
* Reduced or disturbed sleep due to the eyes not fully closing during sleep.

Investigations

The goal of the investigations is to determine the underlying cause of lagophthalmos and its severity.
* The eye care provider will begin by taking a detailed medical history. They will inquire about the onset of lagophthalmos, any associated symptoms, any recent facial trauma or surgeries, and any underlying medical conditions, such as thyroid disorders.
* A thorough physical examination of the eyes, eyelids, and facial muscles will be conducted. The practitioner will assess the degree of lagophthalmos, any signs of facial nerve paralysis, and any other abnormalities.
* Since facial nerve paralysis is a common cause of lagophthalmos, a neurological examination may be performed to assess the function of the facial nerve and rule out neurological conditions.
* The practitioner will assess the health of the cornea, conjunctiva, and other eye structures.
* The degree of lagophthalmos can be quantified by measuring the gap between the upper and lower eyelids when the patient tries to close their eyes forcefully.
* Schirmer's test to measure tears production and can help determine if the eyes are excessively dry due to incomplete eyelid closure. In cases of lagophthalmos, dry eyes are a common concern.

Management

Treatment of lagophthalmos depends on the underlying cause and the severity of the condition. Some common management approaches include:
* Lubricating eye drops or ointments can help keep the eye moist and prevent dryness.
* In milder cases, eyelid taping with specialized medical tape can help partially close the eyelids during sleep.
* Small weights can be attached to the upper eyelid to help it close more effectively.
* In cases of severe or persistent lagophthalmos, surgical procedures may be necessary. These can involve various techniques to improve eyelid closure and protect the eye.
* If lagophthalmos is caused by an underlying medical condition, such as Bell's palsy or thyroid eye disease, the treatment plan will also address that condition.

TRICHIASIS

Condition

Trichiasis (**Fig. 1.8**) is a condition that affects the eyes, specifically the eyelashes and their alignment. It occurs when the eyelashes grow in an abnormal direction, causing them to rub against the surface of the eye. The misdirected lashes may be diffused across the entire lid or in a small segmental distribution. The misdirected lashes may cause constant friction can lead to various eye problems and discomfort.

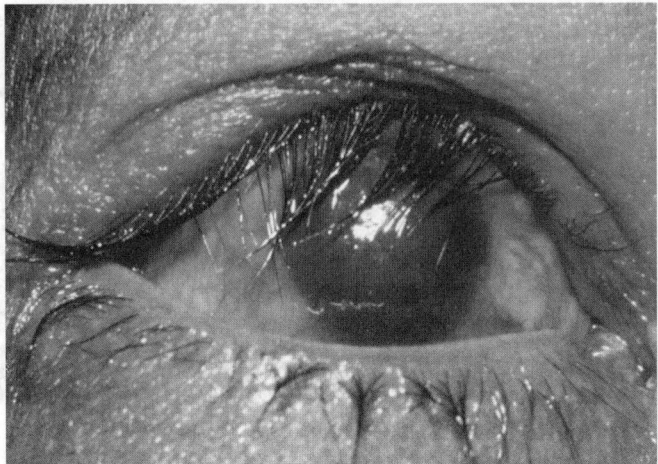

Fig. 1.8: Trichiasis.

Causes

The common causes of trichiasis include:
- Malformation or scarring of the eyelids can cause the eyelashes to turn inward.
- Conditions like trachoma, a contagious eye infection caused by the bacterium Chlamydia trachomatis, can lead to trichiasis.
- Chronic inflammation of the eyelid margin, known as blepharitis, can result in the misalignment of eyelashes.
- Trauma to the eye or eyelid can sometimes cause the eyelashes to grow abnormally.
- Natural aging processes can cause changes in the eyelids and their alignment, leading to trichiasis.

Signs and Symptoms

The symptoms of trichiasis may include:
- Eye irritation
- Redness
- Tearing
- Foreign body sensation
- Light sensitivity
- Corneal abrasions or ulcers

Investigations

The steps typically involved in investigating trichiasis are:
- The practitioner will begin by taking a detailed medical history, which may include asking about any eye-related symptoms, previous eye conditions or surgeries, and any relevant medical conditions.
- The practitioner will examine the external structures of the eye, including the eyelids, eyelashes, and surrounding tissues. They will look for signs of trichiasis, such as misaligned or ingrown eyelashes.
- A slit lamp biomicroscope may be used to get a closer and more detailed view of the eye's anterior structures.

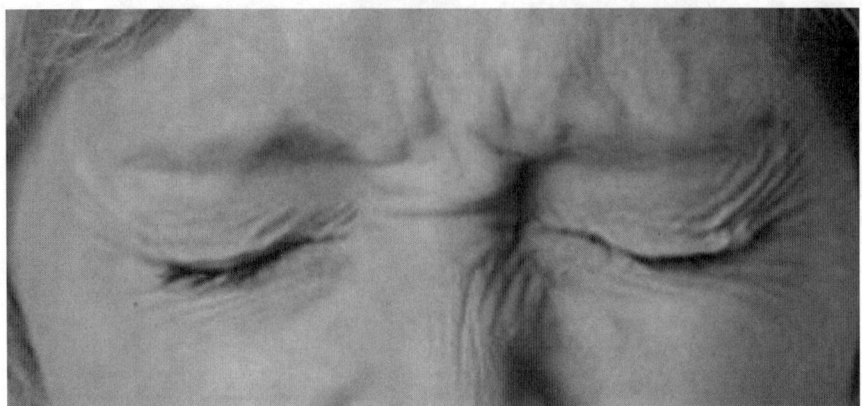

Fig. 1.9: Blepharospasm.

- A visual acuity test may be performed to assess the patient's vision and to check for any vision-related issues that may be associated with trichiasis.
- Fluorescein dye may be applied to the eye's surface to check for any corneal abrasions or ulcers caused by the rubbing of misaligned eyelashes.
- The practitioner may gently evert the eyelids to examine the inner surface of the eyelids for signs of trichiasis or other eye conditions.
- If trichiasis is identified, the practitioner may investigate the underlying cause, which could include conditions like blepharitis, trachoma, or eyelid malformations.

Management

If left untreated, trichiasis can lead to serious eye complications, such as corneal damage and vision loss. Treatment options for trichiasis may include:
- Manual epilation is one of the useful management. This involves the removal of ingrown or misaligned eyelashes by an eyecare practitioner.
- Electrolysis is another useful management that uses a small electrical current to destroy the hair follicles of misaligned eyelashes, preventing them from regrowing.
- Cryotherapy can be recommended to the affected eyelid area to destroy the hair follicles.

BLEPHAROSPASM

Condition

Blepharospasm (**Fig. 1.9**) is a medical condition characterized by involuntary, repetitive, and uncontrollable contractions or spasms of the muscles around the eyelids. These spasms can cause the affected individual to repeatedly blink or close their eyes, and in severe cases, it can lead to functional blindness. The spasms can range from mild and occasional to severe and persistent, significantly affecting a person's quality of life.

Causes

The exact cause of blepharospasm is not always clear, but it is believed to be related to a combination of genetic, environmental, and neurological factors. Stress and fatigue can exacerbate symptoms.

Signs and Symptoms

The primary symptom is the involuntary closure of the eyelids. The spasms may start in one eye but often progress to affect both eyes. Some individuals may experience light sensitivity as well.

Investigations

A diagnosis of blepharospasm is typically made based on a physical examination and a review of the patient's medical history. Sometimes, additional tests like electromyography (EMG) or imaging studies may be conducted to rule out other potential causes of eyelid spasms.

Management

The treatment of blepharospasm primarily involves relieving the symptoms. Options include: Botulinum toxin (Botox) injections can temporarily paralyze the muscles responsible for the eyelid spasms and are often effective.

Some drugs, such as muscle relaxants or anticholinergic medications, may provide relief for some individuals.

In severe cases that do not respond to other treatments, surgical procedures like myectomy (removing a portion of the muscles responsible for the spasms) may be considered.

Living with blepharospasm can be challenging, but support groups and lifestyle modifications can help individuals cope with the condition. Managing stress and getting enough sleep are important steps in symptom management.

ENTROPION

Condition

Entropion **(Fig. 1.10)** is a medical condition that affects the eyelids, specifically the lower eyelid. It occurs when the edge of the eyelid usually the lower one turns inward, causing the eyelashes and the skin to rub against the surface of the eye. This condition can be painful and uncomfortable, and it can lead to various eye problems if left untreated.

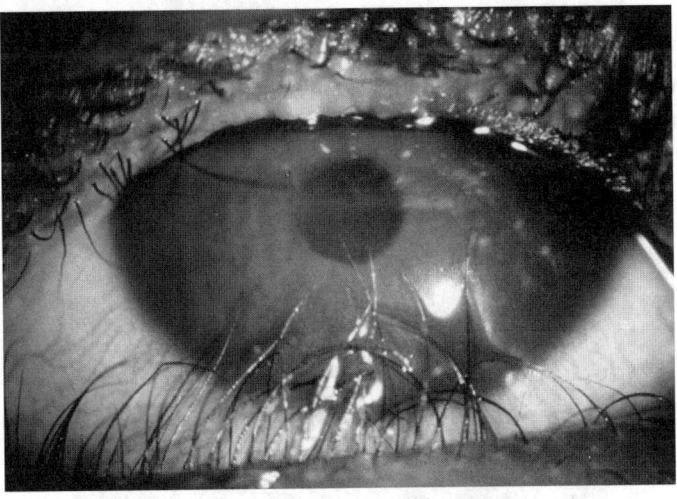

Fig. 1.10: Entropion.

Causes

Entropion can be caused by various factors, including age-related changes in the eyelid tissues, scarring from injury or surgery, muscle weakness, or congenital conditions. In some cases, it can be the result of spasms in the muscles surrounding the eye.

Signs and Symptoms

The most common symptoms of entropion include:
- Foreign body sensation
- Reflex epiphora
- Ocular discharge
- Eye redness and irritation
- Photophobia (sensitivity to light)
- Superficial keratopathy

Investigations

An eye care specialist, such as an ophthalmologist, can diagnose entropion through a physical examination of the eyelids and an assessment of the eye's condition.

Management

Treatment for entropion depends on its cause and severity. Some common approaches include:
- Artificial tears can help alleviate eye irritation and keep the eye moist.
- Eyelid taping may help to support the eyelid's position.
- In some cases, Botox injections may be used to temporarily relax the muscles around the eye.
- Surgery is often required to fix the eyelid's position permanently. The specific surgical procedure used will depend on the individual case and the underlying cause of entropion.
- If left untreated, entropion can lead to corneal ulcers and vision problems. The constant rubbing of the eyelashes against the cornea can cause damage to the clear front surface of the eye.

ECTROPION

Condition

Ectropion (**Fig. 1.11**) is a condition that affects the eyelids, specifically the lower eyelid. It occurs when the edge of the eyelid, typically the lower one, turns outward, away from the eye. This

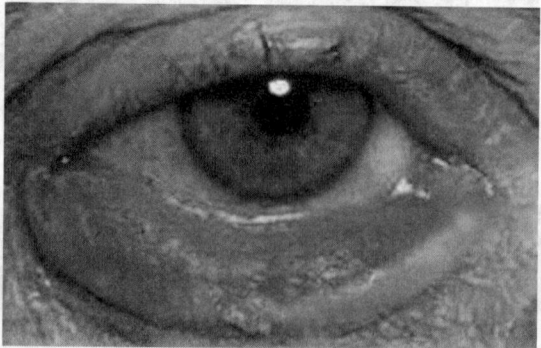

Fig. 1.11: Ectropion.

results in the inner surface of the eyelid being exposed, which can lead to various eye problems and discomfort. Ectropion can affect one or both eyes and is often associated with aging.

Causes

The most common cause of ectropion is age-related changes in the eyelid tissues. The skin and muscles that support the lower eyelid become lax over time, allowing the eyelid to turn outward. Other potential causes of ectropion include facial nerve palsy, scarring from injury or surgery, or congenital conditions.

Signs and Symptoms

Ectropion can cause several symptoms, including:
- Eye redness and irritation
- Sensation of dryness and foreign body in the eye
- Excessive tearing (epiphora)
- Increased sensitivity to wind, light, or dust
- Corneal exposure, which can lead to corneal damage if not addressed

Investigations

An ophthalmologist can diagnose ectropion through a physical examination of the eyelids and an assessment of the eye's condition. They will evaluate the eyelid's position and its impact on the eye's health.

Management

Treatment for ectropion depends on its underlying cause and severity. Some common approaches include:
- Artificial tears can help alleviate eye dryness and irritation.
- Eyelid taping may help to support the eyelid's position.
- Lubricating ointments and eye drops can be prescribed to manage dry eye symptoms.
- In most cases, surgical correction is necessary to reposition the eyelid. The specific surgical technique used will depend on the individual case and the underlying cause of ectropion.
- If left untreated, ectropion can lead to corneal ulcers, eye infections, and vision problems due to the constant exposure of the eye's surface.

DISEASES OF CONJUNCTIVA

Conjunctiva is the thin, transparent membrane that covers the sclera and lines the inside of the eyelids. It plays a crucial role in protecting the eye by producing mucus and tears, which help keep the eye moist and lubricated. The conjunctiva can become inflamed, which is characterized by redness, itching, and discharge from the eye.

CONJUNCTIVITIS

Condition

Conjunctivitis as shown in **Figure 1.12** is commonly known as pink eye. It is an inflammation from infection or allergies. The condition can affect one or both eyes. Conjunctivitis is typically of three types as shown in **Table 1.5**.

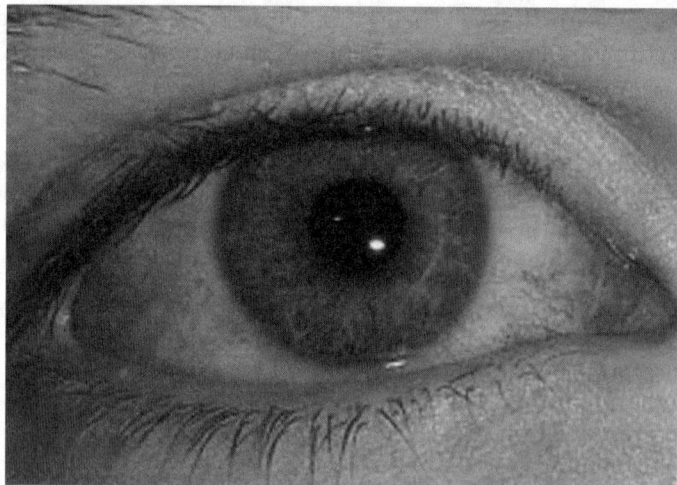

Fig. 1.12: Conjunctivitis.

Table 1.5: Types of conjunctivitis.		
Infectious conjunctivitis	*Allergic conjunctivitis*	*Non-infectious conjunctivitis*
This type of conjunctivitis is caused by bacteria or viruses. Common viral causes include adenoviruses (associated with the common cold), while bacterial conjunctivitis can result from various bacterial strains. It is highly contagious.	Allergies to substances like pollen, pet dander, dust mites, or certain foods can lead to allergic conjunctivitis. This type of conjunctivitis is not contagious and can be triggered by exposure to allergens.	This form of conjunctivitis can result from irritation due to factors such as exposure to chemicals (e.g., chlorine from swimming pools), smoke, air pollution, or foreign objects in the eye. This type of conjunctivitis is not contagious.

Causes

There are several potential causes of conjunctivitis, which may include:
- Viruses, such as the adenovirus, are a common cause of viral conjunctivitis.
- Bacterial conjunctivitis is usually caused by bacteria like *Staphylococcus aureus* or *Streptococcus pneumoniae*. It can result from an eye injury, contact with contaminated surfaces or personal items, and poor hygiene.
- Allergic conjunctivitis occurs when the eyes react to allergens like pollen, dust mites, pet dander, or certain foods. It can be seasonal or perennial, depending on the allergen.
- Exposure to irritants like smoke, chemicals, or foreign bodies can cause irritant conjunctivitis.
- Contact with harsh chemicals or environmental pollutants can lead to chemical conjunctivitis, which can be painful and should be treated promptly.
- Certain autoimmune diseases, such as rheumatoid arthritis or systemic lupus erythematosus, can cause chronic conjunctivitis.
- Improper use or maintenance of contact lenses can lead to contact lens-associated conjunctivitis. Bacterial and fungal infections can develop when lenses are not cleaned or stored properly.
- Newborns can develop a form of conjunctivitis due to exposure to bacteria during birth, known as neonatal conjunctivitis.
- Sexually transmitted infections, particularly chlamydia and gonorrhea, can lead to a form of conjunctivitis in adults.

- Injuries to the eye, such as scratches, foreign bodies, or blunt trauma, can cause traumatic conjunctivitis.

Signs and Symptoms

Some common signs and symptoms associated with conjunctivitis are listed below:
- Diffuse of patchy redness
- Itchy eyes are a common symptom, especially in cases of allergic conjunctivitis.
- Excessive tearing or watery discharge from the eyes is often present, particularly in cases of viral and allergic conjunctivitis.
- Viral conjunctivitis characterize by a clear, watery discharge that may become thicker over time whereas bacterial conjunctivitis may show a thicker, yellow or greenish discharge that can cause the eyelids to stick together, especially after sleep. In case of allergic conjunctivitis a thin, watery discharge may be observed.
- Many people with conjunctivitis experience a feeling of having sand or grit in their eyes.
- There may be a burning or stinging sensation in the eyes, especially in cases of viral and allergic conjunctivitis.
- Photophobia, or sensitivity to light, can be a symptom of conjunctivitis, particularly in severe or allergic cases.
- Swelling of the eyelids and the conjunctiva may occur in some cases, especially with allergic conjunctivitis.
- Vision can be temporarily blurred due to excessive tearing, discharge, or other eye discomfort.
- In bacterial conjunctivitis, the discharge can dry and cause the eyelids to crust, especially upon waking in the morning.
- The eyes may feel irritated, sore, or tender to the touch.
- In some cases of viral or bacterial conjunctivitis, the lymph nodes near the ear or jaw may become enlarged and tender.

Investigations

Typically, an ophthalmologist conducts an investigation to determine the cause of the conjunctivitis. The goal of the investigation is to identify whether the conjunctivitis is viral, bacterial, allergic, or related to an irritant.

The investigation starts with detailed medical history, including information about the patient's symptoms, the duration of symptoms, any recent eye injuries or exposure to irritants, previous episodes of conjunctivitis, and any relevant medical conditions or allergies.

A thorough examination of the eyes and eyelids will be conducted. The examiner looks for signs of redness, swelling, discharge, and any other visible symptoms. He also checks for any enlargement of the lymph nodes near the ear or jaw, which can be a sign of viral or bacterial conjunctivitis.

In cases of suspected bacterial conjunctivitis, a sample of the eye discharge may be collected using a sterile swab. This sample can be sent to a laboratory for culture and sensitivity testing to identify the specific bacteria causing the infection and determine the most effective antibiotic treatment.

If allergic conjunctivitis is suspected, the healthcare provider may inquire about potential allergens and may recommend allergy testing to identify specific triggers.

In some cases, particularly if there is a high suspicion of a viral cause, specialized testing may be performed to identify the specific virus.

If the patient uses contact lenses, the healthcare provider will inquire about lens use and care practices. Contact lens-related conjunctivitis may be due to improper lens hygiene.

The examiner may also assess for any underlying medical conditions or factors that could be contributing to conjunctivitis, such as autoimmune diseases, sexually transmitted infections, or systemic conditions.

Management

Once the investigation is complete, the examiner may make a diagnosis based on the findings and determine the appropriate treatment. Treatment options may include antibiotics for bacterial conjunctivitis, antihistamines for allergic conjunctivitis, or supportive care for viral conjunctivitis. He may also recommend health hygiene to prevent the spread of infectious conjunctivitis and to alleviate symptoms. If symptoms persist or worsen, a follow-up visit may be necessary.

PTERYGIUM

Condition

A pterygium **(Fig. 1.13)** is a growth of pink, fleshy tissue on the conjunctiva, which is the clear, thin membrane that covers the sclera. This growth may start in the corner of the eye and spread to the cornea. Pterygia often look like raised, or triangular shaped growths on the eye. They may be pink, red, or even yellowish.

Causes

Pterygia are commonly associated with prolonged exposure to ultraviolet (UV) light, such as sunlight. Dry, dusty, or windy environments may also increase the risk. Over time, these factors can lead to the development of pterygia.

Signs and Symptoms

Pterygia can cause symptoms such as eye redness, irritation, foreign body sensation, and blurred vision. In severe cases, they may interfere with vision by encroaching on the cornea.

Investigations

The examiner will evaluate the condition of the conjunctiva, cornea, and other ocular structures to determine if the pterygium is affecting your eye health or causing symptoms like redness, irritation, or blurred vision.

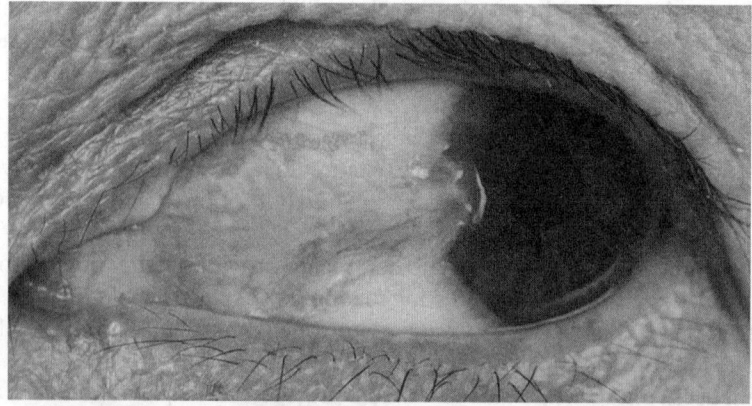

Fig. 1.13: Pterygium.

Management

Mild cases of pterygium may not require treatment and can be managed with lubricating eye drops. In more severe cases, or if the growth causes discomfort or visual disturbances, surgical removal may be necessary. After surgery, pterygia can recur, so close follow-up and protective measures like sunglasses and artificial tears are often recommended.

PINGUECULA

Condition

A pinguecula **(Fig. 1.14)** is a common, non-cancerous growth or lesion on the conjunctiva. Pingueculae are typically found on the side of the eye closer to the nose, although they can occur on the outer side as well. They often appear as small, yellowish or white bumps or deposits on the conjunctiva, and they may have a raised, slightly elevated appearance.

Causes

These growths are primarily associated with chronic exposure to environmental elements, such as ultraviolet (UV) light from the sun, wind, and dust. Long-term exposure to these factors can lead to the development of pingueculae.

Signs and Symptoms

In most cases, pingueculae do not cause significant symptoms. However, they can occasionally become irritated, causing dryness, redness, or a gritty feeling in the eye.

Investigations

The examiner evaluates the condition of the conjunctiva, cornea, and other ocular structures to determine if the pinguecula is causing any problems, such as redness or irritation.

Management

In many cases, no specific treatment is needed for pingueculae. Lubricating eye drops may be recommended to relieve any discomfort. Protective measures, such as wearing sunglasses that block UV light, can help prevent further growth or irritation. Pingueculae are typically

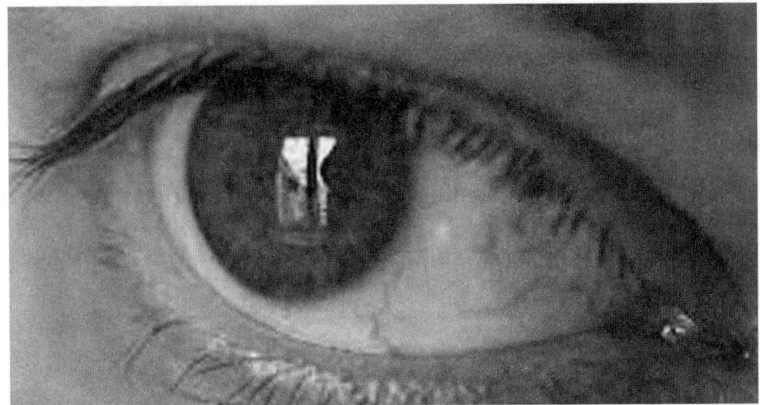

Fig. 1.14: Pinguecula.

benign and do not require surgical removal. However, if they become consistently irritated or are associated with significant discomfort, they may be excised through a minor surgical procedure.

RED EYES

Condition

Red eyes occur when the blood vessels on the surface of the eye (conjunctiva) become enlarged and dilated. Red eye is a descriptive term. Our task is to determine the cause of the redness, so that appropriate treatment can be initiated.

Causes

There are several causes of red eye with conjunctivitis is the most common among all. There may be other causes, such as:
- Lid diseases
- Trauma
- Corneal infection
- Structural change
- Inflammation of intraocular structure
- Acute glaucoma
- Uveitis
- Immune reactions
- Neoplasm
- Subconjunctival hemorrhage
- Dry eyes
- Lack of sleep or fatigue
- Environmental factor

Signs and Symptoms

- Foreign body sensation
- Discharge
- Itching
- Light sensitivity
- Tearing
- Pain
- Puffy eyes

Investigations

The examiner starts with extensive history taking that may include questions about family history, contact lens use, and use of topical and systemic medication, recent trauma, associated systemic illness and then continue examining the different structures of the eye including:
- Eye lid involvement
- Pupils
- Cornea
- Red reflex
- Posterior pole and optic nerve

Management

The treatment and management of red eyes depend on the underlying cause of the redness. It is essential to identify the cause in order to provide appropriate care. Some of the commonest approaches are listed below:
- Frequent cleaning of the eyes with warm, clean water.
- Avoidance of contact with others to prevent the spread of infection.
- Avoidance of allergens, if possible.
- Cold compresses to reduce swelling and itching.
- Avoidance of environmental factors that worsen dry eye.
- Avoid rubbing your eyes, as this can worsen irritation and potentially introduce infections.
- Maintain good hygiene, including regular handwashing, especially if you have infectious conjunctivitis.
- Protect your eyes from environmental factors like wind, smoke, and excessive sun exposure.
- Discontinuation of contact lenses.

DISEASES OF CORNEA

The cornea is the transparent, front surface of the eye that covers the iris and the pupil. It plays a crucial role in vision by acting as the eye's outermost lens, responsible for focusing light onto the retina. The cornea has a curved shape, similar to a dome, and it is primarily composed of layers of specialized cells and collagen fibers. It is avascular, meaning it lacks blood vessels, and it relies on the aqueous humor and tear film for nourishment and protection.

One of the remarkable features of the cornea is its transparency, allowing light to pass through with minimal distortion. The cornea also serves as a protective barrier against dust, debris, and microbial invaders. It is highly sensitive due to its rich supply of nerves, making it susceptible to irritation and pain when injured or irritated.

KERATITIS

Condition

Keratitis is the inflammation of the cornea. It is characterized by corneal edema, infiltration of inflammatory cells, and ciliary congestion **(Fig. 1.15)**. Keratitis may be associated with infectious as well as non-infectious diseases, which may be systemic or localized.

Causes

- Keratitis can be caused because of direct effect of microbial agent, i.e., bacteria, virus, fungi or protozoa.
- Physical injury to the cornea, such as scratches or foreign objects entering the eye, can lead to keratitis.
- Improper use, cleaning, or hygiene of contact lenses can increase the risk of contact lens-related keratitis, particularly if bacteria or other microorganisms become trapped between the lens and the eye.
- Prolonged periods of dry eye can cause damage to the cornea and lead to keratitis.
- Certain allergies can trigger inflammation in the eye, leading to allergic keratitis.
- Conditions like rheumatoid arthritis or systemic lupus erythematosus can affect the cornea and lead to keratitis.

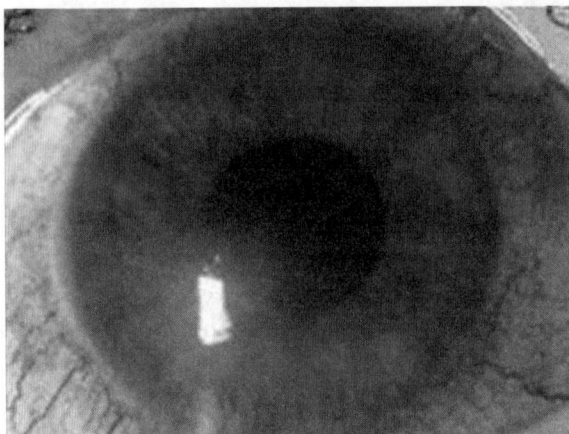

Fig. 1.15: Keratitis.

Signs and Symptoms

- Stromal infiltrates with overlying epithelial defect
- Severe bulbar conjunctival redness
- Watering and muco-purulent discharge
- Inflammation
- Localized epithelial and stromal edema with striae and folds
- Lid swelling
- Foreign body sensation
- Severe pain
- Redness
- Light sensitivity
- Vision disturbances

Investigations

The investigation of keratitis typically involves a series of diagnostic tests and examinations by an ophthalmologist. The purpose of these investigations is to determine the underlying cause of keratitis and its severity so that appropriate treatment can be prescribed. The specific diagnostic tests and procedures used will depend on the clinical presentation of the keratitis and the suspected underlying cause. The investigation starts with history taking and is then followed up by following set of examinations:

- Visual acuity test.
- Slit lamp examination of cornea, as well as other structures in the eye, in detail.
- Fluorescein staining.
- If an infectious cause is suspected, a swab or scraping of the affected area may be collected for microbiological culture to identify the specific pathogen responsible for the keratitis.
- Measuring the intraocular pressure is important, as high intraocular pressure may suggest secondary glaucoma as a complication of keratitis.
- In cases of suspected systemic diseases or autoimmune conditions, blood tests may be ordered to identify underlying causes.
- Anterior segment optical coherence tomography (AS-OCT) or confocal microscopy may be used to obtain detailed images of the cornea.

Management

Keratitis is a serious condition that can potentially lead to vision loss if not treated promptly. Treatment may include antibiotic or antiviral eye drops, corticosteroids, lubricating eye drops, or other medications, depending on the cause and severity of the keratitis.

CORNEAL ULCER

Condition

Corneal ulcer is potentially sight threatening ocular emergency. It is a defect of corneal epithelium that also involves underlying stroma **(Fig. 1.16)**. The condition is typically characterized by painful, open sore or erosion on the surface of the cornea.

Causes

Corneal ulcers can be caused by different factors, including bacterial, viral, or fungal infections, foreign objects or particles entering the eye, contact lens-related issues, dry eye, and certain systemic diseases.

Signs and Symptoms

Common symptoms of a corneal ulcer include severe eye pain, redness, photophobia, blurred or decreased vision, excessive tearing, and the sensation of having a foreign body in the eye.

Investigations

The investigation of a corneal ulcer typically involves a thorough eye examination, including the use of a slit lamp to visualize the ulcer and determine its size and depth. Fluorescein staining may be used to highlight the ulcer.

Management

Treatment of a corneal ulcer depends on the underlying cause. Bacterial ulcers are typically treated with topical antibiotics, while viral ulcers may require antiviral medications. Fungal ulcers need antifungal treatments. In some cases, corticosteroid eye drops may be used to reduce inflammation, but only when an infectious cause has been ruled out, as steroids can worsen certain infections. Lubricating eye drops or ointments may be used to promote healing.

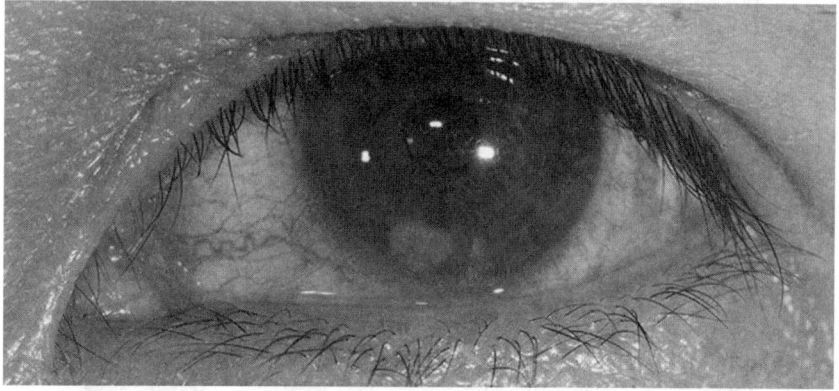

Fig. 1.16: Corneal ulcer.

CORNEAL OPACITY

Condition

Corneal opacity refers to a condition in which the cornea becomes cloudy or loses its transparency **(Fig. 1.17)**. This cloudiness can be partial or complete and is usually caused by various underlying factors or eye conditions. Corneal opacity can significantly impact vision, as it interferes with the passage of light through the cornea and onto the retina.

Causes

The common causes of corneal opacity include:
- Corneal scarring
- Infections, such as bacterial, viral, or fungal keratitis, can lead to inflammation and scarring of the cornea.
- Certain inherited or genetic conditions can lead to progressive clouding of the cornea. Conditions like Fuchs' dystrophy and lattice dystrophy are examples.
- Untreated or severe corneal ulcers may result in scarring and opacity.
- Trauma, foreign objects, or chemical burns to the cornea can cause opacity if not appropriately managed.
- Conditions like keratoconus, which cause the cornea to thin and change shape, can lead to opacity in advanced stages.

Signs and Symptoms

The signs and symptoms of corneal scarring may vary depending on the extent and location of the scar. Some common signs and symptoms of corneal scars may include:
- Reduced visual acuity
- Blurred vision
- Glare and light sensitivity
- In cases where the corneal scarring is associated with underlying conditions like recurrent corneal erosion or inflammation, there may be eye pain and discomfort.
- The eye may appear red or bloodshot due to irritation and inflammation associated with the scar.

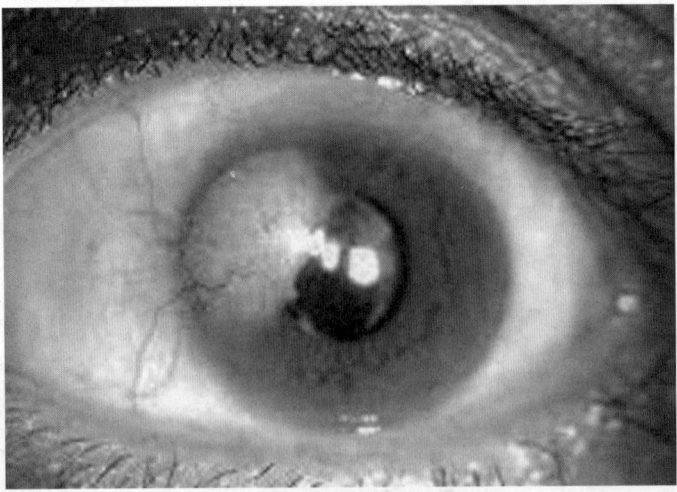

Fig. 1.17: Corneal opacity.

- Scarring can lead to irregularities on the corneal surface, which may be visible during an eye examination.
- Patients may report seeing ghost images or halos around lights, especially in low-light conditions.
- Excessive tearing (epiphora) may occur in response to the irritation and discomfort caused by the scar.

Investigations

A simple visual inspection of the eye can often reveal corneal opacity. It may appear as a white or greyish area on the cornea. Slit lamp can be used to examine the eye's structures in detail. It provides a magnified view of the cornea and allows the examiner to assess the location, size, and extent of the opacity. Corneal opacity may be associated with changes in corneal thickness, which can be detected with pachymetry.

Management

The treatment of corneal opacity depends on its underlying cause, extent, and impact on vision. Phototherapeutic keratectomy (PTK) which is a laser procedure, can be used to remove superficial corneal opacities and irregularities. Corneal transplantation (keratoplasty) may be used in extreme cases. Keratoplasty is a surgical procedure in which the damaged or scarred cornea is replaced with a clear donor cornea. There are different types of keratoplasty procedures, including full-thickness (penetrating) and partial-thickness (lamellar) transplants, depending on the extent of the opacity.

KERATOCONUS

Condition

Keratoconus is a progressive eye disorder in which the cornea gradually thins and bulges into a cone-like shape **(Fig. 1.18)**. This irregular shape of the cornea can cause significant visual distortion, including nearsightedness (myopia) and astigmatism. Keratoconus is a non-inflammatory condition that typically affects both eyes, although it can progress at different rates in each eye.

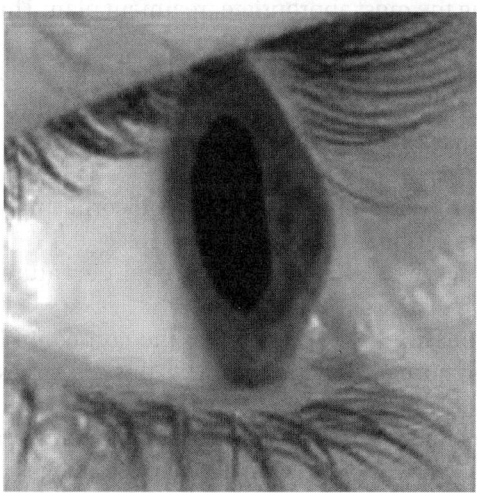

Fig. 1.18: Keratoconus.

Causes

The exact cause of keratoconus is not fully understood, but it is believed to involve a combination of genetic, environmental, and other factors. Some of the possible causes and risk factors associated with keratoconus include:
- One of the most significant factors in the development of keratoconus appears to be genetics. It often runs in families, suggesting that there is a hereditary component. Individuals with a family history of keratoconus are at a higher risk of developing the condition.
- Frequent and vigorous eye rubbing, especially in individuals with allergies or itchy eyes, may increase the risk of keratoconus. The mechanical pressure on the cornea could contribute to the thinning and bulging of the cornea.
- Conditions like atopic dermatitis (eczema) and allergic rhinitis (hay fever) are associated with an increased risk of keratoconus. These conditions may lead to eye rubbing and contribute to the progression of the disease.
- Some rare genetic disorders and conditions that affect connective tissue, such as Ehlers-Danlos syndrome or Marfan syndrome, are associated with a higher risk of keratoconus.

Signs and Symptoms

- The most important sign is the blurry and distorted vision. As the cornea becomes more irregular in shape, it leads to blurred and distorted vision. Straight lines may appear wavy or bent, and vision may be ghosted or double.
- Vision correction with eyeglasses or regular soft contact lenses may become less effective over time, requiring frequent changes in prescriptions.
- People with keratoconus often experience heightened sensitivity to light, making bright lights and glare uncomfortable.
- In advanced cases of keratoconus, tiny cracks or scars can develop in the cornea, further reducing visual acuity.

Investigations

Early diagnosis and management are important to preserve vision and slow the progression of keratoconus. A regular eye examination by an eye care specialist is essential for monitoring the condition and determining the most appropriate treatment plan. The common strategies that may be applied are listed down:
- A standard visual acuity test is conducted to assess the patient's clarity of vision.
- A frequent refraction procedure may be used to determine the patient's prescription for eyeglasses or contact lenses. It helps know the status of myopia or astigmatism that may be present.
- A slit lamp examination is performed to examine the cornea to look for signs of thinning, scarring, and other irregularities.
- Keratometry, may be applied to check the corneal curvature. Keratometry provides quantitative data to help diagnose keratoconus.
- Corneal pachymetry measures the thickness of the cornea. In keratoconus, the cornea tends to be thinner than normal, and measuring its thickness is essential for diagnosis and management.
- Specialized imaging techniques, such as corneal tomography or anterior segment optical coherence tomography (AS-OCT), provide detailed 3D images of the cornea, helping to assess its shape and thickness more accurately.

- The ophthalmologist may use a scalpel to gently touch the cornea's surface. If the cornea is thin due to keratoconus, it will deform and protrude easily when touched.
- The examiner may use fluorescein staining to highlight irregularities in the corneal surface, such as breaks, scars, or other signs of keratoconus.
- In advanced cases of keratoconus, visual field testing may be conducted to evaluate peripheral vision and assess the impact of the condition on a patient's overall visual field.

Management

Treatment for keratoconus varies based on the severity and progression of the condition. Some common treatment options include:
- In the early stages, eyeglasses or rigid gas-permeable (RGP) contact lenses may be sufficient to correct vision.
- Specially designed contact lenses, such as scleral lenses or hybrid lenses, can provide more stable and comfortable vision correction for those with moderate to advanced keratoconus.
- Corneal cross-linking, a minimally invasive procedure may be used to strengthen the cornea and slow the progression of keratoconus.
- Intacs or corneal rings are small plastic rings inserted into the cornea to flatten the cone shape and improve vision.
- Corneal transplant in severe cases when other treatments are not effective, a corneal transplant may be necessary to replace the irregular cornea with a clear donor cornea.

KERATOPLASTY

Keratoplasty, also known as corneal transplantation, is a surgical procedure in which a damaged or diseased cornea is replaced with a clear, healthy cornea from a donor. The cornea is the clear, front surface of the eye responsible for focusing light onto the retina. Keratoplasty is performed to improve or restore vision in individuals with various corneal conditions that cannot be effectively treated by other means.

There are several types of keratoplasty as shown in **Flowchart 1.2**.

Flowchart 1.2: Different types of keratoplasty.

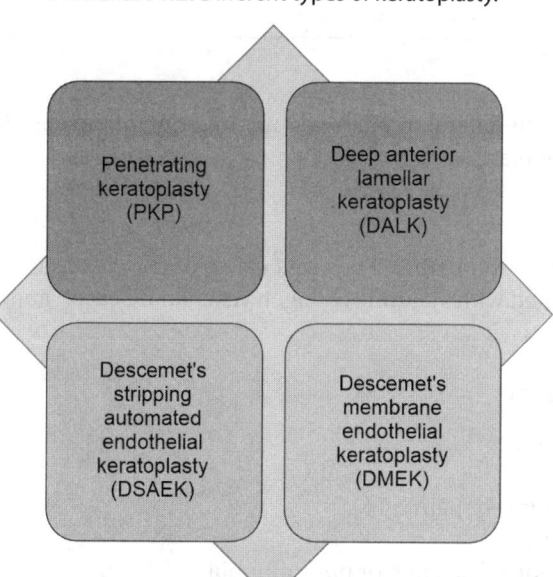

- In penetrating keratoplasty, the entire central cornea is removed and replaced with a donor cornea. This procedure is used for a variety of corneal conditions, including keratoconus, corneal scarring, and corneal dystrophies.
- In case of deep anterior lamellar keratoplasty, the front layers of the cornea are removed and replaced with a donor cornea, while the endothelial layer is left intact. DALK is primarily used when the inner layer of the cornea (endothelium) is healthy, but the anterior layers are affected, as in keratoconus.
- Descemet's stripping automated endothelial keratoplasty (DSAEK) and Descemet's membrane endothelial keratoplasty (DMEK) are specifically aimed at replacing the endothelial layer of the cornea, which is responsible for maintaining corneal transparency. They are used in cases of endothelial dysfunction, such as Fuchs' dystrophy and some cases of corneal edema.

The choice of keratoplasty procedure depends on the specific corneal condition, the depth of corneal involvement, and the health of the different layers of the cornea. The procedure is typically performed under local or general anesthesia, depending on the patient's age and health. After keratoplasty, patients typically go through a recovery period during which vision gradually improves. Visual rehabilitation often involves the use of eyeglasses or contact lenses to achieve the best possible vision. Postoperative care, including the use of medicated eye drops, is essential to prevent infection and promote healing.

Keratoplasty has a high success rate in improving vision and treating corneal conditions. However, it is important to note that there can be risks and complications associated with the procedure, and the long-term success of the transplant depends on various factors, including the patient's overall health and the specific characteristics of the corneal graft. Regular follow-up appointments with an eye care specialist are crucial to monitor the transplanted cornea and manage any potential issues.

DISEASES OF SCLERA

EPISCLERITIS

Condition

Episcleritis is an acute unilateral or bilateral inflammation of the episclera. Episcleritis can be diffuse, sectoral or nodular.

Causes

Episcleritis is most often idiopathic. The exact cause of episcleritis is often unknown, but it is believed to be associated with systemic collagen vascular diseases, autoimmune diseases, and even some infections.

Signs and Symptoms

Patient symptoms include:
- Redness
- Mild ocular discomfort or pain
- Normal visual acuity
- They rarely experience discharge or photophobia

Investigations

The investigation of episcleritis typically involves comprehensive medical history, including any pre-existing medical conditions, medications and whether the similar eye issues had been experienced in the past. Patients will often describe tenderness or mild pain over the affected area but do not exhibit discharge, photophobia, or reduced visual acuity.

The history taking is followed by a comprehensive eye examination to confirm the diagnosis, determine the underlying cause and rule out other more serious eye conditions.

If an underlying systemic condition is suspected, blood tests may be advised to assess your overall health.

Management

Once the diagnosis of episcleritis is confirmed and any underlying causes are identified, the treatment can be executed which may involves the use of lubricating eye drops, artificial tears, or topical anti-inflammatory medications to alleviate the discomfort and reduce inflammation. If there is an underlying systemic condition, the patient may be referred to a specialist for further evaluation and management.

SCLERITIS

Condition

Scleritis is a rare but serious inflammation of the sclera. It is an ocular condition that can cause significant pain and potentially lead to vision loss if left untreated. Scleritis is typically classified into two main categories: anterior scleritis and posterior scleritis. While anterior scleritis affects the front portion of the sclera and is usually more painful and visually threatening, posterior scleritis affects the back portion of the sclera, closer to the optic nerve and retina. It can be associated with less pain but may still result in visual disturbances or complications.

Causes

The exact cause of scleritis is not always clear, but it is often associated with underlying systemic conditions such as autoimmune disorders (e.g., rheumatoid arthritis, systemic lupus erythematosus), infections, or sometimes trauma. Scleritis can be a manifestation of a systemic disease, so a thorough evaluation by a medical professional is essential to identify and treat any underlying conditions.

Signs and Symptoms

Common symptoms of scleritis may include severe eye pain, redness, sensitivity to light, tearing, blurred vision, and sometimes a visible bluish or purplish discoloration of the sclera.

Investigations

Scleritis is a complex condition, and the diagnostic process may vary based on the individual case. Diagnosing scleritis typically involves a combination of clinical evaluation, medical history assessment, and various diagnostic tests. The ophthalmologist may conduct thorough examination to assess the severity of symptoms and identify any visible signs of scleritis, such as redness, swelling, or discoloration of the sclera.

Depending on the underlying systemic conditions or complications associated with scleritis, consultation with other medical specialists, such as rheumatologists or immunologists, may be necessary for further evaluation and management.

Management

Treatment for scleritis typically involves anti-inflammatory medications, such as corticosteroids or nonsteroidal anti-inflammatory drugs (NSAIDs), which may be administered topically, orally, or through injections. Prompt diagnosis and appropriate treatment are crucial to reduce pain and prevent complications. The patient may be referred to seek the other specialized medical services based on diagnosis.

STAPHYLOMA

Condition

A staphyloma is a bulging or protrusion of a part of the eye through an area of weakened tissue or thinning in the eye's structure. Staphylomas can occur in various parts of the eye, and they are usually a result of structural abnormalities, trauma, or underlying eye conditions.

Staphyloma may be of two types—anterior staphyloma and posterior staphyloma as shown in **Table 1.6**.

Causes

Staphylomas are typically caused by structural weaknesses or abnormalities in the eye's tissues. There are several factors and conditions that can contribute to the development of staphylomas, including:

- High myopia is one of the most common risk factors for the development of staphylomas.
- In some cases, individuals may have naturally thin scleral tissue. This thinness can make the eye more susceptible to developing staphylomas.
- Severe eye injuries or trauma, such as a perforating injury or blunt trauma, can weaken the eye's tissues and lead to staphyloma formation.
- Certain inflammatory eye conditions, such as scleritis, can lead to thinning of the sclera and may contribute to staphylomas.
- There may be a genetic component to the development of staphylomas, especially in cases of high myopia.

Investigations

Staphylomas are typically diagnosed through a comprehensive eye examination by an ophthalmologist. Imaging studies, such as optical coherence tomography or ultrasound, may be used to assess the extent and location of the staphyloma and to assess its impact on the retina and surrounding structures.

Management

The management of staphylomas may involve addressing the underlying cause, if possible, and preventing or managing associated complications. It is essential for individuals with risk

Table 1.6: Two types of staphyloma.

Anterior staphyloma	Anterior staphyloma occurs as a response to trauma or infection. The scleral architecture is disturbed and the internal pressure of the eye stretches the weak point causing the protrusion
Posterior staphyloma	Posterior staphylomas occur in the back part of the eye, near the optic nerve and retina. They are often associated with conditions like high myopia in which the elongated eyeball can cause the posterior segment of the eye to bulge

factors, such as high myopia, to have regular eye examinations to monitor for the development of staphylomas and any related issues like retinal detachment or vision changes. If a staphyloma is detected, treatment and management will be determined on a case-by-case basis by an ophthalmologist.

DISEASES OF UVEA

UVEITIS

Condition

Uveitis is the inflammation of the uvea, which is the middle layer of the eye. The uvea consists of the iris, ciliary body, and choroid. Inflammation usually happens when your immune system is fighting an infection. It can also happen when the immune system attacks healthy tissue in your eyes. Uveitis may subside quickly, but it can come back. And sometimes it may turn into chronic. It can affect one or both eyes.

Causes

Uveitis can be a serious eye condition that may result from various causes, including infections, autoimmune diseases, or other underlying health issues.

Signs and Symptoms

Some common symptoms of uveitis include eye redness, pain, light sensitivity, and blurred vision.

Investigations

The investigation of uveitis typically involves a thorough medical evaluation and a series of diagnostic tests to determine the cause, extent, and severity of the condition. The ophthalmologist will start by taking a detailed medical history, including any recent illnesses, medications, allergies, and family history of eye conditions or autoimmune diseases which will be followed by extensive examination of the eye. The ophthalmologist may perform following tests to identify the signs of uveitis:
- Visual acuity testing
- Slit lamp biomicroscopy
- Ophthalmoscopy

More serious tests may be conducted from case to case to that may include blood tests to check the signs of infections, inflammation and autoimmune diseases. In some cases, imaging studies like ultrasound or optical coherence tomography may be used to visualize the internal structures of the eye and assess the severity of uveitis. Fluorescein angiography can be useful for detecting vascular abnormalities associated with uveitis.

Management

Treatment may involve medication, including corticosteroids or immunosuppressive drugs, depending on the cause and type of uveitis.

ENDOPHTHALMITIS

Condition

Endophthalmitis is a severe eye condition characterized by the inflammation and infection of the internal structures of the eye, including the vitreous humor and the surrounding tissues. It is considered a medical emergency and requires prompt diagnosis and treatment to prevent vision loss and further complications.

Signs and Symptoms

- Severe eye pain
- Redness and swelling of the eye
- Decreased vision
- Sensitivity to light (photophobia)
- Excessive tearing
- Floaters (specks or strings in the visual field)
- Reduced or absent pupillary response

Investigations

The diagnosis of endophthalmitis typically involves a comprehensive eye examination and may include additional tests such as:

- Ultrasound may be used to assess the condition of the vitreous and retina when direct visualization is difficult due to inflammation.
- Bacterial or fungal cultures are performed on samples of intraocular fluid to identify the specific causative microorganisms and guide treatment decisions.

Management

Treatment for endophthalmitis is urgent and often involves a combination of the following:

- Antibiotics or antifungal agents are injected directly into the eye to combat the infection within the vitreous humor.
- In cases of endogenous endophthalmitis, oral or intravenous antibiotics are administered to treat the underlying systemic infection.
- In severe cases, surgical intervention may be necessary to drain and remove infected vitreous material (vitrectomy).

PANOPHTHALMITIS

Panophthalmitis is a severe inflammation of the globe. Panophthalmitis can result as a rare complication of ophthalmic surgery. Panophthalmitis usually associated with severe eye pain, reduced visual acuity, chemosis, periorbital swelling, and ptosis. The management of panophthalmitis secondary to IOFB involves both medical and surgical interventions.

DISEASES OF LENS

CATARACT

A cataract is a common eye condition that affects the lens of the eye, causing it to become cloudy or opaque **(Fig. 1.19)**. The lens is normally clear and helps to focus light onto the retina

Normal, clear lens   Lens clouded by cataract

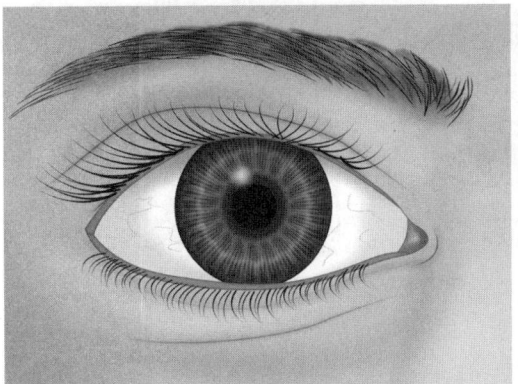
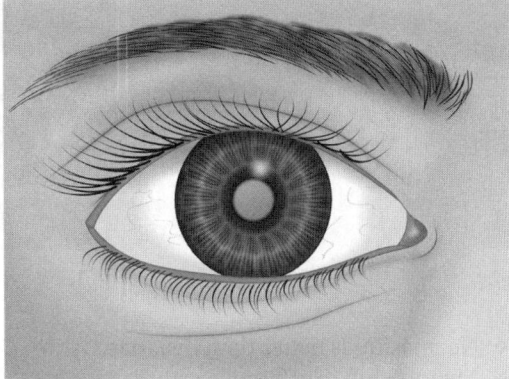

Fig. 1.19: Cataract.

at the back of the eye, which allows us to see sharp and clear images. However, when a cataract forms, it can cause vision problems.

Causes of Cataract

Cataracts typically develop slowly and are most often associated with aging. They can also occur due to other factors, such as:
- Exposure to ultraviolet (UV) radiation from the sun
- Diabetes
- Smoking
- Certain medications
- Eye injuries
- Family history of cataracts

Symptoms of Cataract

The patient who develops cataract usually reports following symptoms:
- Blurry or hazy vision
- Difficulty seeing at night
- Increased sensitivity to glare from lights
- Changes in color perception
- Double vision in one eye
- Frequent changes in eyeglass or contact lens prescription

Types of Cataract

There are mainly three types of cataract as shown in **Figure 1.20**.

Nuclear Cataract

Nuclear cataract is the cloudiness of the nucleus which is the central portion of the lens. As nuclear sclerosis progresses, lens becomes more hardened and opaque. The patient with nuclear cataract shows following symptoms:
- Glare
- Monocular diplopia, worse in dim light

| Cortical cataracts | Nuclear cataracts | Posterior capsular cataracts |

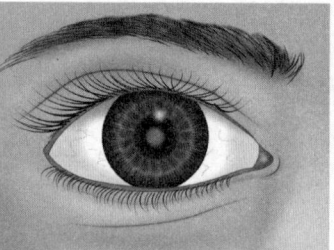
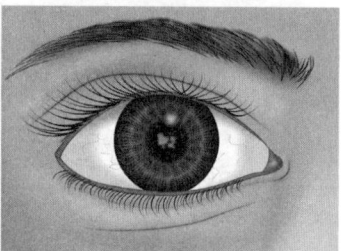

Fig. 1.20: Types of cataract.

- Near vision is better than distance vision
- Myopic shift in refractive error

Cortical Cataract

A cortical cataract begins as whitish, wedge-shaped opacities or streaks on the outer edge of the lens cortex. As it slowly progresses, the streaks extend to the center and interfere with light passing through the center of the lens. The patient with nuclear cataract shows following symptoms:

- Glares
- Light sensitivity
- Problems with depth perception
- Blur vision

The effect of cortical cataract on refractive error is less clear. Cortical cataracts have more astigmatism compare to patients with no cataract which is because of changes in index of refraction in the area of cortical cataract.

Posterior Subcapsular Cataract

Posterior capsular cataracts form faster than the other two types. PSC affect the back of the lens, aside the capsule which holds the lens in place. PSC cataract can form in perfectly normal eyes. The patient with nuclear cataract shows following symptoms:

- Interferes with reading vision
- Reduces your vision in bright light
- Causes glare or halos around lights

Steroids and diabetes are classically known to cause posterior subcapsular cataracts on the back surface of the lens.

LATEST TECHNIQUES IN SURGERY OF CATARACT

Cataract surgery had already evolved significantly, with several advanced techniques and technologies being used to improve patient outcomes and reduce the invasiveness of the procedure. Some of the latest techniques and technologies in cataract surgery are listed below:

Phacoemulsification

Phacoemulsification is the most common and modern technique for cataract surgery. It involves using ultrasound energy to break up the cloudy lens into small fragments, which are then suctioned out of the eye through a small incision. This procedure is minimally invasive and often allows for quicker recovery.

Femtosecond Laser-assisted Cataract Surgery

This advanced technique uses a femtosecond laser to create precise incisions, capsulotomies, and fragment the cataract before traditional phacoemulsification. This technology can enhance the accuracy of the procedure and reduce the risk of complications.

Microincision Cataract Surgery

Microincision cataract surgery (MICS) involves making smaller incisions, typically less than 2.2 mm in size. This minimally invasive approach reduces the risk of complications, such as infection, and speeds up recovery time.

Advanced IOLs

Intraocular lenses have also seen significant advancements. Multifocal and toric IOLs are now available, offering patients the potential for improved near and distance vision or astigmatism correction. Extended depth of focus (EDOF) and accommodating IOLs are also options designed to reduce the need for glasses after cataract surgery.

SUBLUXATION/DISLOCATION OF LENS

Subluxation and dislocation of the lens are medical conditions that involve the displacement of the eye's crystalline lens, which is normally positioned behind the iris and the pupil. These conditions can result from various reasons and can lead to serious complications.

Subluxation refers to the partial displacement or misalignment of the lens within the eye. This condition can be caused by various factors, including trauma, congenital disorders, or connective tissue diseases like Marfan syndrome or Ehlers-Danlos syndrome. When the lens is partially dislocated, it may not cause significant visual disturbances, and the eye may compensate for the displacement.

Dislocation, also known as luxation, refers to the complete displacement of the lens from its normal position within the eye. Lens dislocation can be categorized into two main types: anterior dislocation and posterior dislocation. In case of anterior dislocation, the lens moves forward and may sometimes end up in the anterior chamber of the eye and in case of posterior dislocation, the lens moves backward and may end up in the vitreous cavity at the back of the eye.

The common causes and associated conditions are:
- **Trauma:** A significant injury to the eye can displace the lens, causing subluxation or dislocation.
- **Congenital disorders:** Some individuals may have a genetic predisposition to lens subluxation or dislocation.
- **Connective tissue disorders:** Conditions like Marfan syndrome and Ehlers-Danlos syndrome can weaken the eye's supporting structures, increasing the risk of lens displacement.
- **Cataracts or surgery:** In some cases, surgical procedures on the eye, such as cataract surgery, can lead to lens dislocation.

The patient usually reports following symptoms:
- Visual disturbances, such as blurred or distorted vision.
- Sensitivity to light
- Pain or discomfort in the eye.
- Halos or glare around lights.
- Headaches or eye strain.

The treatment approach depends on the extent of lens displacement and associated symptoms. Surgical intervention may be necessary to reposition or remove the dislocated lens. The specific procedure used depends on the nature of the dislocation and the patient's overall eye health.

DISEASES OF THE ANGLE OF ANTERIOR CHAMBER

GLAUCOMA

Glaucoma is a group of eye conditions that can lead to damage of the optic nerve, which is crucial for transmitting visual information from the eye to the brain. This damage is often associated with elevated intraocular pressure (IOP), but glaucoma can also occur with normal or low IOP. If left untreated, glaucoma can result in vision loss and blindness. Two most common types of glaucoma are:

1. **Open-angle glaucoma:** This is the most common form of glaucoma. It occurs when the drainage system within the eye, known as the trabecular meshwork, becomes less efficient at draining aqueous humor. As a result, the pressure within the eye increases gradually over time, leading to optic nerve damage.
2. **Angle-closure glaucoma:** This type of glaucoma is less common but more acute. It happens when the drainage angle of the eye becomes blocked, causing a sudden increase in intraocular pressure. Angle-closure glaucoma requires immediate medical attention because it can lead to rapid vision loss.

Symptoms

Glaucoma is often called the "silent thief of sight" because it typically progresses slowly and may not cause noticeable symptoms in its early stages. As a result, regular eye exams are crucial for the early detection and management of glaucoma. Common symptoms may include:
- Peripheral vision loss
- Tunnel vision
- Blurred vision
- Halos around lights
- Eye pain or redness in cases of acute angle-closure glaucoma

Causes

The exact causes of glaucoma are not fully understood, but the condition is often associated with elevated intraocular pressure (IOP), which can damage the optic nerve over time. There are several factors that can contribute to the development of glaucoma:
- Elevated intraocular pressure is a significant risk factor for glaucoma. The eye constantly produces a clear fluid called aqueous humor, and it must drain properly to maintain a healthy IOP. When the drainage system becomes less efficient or blocked, the pressure within the eye can increase, leading to optic nerve damage.
- A family history of glaucoma can increase one's risk of developing the condition. Some forms of glaucoma have a genetic component, and specific gene mutations may be associated with the disease.
- The risk of developing glaucoma increases with age. Primary open-angle glaucoma, the most common form, is more common in older individuals, typically over the age of 40.

- Some ethnic groups, particularly African Americans, are at a higher risk for certain types of glaucoma. They tend to develop glaucoma at a younger age and may experience more severe forms of the disease.
- Certain medical conditions, such as diabetes and hypertension, can increase the risk of glaucoma. Additionally, a history of eye injuries or surgeries can also be a risk factor.
- Long-term use of corticosteroid medications, especially in the form of eye drops, can increase the risk of developing a specific type of glaucoma known as steroid-induced glaucoma.
- Individuals with high myopia may have a higher risk of developing glaucoma.
- Certain eye anatomical features, such as a thinner-than-normal or "cupped" optic nerve head, may be associated with a higher risk of glaucoma.
- Angle-closure glaucoma, a less common but more acute form, is associated with anatomical factors where the drainage angle of the eye is narrowed or blocked. Hyperopia (farsightedness) and a shallow anterior chamber of the eye are among the risk factors for this type of glaucoma.
- It is important to note that glaucoma can develop in individuals without any obvious risk factors, and not everyone with elevated IOP will develop the condition.

Investigations

Diagnosing glaucoma typically involves a combination of eye examinations and tests conducted by an eye care professional, such as an ophthalmologist or optometrist. The following are common investigations and tests used in the diagnosis and assessment of glaucoma:
- **Tonometry:** Tonometry measures the intraocular pressure (IOP) of the eye, which is a key risk factor for glaucoma. The most common tonometry test involves using an instrument called a tonometer.
- **Ophthalmoscopy:** Ophthalmoscopy or fundoscopy allows the eye care professional to examine the optic nerve head at the back of the eye. They use a special instrument called an ophthalmoscope to check for signs of optic nerve damage, such as cupping.
- **Perimetry:** Perimetry assesses the visual field, which is the full extent of what can be seen by the eye. This test helps to detect any peripheral vision loss, which is a common sign of glaucoma. Automated visual field testing is often used, and patients are asked to respond to blinking lights in their peripheral vision.
- **Gonioscopy:** Gonioscopy is used to evaluate the drainage angle of the eye, which is important in distinguishing between open-angle and angle-closure glaucoma. A special contact lens with a mirrored surface is placed on the eye to allow the examiner to view the angle.
- **Pachymetry:** Pachymetry measures the thickness of the cornea. Corneal thickness can affect the accuracy of IOP measurements, and it is an important consideration in glaucoma diagnosis and management.
- **Optical coherence tomography (OCT):** OCT is a non-invasive imaging technique that provides high-resolution cross-sectional images of the retinal layers, optic nerve head, and retinal nerve fiber layer. It is valuable in assessing structural changes in the eye related to glaucoma.
- **Photography:** Photographs of the optic nerve head and retina may be taken for documentation and monitoring of glaucoma progression over time.
- **Assessment of anterior chamber depth:** In cases of angle-closure glaucoma, the depth of the anterior chamber of the eye is assessed to determine the risk of angle closure.

The specific tests and frequency of examinations may vary based on the type and severity of glaucoma, the patient's risk factors, and the healthcare provider's judgment.

Management

The treatment and management of glaucoma primarily aim to lower intraocular pressure (IOP) to prevent further damage to the optic nerve. The specific approach to treatment depends on the type of glaucoma, its severity, and the individual patient's needs. The common methods and strategies for managing glaucoma:

- **Eye drops:** Most people with glaucoma are initially prescribed medicated eye drops to lower IOP. There are several types of eye drops, including prostaglandin analogs, beta-blockers, alpha agonists, and carbonic anhydrase inhibitors. Compliance with the prescribed eye drop regimen is essential for effective management.
- **Oral medications:** In some cases, oral medications may be prescribed to complement eye drops and further reduce IOP.
- **Laser trabeculoplasty:** This procedure is often used to treat open-angle glaucoma. It involves using a laser to open drainage channels in the trabecular meshwork, allowing for better fluid outflow.
- **Laser peripheral iridotomy:** This treatment is used for angle-closure glaucoma. A small hole is created in the peripheral iris to improve the drainage of aqueous humor.
- **Trabeculectomy:** In this surgical procedure, a new drainage channel is created to allow excess fluid to drain from the eye.
- **Drainage implant devices:** Devices like glaucoma drainage implants, also known as glaucoma drainage devices or tubes, are implanted in the eye to help control IOP.
- **Combined procedures:** Some individuals with glaucoma may require a combination of treatments, such as eye drops, laser therapy, and surgery, to effectively manage their condition.
- **Regular monitoring:** Glaucoma is a chronic condition, so ongoing monitoring by an eye care specialist is crucial to assess the progression of the disease and the effectiveness of treatment. Monitoring may involve visual field testing, optical coherence tomography (OCT), and periodic measurement of IOP.
- **Lifestyle and dietary modifications:** Although lifestyle changes cannot cure glaucoma, certain habits can help manage the condition and promote eye health. These include maintaining a healthy lifestyle with regular exercise, not smoking, and managing conditions like diabetes and hypertension. Additionally, some studies suggest that a diet rich in antioxidants, like green leafy vegetables and foods with omega-3 fatty acids, may be beneficial.

Glaucoma is a lifelong condition, and management may require adjustments over time. The goal of treatment and management is to preserve vision and slow the progression of the disease. Early diagnosis and consistent follow-up with an eye care professional are crucial for achieving these goals.

DISEASES OF VITREOUS

VITREOUS HEMORRHAGE

Vitreous hemorrhage, also known as vitreous bleeding or bleeding into the vitreous humor, is a medical condition that occurs when blood leaks into the clear gel-like substance that fills the interior of the eye, known as the vitreous humor. The vitreous humor is located behind the lens and in front of the retina. When blood enters the vitreous humor, it can obstruct vision and cause various visual symptoms.

Causes

Vitreous hemorrhage can result from various underlying causes, including:
- Diabetic retinopathy is one of the most common causes of vitreous hemorrhage. In diabetic retinopathy, damage to blood vessels in the retina can lead to bleeding into the vitreous.
- Tears or detachments of the retina can cause bleeding into the vitreous humor.
- Conditions like retinal vein occlusion or retinal artery macroaneurysm can lead to vitreous hemorrhage.
- Eye injuries, such as a direct blow to the eye, can cause bleeding into the vitreous.
- As people age, the risk of vitreous hemorrhage may increase due to the natural aging process and associated changes in the vitreous humor.

Symptoms

The symptoms of vitreous hemorrhage can vary in severity and may include:
- Sudden onset of floaters (dark spots or specks that appear to drift across your field of vision).
- Blurred or reduced vision.
- Flashes of light.
- Loss of peripheral vision.
- Reddish or hazy appearance in the affected eye.

Investigations

The investigation of vitreous hemorrhage typically involves a series of steps to determine the underlying cause.

The first step is a thorough medical history and physical examination, during which your ophthalmologist will ask you about your symptoms and any relevant medical conditions. They will also assess your visual acuity and perform a basic eye examination.

A dilated eye examination is a crucial part of the evaluation. During this exam, the ophthalmologist will use eye drops to dilate your pupils, allowing a more comprehensive view of the inside of the eye. This will help them identify the source and extent of the vitreous hemorrhage and any associated retinal or vitreous issues.

Depending on the findings, the ophthalmologist may order additional tests to determine the underlying cause of the vitreous hemorrhage. These tests may include:
- **Fluorescein angiography:** This test involves injecting a fluorescent dye into your bloodstream and taking photographs of the retinal blood vessels. It helps to identify abnormalities in blood vessel structure and blood flow.
- **Optical coherence tomography (OCT):** OCT is a non-invasive imaging technique that provides detailed cross-sectional images of the retina and can help assess retinal thickness and other structural changes.
- **B-scan ultrasonography:** Ultrasound imaging may be used to evaluate the extent of the vitreous hemorrhage and to detect any retinal detachments or other abnormalities that are not visible through a dilated eye exam.

Management

The choice of treatment depends on the underlying cause and the severity of the vitreous hemorrhage. Treatment options may include:
- **Observation:** If the hemorrhage is small, and there are no signs of a serious underlying condition, your doctor may recommend a period of observation to see if the hemorrhage resolves on its own.

- **Control of underlying conditions:** If the vitreous hemorrhage is related to an underlying condition, such as diabetic retinopathy, treatment of that condition (e.g., laser therapy or intravitreal injections) may be necessary to prevent further bleeding.
- **Vitrectomy:** In cases of extensive or non-resolving vitreous hemorrhage, the ophthalmologist may recommend a vitrectomy. This surgical procedure involves the removal of the vitreous humor and any blood within it. The vitreous is then replaced with a clear solution. Vitrectomy is often performed when there is a retinal tear, detachment, or other serious issues contributing to the bleeding.
- **Cryotherapy or laser photocoagulation:** These procedures may be used to treat underlying retinal tears or detachments.

VITREOUS OPACITIES

Vitreous opacities refer to the presence of cloudy or hazy areas in the vitreous humor, which is the clear gel-like substance that fills the space between the lens and the retina in the eye. These opacities can manifest as floaters, specks, cobwebs, or other shapes that appear to drift across your field of vision. The vitreous humor is mostly composed of water, collagen fibers, and other substances, and as the eye ages, the vitreous gel can undergo changes that lead to the development of opacities.

Causes

The common causes of vitreous opacities include:
- Age-related changes can make vitreous more liquid and develop clumps of cells or debris, causing floaters.
- Posterior vitreous detachment occurs when the vitreous humor separates from the retina. This separation can cause the release of cells and debris into the vitreous cavity, leading to floaters.
- Inflammatory conditions affecting the eye, such as uveitis, can cause the release of inflammatory cells into the vitreous, leading to opacities.
- Conditions such as diabetic retinopathy or trauma can cause bleeding in the vitreous, leading to the appearance of opacities.
- In some cases, vitreous opacities can be associated with retinal tears or detachment, which may require prompt medical attention.

Signs and Symptoms

Vitreous opacities, commonly known as floaters, can manifest with various signs and symptoms, the common among them are:
- The most common and noticeable symptom is the presence of floaters. These are small, dark specks, cobwebs, or other irregular shapes that seem to float across your field of vision. Floaters are more noticeable against a bright background, such as a clear sky or a white wall.
- Some people with vitreous opacities may also experience flashes of light, especially when they move their eyes quickly. These flashes can be a result of the vitreous tugging on the retina during eye movement.
- In some cases, vitreous opacities may cause temporary blurring of vision, particularly if the floaters are located near the center of your visual field.
- While floaters are often a natural part of the aging process, a sudden increase in their number or the onset of new floaters may indicate a more serious condition, such as a retinal tear or detachment. This requires prompt medical attention.

- Depending on the location and size of the vitreous opacities, you may experience visual disturbances, such as difficulty focusing on objects or seeing clearly.

Investigations

The investigation of vitreous opacities typically involves a thorough eye examination by an ophthalmologist. Here are the steps involved in investigating vitreous opacities:
- **Comprehensive eye examination:** The comprehensive eye examination includes visual acuity test, slit lamp examination and dilated pupil examination to examine the retina and vitreous humor more thoroughly.
- **Retinal examination:** Funduscopy to examine retina using an ophthalmoscope after pupil dilation and optical coherence tomography that provides detailed cross-sectional images of the retina may be recommended.
- **Fluorescein angiography:** If retinal vascular abnormalities are suspected, fluorescein angiography may be performed to assess blood flow in the retina.
- **Ultrasound imaging:** B-scan ultrasonography may be used to visualize the structures of the eye, especially if the view is obstructed by opacities.

Management

- **Observation:** If the vitreous opacities are benign and not causing significant visual impairment, observation may be recommended.
- **Surgery (vitrectomy):** In cases where floaters significantly affect vision or are associated with retinal issues, a vitrectomy may be considered. During this procedure, the vitreous humor is removed and replaced with a clear solution.
- **Laser therapy:** In certain cases, laser therapy may be used to treat underlying retinal issues or to break apart large floaters.

Regular follow-up appointments may be scheduled to monitor the condition and ensure there are no complications.

Addressing Underlying Causes

If the vitreous opacities are symptom of an underlying condition such as diabetic retinopathy or uveitis, the primary condition needs to be addressed through appropriate medical or surgical interventions.

Patients should be educated about the benign nature of most floaters and the importance of seeking prompt medical attention if there are sudden changes in floaters, flashes of light, or other visual symptoms.

VITRECTOMY

A vitrectomy is a surgical procedure in which the vitreous humor, the gel-like substance inside the eye, is removed. This procedure is often performed by an ophthalmologist and is used to treat various eye conditions, including those associated with vitreous opacities (floaters) or retinal issues.

Indications for Vitrectomy

- **Vitreous opacities (floaters):** When floaters significantly impair vision and affect daily activities.
- **Retinal detachment or tears:** To repair and stabilize the retina.
- **Diabetic retinopathy:** In advanced cases with vitreous hemorrhage or traction on the retina.

- ❖ **Macular hole or epiretinal membrane:** To improve vision and restore retinal anatomy.
- ❖ **Endophthalmitis:** Infections inside the eye.
- ❖ **Complications of previous eye surgery:** Such as complications from cataract surgery.

Vitrectomy Procedure

The patient is typically given local anesthesia to numb the eye. In some cases, the procedure may be performed under general anesthesia, especially for more complex cases.

Small incisions are made in the eye to allow the introduction of microsurgical instruments.

The vitreous humor is carefully removed using a vitrectomy probe, which simultaneously cuts and suctions the gel.

The surgeon replaces the removed vitreous with a clear saline solution or a temporary gas or silicone oil bubble to maintain the eye's shape during the procedure.

Postoperative Care

Patients are typically monitored closely in the immediate postoperative period. Depending on the specific case, patients may need to maintain a face-down position for a certain period to facilitate the proper positioning of a gas or oil bubble.

DISEASES OF RETINA

DIABETIC AND HYPERTENSIVE RETINOPATHY

Diabetic retinopathy and hypertensive retinopathy are two distinct eye conditions that can affect individuals with diabetes and hypertension, respectively.

Diabetic Retinopathy

Diabetic retinopathy is a complication of diabetes that affects the eyes. It occurs when high levels of blood sugar damage the blood vessels in the retina. It can be non-proliferative diabetic retinopathy (NPDR) which is the early stage with mild blood vessel damage or proliferative diabetic retinopathy (PDR) which is advanced stage where new blood vessels grow, but they are fragile and can bleed into the eye.

Causes

Prolonged periods of high blood sugar can weaken and damage the small blood vessels in the retina, leading to various changes in the eyes.

Symptoms

- ❖ Blurred or distorted vision
- ❖ Floaters or spots in the field of vision
- ❖ Difficulty seeing at night
- ❖ Gradual vision loss

Prevention and Management

- ❖ Tight control of blood sugar levels
- ❖ Regular eye exams to detect and treat retinopathy early
- ❖ Blood pressure control
- ❖ Laser therapy or surgery in advanced cases

Hypertensive Retinopathy

Hypertensive retinopathy is a condition where high blood pressure damages the small blood vessels in the retina. It is a complication of long-term or severe hypertension. There are stages of hypertensive retinopathy. Grade I is characterized by mild narrowing of the arteries, Grade II is characterized by moderate narrowing with changes in the appearance of the optic nerve, Grade III shows severe narrowing, copper or silver wire arterioles and Grade IV shows the signs of Grade III with swelling of the optic nerve.

Causes

Prolonged high blood pressure can cause the blood vessels in the retina to narrow, leak, or become blocked.

Symptoms

- Blurred or decreased vision
- Headaches
- Hypertensive emergencies may cause more severe symptoms like visual disturbances and swelling of the optic nerve

Prevention and Management

- Control blood pressure through lifestyle changes and medications.
- Regular eye exams to monitor retinal health.
- Address underlying causes of hypertension, such as diet, exercise, and stress management.

Both diabetic and hypertensive retinopathy emphasize the importance of managing the underlying conditions to prevent or slow the progression of retinal damage. It is crucial for individuals with diabetes or hypertension to have regular check-ups with healthcare professionals, including eye exams, to detect and manage any complications early.

RETINAL DETACHMENT

Retinal detachment is a medical emergency. It is an eye problem that happens when the retina is pulled away from its normal position at the back of your eye. This separation can lead to a loss of vision if not promptly treated.

There are three main types of retinal detachment:

1. **Rhegmatogenous retinal detachment:** This is the most common type and is often caused by a tear or hole in the retina that allows fluid to pass through and accumulate between the retina and the underlying tissues.
2. **Tractional retinal detachment:** This occurs when scar tissue on the retina's surface contracts and causes the retina to pull away from the underlying tissue.
3. **Exudative (serous) retinal detachment:** This type involves the accumulation of fluid beneath the retina, but without a tear or hole. It is usually associated with conditions that cause fluid to seep into the retina.

Symptoms

If only a small part of the retina detaches, the subject may not have any symptoms. But if significant part of retina is detached, you may not be able to see as clearly as normal, and you may notice other sudden symptoms, including:

- A lot of new floaters (small dark spots or squiggly lines that float across your vision)
- Flashes of light in the affected eye

- A dark shadow or "curtain" on the sides or in the middle of your field of vision
- Blurred or reduced vision

Causes

Rhegmatogenous retinal detachment is the most common type of retinal detachment and is often associated with a tear or hole in the retina. The causes include:
- As people age, the vitreous gel inside the eye may become more liquid and shrink, increasing the risk of retinal tears.
- Injuries to the eye can lead to retinal tears or detachments.
- Individuals with high myopia are at an increased risk due to elongation of the eyeball.

Scar tissue on the retina's surface can contract and cause the retina to be pulled away from the underlying tissue. The causes include:
- Abnormal blood vessel growth in the retina associated with diabetes can lead to scar tissue formation.
- Premature infants may develop abnormal blood vessels and scar tissue.

Exudative (serous) retinal detachment involves the accumulation of fluid beneath the retina without a tear. The causes include:
- Conditions like uveitis can lead to fluid accumulation.
- Tumors behind the eye can produce fluid and cause detachment.
- In some cases, AMD can be associated with fluid accumulation.

There are other factors that are associated with retinal detachment:
- A family history of retinal detachment may increase the risk.
- Individuals who have had cataract surgery or other eye surgeries may be at a slightly increased risk.
- Certain eye conditions, such as lattice degeneration or retinoschisis, can predispose individuals to retinal detachment.

Investigations

Diagnosing retinal detachment typically involves a comprehensive eye examination by an eye care professional. The following are common methods used in the investigation of retinal detachment:
- Medical history and visual acuity test
- Slit lamp examination and retinal examination
- Ultrasound imaging
- Visual field examination
- Optical coherence tomography (OCT)
- Fluorescein angiography
- Electroretinogram (ERG)

Management

If retinal detachment is suspected based on these investigations, prompt treatment is crucial to prevent further vision loss. Treatment options often involve surgery, and the choice of procedure depends on the type and severity of the detachment. Treatment options often involve surgery, such as pneumatic retinopexy, scleral buckle, or vitrectomy, depending on the type and severity of the detachment.

CENTRAL SEROUS RETINOPATHY

Central serous retinopathy (CSR) is characterized by the accumulation of fluid underneath the central part of the retina, known as the macula. This can lead to distorted or blurred vision in the affected eye.

Symptoms
- Blurred or distorted central vision
- A blind spot or dark area in the central vision
- Reduced color perception
- Objects appearing smaller or farther away than they are

Causes
Exact cause of CSR is not fully understood, but it is often associated with stress and an overactive response of the body's cortisol (a stress hormone) levels. The common causes are listed down:
- Stress is often considered a major contributing factor.
- The use of systemic or local corticosteroids has been associated with an increased risk of CSR. These medications can affect the balance of fluid in the body and may contribute to the accumulation of fluid under the retina.
- High blood pressure has been identified as a potential risk factor for CSR. Elevated blood pressure may affect the integrity of the blood vessels in the choroid.
- There may be a genetic component, as some cases of CSR appear to run in families.
- Dysfunction in the immune system or inflammatory processes may contribute to CSR in some cases.

Investigations
The investigation of CSR typically involves a combination of clinical examination and imaging studies that may include:
- An ophthalmologist will conduct a comprehensive eye examination, including a detailed history and a thorough examination of the retina to assess the extent of the fluid accumulation.
- Measurement of visual acuity is essential to determine the impact of CSR on central vision.
- Fluorescein angiography involves injecting a dye into a vein in the arm and taking photographs as the dye passes through the blood vessels in the retina. This helps identify areas of leakage and pinpoint the source of fluid accumulation.
- Optical coherence tomography is a non-invasive imaging technique that provides high-resolution cross-sectional images of the retina. It is particularly useful in assessing the extent and location of fluid accumulation and monitoring changes over time.

Management
In many cases, CSR resolves spontaneously without specific treatment. Observation and monitoring of visual symptoms may be recommended initially.
- Stress reduction and lifestyle changes may be advised, as stress is considered a potential trigger for CSR.
- If the patient is using systemic or local corticosteroids, discontinuing or reducing their use may be considered under the guidance of a healthcare professional.
- Photodynamic therapy involves using a light-activated drug (verteporfin) and a low-power laser to selectively target and treat abnormal blood vessels in the retina. This may be considered in persistent cases.

- Laser treatment may be used to seal leaking blood vessels and reduce fluid accumulation.
- Anti-vascular endothelial growth factor (anti-VEGF) drugs, such as ranibizumab, have been investigated as potential treatments for CSR, although their use is not yet standard.
- In some cases, oral medications such as mineralocorticoid receptor antagonists may be prescribed to reduce fluid leakage.

CYSTOID MACULAR EDEMA

Cystoid macular edema (CME) is a condition characterized by the presence of fluid-filled cyst-like spaces in the macula. This accumulation of fluid can lead to swelling and thickening of the macula, causing vision distortion and impairment. The associated causes may be diabetic macular edema, uveitis, retinal vascular diseases, age-related macular degeneration (AMD) or any condition that causes leakage from retinal blood vessels. Optical coherence tomography (OCT) is a key to diagnose CME. Besides, fluorescein angiography may be considered. Injections of anti-vascular endothelial growth factor (VEGF) drugs, such as ranibizumab or bevacizumab, are commonly used to reduce vascular leakage and improve CME associated with conditions like DME or neovascular AMD. Intravitreal corticosteroid injections or sustained-release implants can be used to reduce inflammation and edema.

RETINOBLASTOMA

Retinoblastoma is a rare and potentially life-threatening eye cancer that primarily affects the retina of the young children under the age of 5, and it can occur in one or both eyes.

Signs and Symptoms

- Leukocoria (white eye reflex) is often the first noticeable sign. When light is shone into the affected eye, instead of the normal red-eye reflection seen in photographs, a white glow or white pupil may be observed.
- The affected eye may turn inward or outward.
- Children with retinoblastoma may experience redness and irritation in the affected eye.
- The child may have problems with vision in the affected eye.

Investigations

If retinoblastoma is suspected, an eye examination and imaging studies, such as ultrasound or MRI, may be conducted to confirm the diagnosis and determine the extent of the disease.

Management

The management for retinoblastoma may include chemotherapy, laser therapy, cryotherapy, radiation therapy, and in some cases, surgery. The choice of treatment depends on the size and location of the tumor, whether it has spread, and the overall health of the child.

CENTRAL RETINAL ARTERY OCCLUSION

Central retinal artery occlusion (CRAO) is a medical condition that occurs when the central retinal artery, the blood vessel that supplies blood to the retina, becomes blocked. This blockage can lead to a sudden and severe loss of vision in the affected eye. The symptoms of CRAO include sudden, painless vision loss in one eye. The affected eye may also appear pale or cloudy, and the person may experience a sudden onset of blindness. Immediate medical attention is crucial in cases of CRAO to attempt to restore blood flow to the retina and minimize potential vision loss. The treatment options for CRAO may include intraocular pressure reduction, ocular massage or retinal artery bypass surgery. Early diagnosis and prompt treatment are critical in maximizing the chances of preserving vision in cases of CRAO.

CENTRAL RETINAL VEIN OCCLUSION

Central retinal vein occlusion (CRVO) is a condition that occurs when the central retinal vein, a blood vessel that drains blood from the retina, becomes blocked. This blockage can lead to the backup of blood in the retina, causing swelling and potential damage to retinal cells. The symptoms of CRVO may include sudden, painless vision loss or blurring in one eye, distorted or wavy vision, floaters in the field of vision. Laser photocoagulation may be used to treat complications such as macular edema and neovascularisation. In some cases, vitrectomy may be considered for severe cases of CRVO.

BRANCH RETINAL ARTERY OCCLUSION

Branch retinal artery occlusion (BRAO) is a medical condition where one of the smaller arteries that supply blood to a portion of the retina becomes blocked. This blockage can lead to a sudden and localized loss of vision in the affected area of the retina. The severity of vision loss depends on the size and location of the blocked artery. The patient reports sudden and painless vision loss in a specific area of the visual field. The specific treatment approach depends on the underlying cause and the individual's overall health. Gentle massage of the eyeball, lowering of intraocular pressure and systemic anticoagulation medication may be prescribed to manage the case.

BRANCH RETINAL VEIN OCCLUSION

BRVO stands for Branch Retinal Vein Occlusion, a condition in which one of the branches of the central retinal vein becomes blocked. This blockage can lead to blood and fluid backup in the affected area of the retina, causing vision problems. Controlling systemic conditions such as hypertension and diabetes is essential in managing BRVO.

EALE'S DISEASE

Eale's disease, also known as Eale's syndrome, is a rare idiopathic inflammatory disorder that primarily affects the peripheral retina, particularly the veins. It is characterized by retinal inflammation, ischemia, and the formation of abnormal new blood vessels. Eale's disease typically occurs in young adults, and is more prevalent in certain geographic regions, including India. The management of Eale's disease is tailored to the specific stage and manifestations of the disease. Regular follow-up with an ophthalmologist is essential to monitor the progression of the condition and to intervene promptly if complications arise.

DISEASES OF OPTIC NERVE

OPTIC NEURITIS

Optic neuritis is a condition characterized by inflammation of the optic nerve, which is the bundle of nerve fibers that transmits visual information from the eye to the brain. This inflammation can cause a variety of symptoms related to vision. The exact cause of optic neuritis is not always clear, but it is often associated with autoimmune diseases such as multiple sclerosis (MS). In fact, optic neuritis is sometimes considered an early sign of MS. Other potential causes include infections, such as viral or bacterial infections, and inflammatory disorders. Diagnosis is typically based on a combination of clinical symptoms, a thorough eye examination, and often imaging studies such as magnetic resonance imaging (MRI) to assess the optic nerve and rule out other potential causes. Treatment may involve addressing the underlying cause, such as treating an underlying infection or managing an autoimmune condition. In some cases, corticosteroids may be prescribed to reduce inflammation and speed up recovery.

PAPILLEDEMA

"Papilledema" refers to the swelling of the optic nerve head (also known as the optic disc) due to increased intracranial pressure. The optic nerve head is the part of the optic nerve that enters the eye and is visible during an eye examination. Papilledema is not a disease itself but rather a sign of an underlying problem that is causing increased pressure within the skull. The optic nerve head is normally not visible during a routine eye examination because it is covered by the nerve fibers of the retina. When there is increased pressure within the skull, the optic nerve head becomes swollen, and this can be observed during an eye exam. The swelling is a result of the transmission of pressure from the brain to the optic nerve. Symptoms of papilledema can include visual disturbances, headaches (often worse in the morning), and nausea. Treatment aims at addressing the underlying cause of increased intracranial pressure.

OPTIC ATROPHY

Optic atrophy refers to the loss or degeneration of the optic nerve, which can lead to a gradual or sudden loss of vision. The optic nerve is crucial for transmitting visual information from the eyes to the brain. When the optic nerve is damaged and atrophied, it can result in permanent vision impairment. The symptoms of optic atrophy include a gradual or sudden decrease in vision, changes in color vision, and a pale appearance of the optic disc during an eye examination. Treatment options for optic atrophy depend on the underlying cause. Unfortunately, in many cases, the damage to the optic nerve is irreversible, and the goal of treatment is often to address the underlying condition and prevent further deterioration.

DESTRUCTIVE SURGERIES OF EYEBALL

There are certain surgical procedures that may be considered destructive in the sense that they involve removal or alteration of eye tissues. It is important to note that these procedures are typically reserved for specific medical conditions and are not undertaken lightly. These procedures are performed by ophthalmic surgeons, and the decision to undergo such surgeries is made after careful consideration of the individual's medical condition, the potential benefits, and the risks involved. Patients undergoing these procedures may require postoperative care, including rehabilitation and psychological support.

Three common types of destructive surgeries are:
- Enucleation
- Evisceration
- Orbital exenteration

ENUCLEATION

Enucleation is the surgical removal of the entire eyeball. This procedure is usually performed in cases of severe eye trauma, malignant eye tumors, or to manage end-stage eye diseases. In some cases, individuals may experience severe and intractable pain in the eye that cannot be alleviated through other means. Enucleation may be considered as a last resort to relieve pain. After enucleation, a prosthetic eye may be fitted to improve the cosmetic appearance.

EVISCERATION

Evisceration is a surgical procedure that involves the removal of the contents of the eyeball while leaving the outer shell (sclera) intact. This procedure is distinct from enucleation, which involves the complete removal of the entire eyeball, including the sclera. Evisceration is often chosen in certain situations where preservation of the eye's external structure is desired for cosmetic reasons. Similar to enucleation, after evisceration, a prosthetic eye (ocular prosthesis) may be fitted to improve the cosmetic appearance of the eye socket. The prosthetic eye may be custom-made to match the remaining eye, providing a natural-looking appearance.

ORBITAL EXENTERATION

Orbital exenteration is an extensive surgical procedure where the entire contents of the eye socket including the eyeball, surrounding tissues, and sometimes parts of the bony orbit are removed. This procedure is typically reserved for cases of advanced cancer that involves the eye socket or surrounding structures.

STRABISMUS

Strabismus is a condition in which eyes are misaligned and the visual axis of the eyeball is not parallel when an object is looked at **Figure 1.21**. The misaligned may affect one or both eyes and it may be constant or intermittent. Broadly, strabismus is of two types—paralytic and non-paralytic.

PARALYTIC SQUINT

Paralytic squint typically refers to a type of strabismus that is caused by paralysis or weakness of the muscles responsible for controlling eye movement. Paralytic squint can be caused by damage or dysfunction of the nerves that control the extraocular muscles, leading to paralysis or weakness in one or more of these muscles. The common causes include trauma, inflammation, vascular issues, or compression of the nerves. The patient suffering from paralytic squint may show reduced ability to turn the eye in the direction of normal action of the muscle. Diplopia occurs over the part of the field of fixation towards which the affected muscle move the eye.

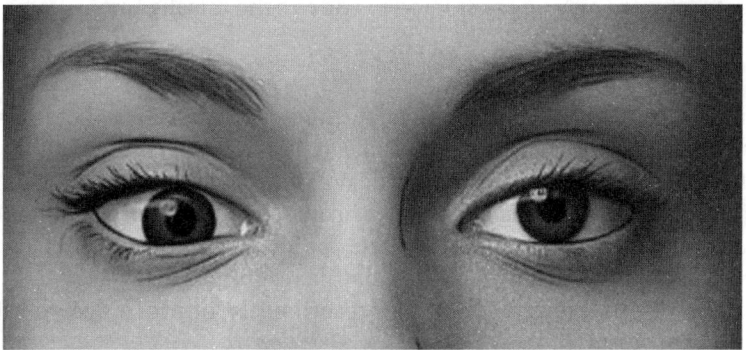

Fig. 1.21: Right eye—strabismus.

The patient may show the tendency to hold his head so that his face is turned in the direction of paralyzed muscle. This is done to lessen the diplopia. False orientation or projection and vertigo are also seen in patient having paralytic squint. The diagnosis is typically made through a comprehensive eye examination, which may include assessing eye movements, measuring visual acuity, and determining the extent of misalignment. The treatment is directed to the cause of the palsy or symptomatic treatment may be resorted to, i.e., correcting diplopia through prism, orthoptic exercise or if necessary surgery.

NON-PARALYTIC SQUINT

Non-paralytic squint, also known as concomitant squint refers to a misalignment of the eyes that is not caused by paralysis or weakness of the eye muscles. The misalignment of the eyes remains constant regardless of the direction of gaze. Unlike paralytic squint, where the misalignment may vary depending on the direction of gaze, concomitant squint is characterized by a consistent deviation of the eyes in direction of gaze. The extraocular muscles responsible for eye movement are typically functioning normally, but there is a lack of coordination between the eyes. There are two types of concomitant squint:
1. Latent squint (heterophoria)
2. Manifest squint (heterotropia)

Latent Squint

Latent squint, also known as heterophoria is the misalignment of the eyes that is not always present and may occur in certain conditions. The eyes are typically aligned when both eyes are used together, but the misalignment becomes apparent when binocular vision is disrupted, or during periods of fatigue, illness, etc. The squint is latent and can be made manifest when fusion is impossible as by covering one eye. The subject having latent squint may show following symptoms:
- Eye strain
- Blurring or running of letters after certain hours of continuous reading
- Intermittent diplopia

The diagnosis of latent squint may require specialized testing, such as the cover-uncover test and the alternate cover test, to detect the misalignment under specific conditions. The treatment approach for latent squint depends on the severity and impact on the individual's vision and daily life:
- Correction of refractive errors with glasses may be recommended.
- Vision therapy or eye exercises may be prescribed to improve eye coordination and strengthen the eye muscles.
- In some cases, surgery may be considered to address the misalignment.

Manifest Squint

Manifest squint, also known as heterotropia, refers to the type of strabismus where the misalignment of the eyes is consistently present and noticeable, regardless of the direction of gaze or other conditions. The eyes are visibly misaligned and do not work together as a team. The misalignment is typically noticeable to others and may be evident in photographs or during routine observations. The treatment for manifest squint depends on the type and underlying cause:
- Correction of refractive errors with glasses may be recommended.
- Vision therapy or eye exercises may be prescribed to improve eye coordination and strengthen eye muscles.
- In some cases, surgery may be considered to realign the eyes.

Strabismus can be classified into four main types based on the direction of eye deviation. These types are:
1. **Esotropia:** In esotropia, one eye deviates inward, towards the nose, while the other eye remains aligned or may also turn inward. Esotropia is often referred to as "cross-eyed" or "crossing of the eyes."
2. **Exotropia:** Exotropia is characterized by one eye turning outward, away from the nose, while the other eye remains straight or may also turn outward. Exotropia is commonly known as "wall-eyed" or "wandering eye."
3. **Hypertropia:** Hypertropia involves one eye deviating upward, while the other eye remains straight or may have a different degree of upward deviation. It is often called "vertical strabismus" or "hyperdeviation."
4. **Hypotropia:** Hypotropia is characterized by one eye deviating downward, while the other eye remains straight or may have a different degree of downward deviation. It is another form of "vertical strabismus" or "hypo-deviation."

The classification based on the direction of deviation helps describe and identify the specific type of strabismus a person may have. Each type may have different underlying causes, and the treatment approach can vary depending on factors such as the type and severity of strabismus, age of onset, and overall eye health.

It is important to note that there are also terms such as "intermittent" or "manifest" that describe whether the misalignment is consistently present (manifest) or only occurs at certain times (intermittent). Additionally, terms like "concomitant" or "non-concomitant" describe whether the misalignment remains consistent regardless of gaze direction (concomitant) or varies with different gaze directions (non-concomitant).

Investigation of Strabismus

Strabismus of larger degree can be diagnosed by inspection. Cover test can be used to diagnose the smaller degree of strabismus both for distance vision and near vision to detect the presence and type of squint. The complete strategy for investigation of squint may include following examinations:
- Examination of ocular movement
- Examination of papillary reaction
- Examination of visual acuity
- Examination of angle of deviation
- Examination under full mydriasis
- Estimation for state of binocular vision

Treatment

There are four modes of treatment that can be applied to treat strabismus:
1. Correction of refractive error
2. Occlusion treatment
3. Orthoptic exercise
4. Surgical treatment

The general line of treatment is as follows:
Mydriatics are instilled to examine ocular media and fundus, and estimation of refractive error. If gross refractive error is present, correct the refractive error. If no refractive error is found, occlusion of non-squint eye to improve the vision of the squint eye is recommended followed by orthoptics treatment. In severe cases surgery is recommended which is followed by orthoptics treatment.

DISEASES OF ORBIT

PROPTOSIS

Proptosis refers to the displacement or protrusion of the eye, from its normal position within the eye socket. It is often used to describe bulging or protruding eyes. Proptosis can be caused by various medical conditions and can affect one or both eyes. Some common causes of proptosis include:
- Graves' disease
- Orbital cellulitis
- Orbital tumors
- Trauma
- Vascular abnormalities

The treatment of proptosis depends on the underlying cause. In some cases, addressing the primary condition may help reduce or resolve proptosis. Treatment options may include medications, surgery, or other interventions depending on the specific diagnosis.

ORBITAL FRACTURE

Orbital fracture refers to a break or cracks in one or more of the bones that form the eye socket (orbit). The orbit is a bony structure that surrounds and protects the eye. Orbital fractures can result from various causes, including trauma to the face. Common causes of orbital fractures include trauma, falls, industrial accidents and penetrating injuries.

ORBITAL CELLULITIS

Orbital cellulitis is a serious infection involving the soft tissues within the eye socket (orbit). It can be a potentially sight-threatening condition and requires prompt medical attention. This condition typically arises from a bacterial infection, often originating from nearby structures such as the sinuses or eyelids. Orbital cellulitis can affect both adults and children. Common causes and risk factors for orbital cellulitis include sinus infection, dental infection, eyelid infections, injuries, etc. The symptoms of orbital cellulitis may include:
- Swelling and redness around the eye
- Pain, especially with eye movement
- Restricted eye movement
- Pus or discharge from the eye
- Fever
- Vision changes

Treatment often involves hospitalization and intravenous antibiotics to effectively combat the bacterial infection. In severe cases, surgical drainage may be necessary to remove accumulated pus and relieve pressure within the orbit. The goal of treatment is to control the infection, prevent complications, and preserve vision.

COMMUNITY OPHTHALMOLOGY

BLINDNESS—VARIOUS PROGRAMS RELATED OF BLINDNESS

Community ophthalmology is a branch of medicine that focuses on providing eye care services at the community level. It aims to prevent and manage eye diseases and promote eye health within communities. In the context of blindness prevention, various programs are implemented to address different aspects of eye care. There are several programs that were launched that were related to community ophthalmology and blindness prevention, some of the popular among them are:

Eye Screening Programs

Regular organizing of eye screening programs in communities to detect common eye conditions early on. This includes screenings for conditions like glaucoma, diabetic retinopathy, and refractive errors.

Cataract Surgery Campaigns

Cataracts are a leading cause of blindness worldwide. Community ophthalmology programs often include campaigns to identify individuals with cataracts and provide them with access to cataract surgery.

School Eye Health Programs

Implement eye health programs in schools to identify and address vision problems in children. This includes vision screenings, provision of eyeglasses, and education on eye health.

Community-based Rehabilitation Services

Develop rehabilitation services for individuals who are visually impaired or blind. This includes training programs to enhance their independent living skills and facilitate their integration into the community.

Training and Capacity Building

Provide training to healthcare professionals, community health workers, and volunteers to enhance their knowledge and skills in diagnosing and managing eye conditions.

In India, where the burden of blindness is significant, several programs and initiatives have been implemented to address eye health at the community level. Some of the key among them are:

Indian National Trachoma Control Programme (1955)

Indian National Trachoma Control Programme was one of the earliest initiatives after independence. Trachoma, caused by a bacterial infection, is a leading cause of preventable blindness. This program likely played a crucial role in addressing this specific issue.

Vitamin A Supplementation and Antibiotic Eye Drops

The inclusion of vitamin A supplementation and antibiotic eye drops in the National Family Planning and Welfare Programme, later integrated into the Reproductive and Child Health Programme, reflects a comprehensive approach to combat nutritional blindness and prevent ophthalmia neonatorum, an eye infection in newborns.

National Programme for Control of Blindness (NPCB, 1976)

The NPCB, initiated in 1976, marked a significant turning point in community eye care in India. The program's evolution from the "Eye Camp Approach" to "Comprehensive Eye Health Care

Camps" and the "Base Camp Approach" showcases a dynamic and adaptable strategy to reach diverse populations.

Centers of Excellence and Regional Institutes

The involvement of prestigious institutions like the Dr Rajendra Prasad Centre for Ophthalmic Sciences and 20 Regional Institutes, along with collaborations with organizations like Aravind Eye Care System, LV Prasad Eye Institute, and Sankara Nethralaya, indicates a strong commitment to advanced research, training, and treatment of eye diseases.

Diverse Eye Care Delivery Systems

The presence of various eye care delivery systems, including optometrists, ophthalmic assistants, individual and group practices, charitable hospitals, Lions Club Eye Hospitals, and private and corporate hospitals, highlights the multi-faceted approach to addressing eye health. This diversity is essential to cater to the varied healthcare needs of the population.

Government and Private Medical College Hospitals

The involvement of both government and private medical college hospitals underscores a collaborative effort between the public and private sectors. This collaboration is crucial for widespread coverage and accessibility of eye care services.

Advanced Centers for Eye Diseases

The designation of certain institutions as WHO Collaborative Advanced Centres demonstrates India's commitment to staying at the forefront of eye care management with state-of-the-art tools and technology.

Overall, the comprehensive nature of these programs and the integration of various delivery systems contribute to the success of India's initiatives in preventing blindness and promoting eye health at the community level. Ongoing collaborations, research, and adaptability to emerging challenges will continue to shape the future of eye care in the country.

MISCELLANEOUS

VITAMIN A DEFICIENCY

Vitamin A deficiency is a nutritional disorder that occurs when there is an insufficient intake or absorption of vitamin A, an essential fat-soluble vitamin. Vitamin A plays a crucial role in maintaining the health of the skin, vision, immune system, and various other physiological functions. Lack of an adequate amount of vitamin A can lead to a range of health problems. Vitamin A is essential for maintaining the health of the eyes, particularly the functioning of the retina and other structures involved in vision. The key implications of vitamin A deficiency for eye health:

Night Blindness (Nyctalopia)

Vitamin A is critical for the production of rhodopsin, a light-sensitive pigment in the retina. Rhodopsin is essential for low-light vision. Vitamin A deficiency can lead to night blindness, where individuals have difficulty seeing in low-light conditions.

Xerophthalmia

In more severe cases of vitamin A deficiency, a condition known as xerophthalmia can develop. This condition is characterized by dryness of the conjunctiva and cornea. Xerophthalmia can progress to more severe forms, including corneal ulcers and blindness if not addressed.

Increased Susceptibility to Infections

Vitamin A plays a crucial role in maintaining the integrity of the epithelial cells in the eyes and other mucous membranes. These cells act as a barrier against infections. Vitamin A deficiency can compromise the barrier function, leading to an increased susceptibility to infections, particularly in the eyes.

Impaired Conjunctival Function

The conjunctiva, the thin membrane covering the front surface of the eye and the inside of the eyelids, is also affected by vitamin A deficiency. Conjunctival issues can contribute to dryness, redness, and an increased risk of infections.

Corneal Health

The cornea is the transparent front part of the eye that plays a crucial role in focusing light. Vitamin A deficiency can affect the health of the cornea, leading to a condition called keratomalacia, which involves softening and damage to the cornea.

IMPAIRED TEAR PRODUCTION

Vitamin A is involved in the production of tears, and deficiency can lead to dry eyes. Dry eyes can contribute to discomfort, irritation, and an increased risk of corneal abrasions.

Blindness

Severe and prolonged vitamin A deficiency can result in irreversible damage to the eyes, leading to blindness. This is particularly significant in populations where vitamin A deficiency is prevalent, especially in developing countries. **Table 1.7** shows the sources of Vitamin A.

LOW VISION AIDS

Low vision aids are devices and tools designed to help individuals with low vision make the most of their remaining vision. Low vision is a visual impairment that cannot be fully corrected with regular eyeglasses, contact lenses, medication, or surgery. The goal of low vision aids is to enhance visual function, improve independence, and facilitate daily activities. Some common types of low vision aids:

Table 1.7: Sources of vitamin A.

Animal products	Fruits	Vegetables
• Liver • Fish • Dairy products • Eggs	• Mangoes • Papayas • Watermelon • Red and pink grapefruits • Oranges	• Carrots • Sweet potatoes • Butternut squash • Spinach • Kale • Broccoli • Red and yellow peppers

Magnifiers

Two common types of magnifiers are commonly used as low vision aids—handheld magnifiers and stand magnifiers.

Handheld magnifiers are portable devices that can be held close to the reading material to magnify text or images and stand magnifiers are designed to stand on a surface, allowing hands-free use while reading.

Telescopic Aids

Monocular telescopes are small telescopes that are used for distance viewing, such as watching television or looking at a whiteboard in a classroom. Bioptic telescopes are mounted on eyeglasses and can be flipped down when needed for tasks like reading signs or recognizing faces at a distance.

Closed-circuit Television

Closed-circuit television (CCTV) systems use cameras and video displays to magnify and display printed material or objects on a screen. They can provide variable magnification and color contrast options.

Reading Glasses with High-power Lenses

Some individuals with low vision may benefit from reading glasses with high-power lenses, designed to magnify close-up objects.

Filters and Tinted Lenses

Colored filters or tinted lenses can help improve contrast and reduce glare, making it easier for individuals with low vision to see objects more clearly.

Large Print Materials

Large print books, calendars, and other materials with enlarged text can be helpful for reading.

Electronic Devices and Apps

The devices like screen magnification, voice input, and text-to-speech capabilities and specialized apps are apps designed for magnification, contrast enhancement, and voice assistance that can be installed on smart phones or tablets for low vision patients.

Talking Products

Talking watches and clocks are used that announce the time audibly.

Braille Devices

Braille displays convert digital text into Braille, providing access to electronic information. Braille notetakers are portable devices that allow users to take notes, read, and write in Braille.

White Canes and Mobility Aids

White canes help individuals with low vision navigate their surroundings by detecting obstacles and providing tactile feedback.

FIRST-AID IN OCULAR INJURIES

First-aid for ocular injuries involves providing immediate care to someone who has sustained an injury to the eye. Quick and appropriate first aid measures can help minimize damage, reduce the risk of complications, and promote the best possible outcome. The common first aid steps for common ocular injuries are listed below:

Chemical Burns

If the eye comes into contact with a chemical substance, immediately rinse the affected eye with copious amounts of lukewarm, clean water. Hold the eyelids open while rinsing to ensure thorough flushing. Continue rinsing for at least 15 minutes.

Foreign Object in the Eye

Advise the person not to rub the eye, as this can cause further damage. Encourage blinking and tearing to help naturally flush out the foreign object. If the object does not come out with blinking, use clean water to irrigate the eye gently. Do not use sharp objects to remove the object.

Blows to the Eye

Apply a cold compress or ice pack wrapped in a cloth to the injured eye to help reduce swelling and minimize pain. Avoid applying pressure to the eye or surrounding areas.

Cut or Puncture Wounds

Do not attempt to remove an object that has penetrated the eye. Protect the eye by placing a protective covering, such as a paper cup or the bottom of a plastic container, around the object.

Embedded Objects

Do not attempt to remove an embedded object. Protect the eye by placing a protective covering, such as a paper cup, around the object. Arrange for prompt transportation to the nearest emergency medical facility.

Burns

For thermal burns (heat burns), gently cool the affected eye with a clean, damp cloth or cool, but not cold, water. Do not use ice or very cold water, as extreme cold can cause further damage. Seek immediate medical attention for any eye burn.

Eye Contusions (Black Eye)

Apply a cold compress or ice pack wrapped in a cloth to the injured eye to help reduce swelling and minimize pain. Over-the-counter pain relievers may be used according to package instructions.

In all cases of ocular injury, it is essential to seek prompt medical attention, especially for injuries involving chemical exposure, embedded or penetrating objects, or burns. These first aid measures are intended to provide immediate care until professional medical help is obtained.

AMBLYOPIA

Amblyopia, commonly known as "lazy eye," is a vision development disorder that typically begins in childhood. It occurs when one eye has better focus and alignment than the other, leading the brain to favour the clearer eye and ignore signals from the weaker or misaligned eye. This can result in reduced vision in the weaker eye. The most common causes of amblyopia include strabismus and uncorrected refractive errors. Significant differences in the prescription between the two eyes, such as one eye being more nearsighted, farsighted, or having astigmatism is also one of the common causes of amblyopia. Amblyopia often does not cause noticeable symptoms. The brain effectively suppresses the input from the weaker eye. In some cases, signs may include poor depth perception, squinting, or the child consistently favouring one eye. Amblyopia is usually diagnosed through a comprehensive eye examination, which may include visual acuity testing, refraction, and an assessment of eye alignment. The primary goal of amblyopia treatment is to strengthen and improve the vision in the weaker eye. Treatment options may include corrective lenses if refractive errors are present, patching of the stronger eye to encourage the use and strengthening of the weaker eye and vision therapy which includes eye exercises and activities designed to improve eye coordination and visual acuity. In some cases, surgery for strabismus or other structural issues affecting eye alignment may be resorted to.

Treatment of amblyopia is most effective when started early, preferably during the critical period of visual development in childhood. If the amblyopia is left untreated it can lead to permanent vision impairment in the affected eye.

While the critical period for optimal treatment outcomes is in early childhood, interventions can still be beneficial for older children and adults. It may be more challenging to achieve significant improvement in visual acuity compared to early intervention, but some degree of improvement is still possible. The success of treatment in older individuals depends on factors such as the severity of amblyopia, the underlying cause, and the individual's motivation and compliance with treatment.

COLOR BLINDNESS

INTRODUCTION

Color blindness, also known as color vision deficiency, is a visual impairment that affects a person's ability to perceive certain colors accurately. This condition is often inherited and more common in males.

The most common form of color blindness is red-green color blindness, where individuals have difficulty distinguishing between red and green hues. Blue-yellow color blindness and total color blindness (seeing only shades of gray) are less common.

Color blindness is often inherited and linked to the X chromosome. The genes responsible for normal color vision are located on the X chromosome, and certain variations in these genes can lead to color vision deficiencies.

Since males have one X and one Y chromosome, a single inherited color vision gene mutation on their X chromosome can result in color blindness. Females, with two X chromosomes, are more likely to be carriers but may not experience color blindness unless both X chromosomes carry the mutation.

Types of Color Blindness

- **Red-green color blindness:** This is the most common type and includes protanopia (lack of red cones) and deuteranopia (lack of green cones).
- **Blue-yellow color blindness:** This less common type includes tritanopia (lack of blue cones).
- **Total color blindness:** Extremely rare, individuals with total color blindness see the world in shades of gray.

Symptoms

Color blindness can affect daily activities such as reading maps, traffic signals, and identifying ripe fruits. Some professions, like those involving electrical wiring or certain aspects of graphic design, may be challenging for individuals with color vision deficiencies. The individual having color deficiency shows following symptoms:
- Difficulty distinguishing between certain colors, especially red and green.
- Seeing colors as less vibrant or appearing similar.
- Inability to perceive specific color combinations.

Diagnosis

Color blindness can be diagnosed through various color vision tests, such as the Ishihara Color Test, which involves identifying numbers within colored circles.

Management and Support

There is currently no cure for color blindness. However, individuals can learn to adapt and compensate for their color vision deficiency.

2 CHAPTER

Nursing Procedures like Vital Recording, IM/IV/SC Injection, Oxygen Therapy, Nebulization and IV Infusion

Ajay Kumar Bhootra, Sumitra Agarwal

TEMPERATURE MONITORING AND FEVER

Monitoring temperature and identifying fever are important aspects of healthcare, especially in the context of infectious diseases. Fever is generally considered a body temperature of 100.4°F (38°C) or higher.

METHODS OF MEASUREMENT

Table 2.1 shows the different methods of measuring temperature.

NORMAL BODY TEMPERATURE

Table 2.2 shows the normal body temperature and threshold limits for consideration for fever. The temperature is little lower in the morning and higher in the late afternoon. Children generally have higher baseline temperatures. Physical activity and menstrual cycle for women affect body temperature.

Table 2.1: Different methods of temperature measurement.

Methods to measure temperature	
Oral thermometers	Placed under the tongue
Rectal thermometers	Inserted into the rectum
Ear (tympanic) thermometers	Measure infrared radiation inside the ear
Forehead thermometers	Scan the temporal artery on the forehead
Infrared thermometers	Measure body temperature without direct contact

Table 2.2: Normal body temperature.

Methods of measurement	*Normal body temperature*	*Consideration for fever*
Oral thermometers	98.6°F (37°C)	100°F or 37.8°C
Rectal thermometers	98.6°F (37°C)	100.4°F or 38°C
Ear (tympanic) thermometers	98.6°F (37°C)	100.4°F or 38°C
Forehead thermometers	98.6°F (37°C)	100.4°F or 38°C
Infrared thermometers	98.6°F (37°C)	100.4°F or 38°C

Causes of Fever

The common causes of fever are listed below:
- Infections (viral, bacterial, fungal)
- Inflammatory conditions
- Some medications
- Heat-related illnesses

Signs and Symptoms

The common symptoms of fever are listed down:
- Elevated body temperature
- Sweating
- Shivering
- Increased heart rate and breathing

When to Seek Medical Attention?

Seeking medical attention for fever is greatly age related. While the adults may delay seeking medical attention, children and adults may need to seek medical attention a little quickly. In general, the following situation calls for immediate medical attention:
- Persistent fever without an obvious cause
- High fever (above 104°F or 40°C)
- Seizures
- Difficulty breathing
- Persistent vomiting
- Pain with urination or pain in the back

Management

The management of fever is usually started with self-treatment which may include following steps:
- Take paracetamol or ibuprofen, it can help reduce fever.
- Drink plenty of fluids, particularly water.
- Take rest to recover.
- Avoid alcohol, tea and coffee to avoid dehydration.
- Sponge exposed skin with tepid water.
- Avoid taking cold baths or showers. Skin reacts to the cold by constricting its blood vessels, which will trap body heat. The cold may also cause shivering, which can generate more heat.

Prevention

Limiting exposure to infectious agents is one of the best ways to prevent a fever. The other tips that can help reduce your exposure are:
- Proper hygiene to prevent infections
- Vaccinations
- In certain situations, prophylactic use of antipyretics
- Avoid sharing cups, glasses, and eating utensils with other people.

Regular temperature monitoring is a simple yet crucial tool for assessing health. While fever is often a sign of an underlying issue, it is important to consider other symptoms and seek medical advice when needed. In the context of infectious diseases, monitoring and early detection of fever can play a significant role in controlling the spread of illnesses.

PULSE MONITORING

Pulse monitoring refers to the measurement and tracking of a person's pulse, which is the rhythmic beating of the heart. The pulse is typically measured as the number of heart beats per minute (bpm). Monitoring the pulse can provide valuable information about a person's cardiovascular health and fitness level.

NORMAL RESTING HEART RATE

The normal resting heart rate for adults is typically between 60 and 100 beats per minute. Factors such as age, fitness level, and overall health can influence the resting heart rate.

METHODS OF PULSE MONITORING

Manual Pulse Measurement

This is often done by placing the fingertips on certain pulse points, such as the radial artery on the wrist or the carotid artery in the neck and counting the number of beats in a set time period (usually 15 or 30 seconds) and then multiplying to get beats per minute.

Heart Rate Monitors

These electronic devices are designed to measure and display the heart rate in real-time. They can be worn on the wrist (like fitness trackers) or as chest straps during exercise.

Exercise and Pulse Monitoring

Monitoring pulse during exercise is crucial for assessing the intensity of the workout. It helps individuals stay within their target heart rate zone for optimal cardiovascular fitness and safety.

Wearable Technology

Many modern fitness trackers and smart watches come with built-in heart rate monitoring features. These devices often use optical sensors to detect blood flow and calculate heart rate.

Medical Applications

In medical settings, pulse monitoring is a standard practice. It helps healthcare professionals assess the cardiac function, detect irregularities, and monitor patients during surgery or recovery.

Pulse Oximetry

This measures the oxygen saturation of the blood, usually through a device that clips onto a person's fingertip. It provides additional information about respiratory and circulatory health.

While pulse monitoring is a useful tool, it's important to note that it is not a standalone diagnostic tool. Other factors and assessments may be necessary for a comprehensive understanding of cardiovascular health.

BLOOD PRESSURE MONITORING

Blood pressure is the force of blood against the walls of arteries as the heart pumps it around the body, vital for delivering oxygen and nutrients to tissues and organs. It's measured in millimeters of mercury (mm Hg) and recorded as two numbers. Monitoring blood pressure is crucial for maintaining cardiovascular health.

Systolic Pressure

The higher number, representing the pressure in the arteries when the heart contracts or beats, pumping blood into the arteries.

Diastolic Pressure

- The lower number, representing the pressure in the arteries when the heart is at rest between beats.
- The standard blood pressure reading is written as systolic over diastolic, such as 120/80 mm Hg.

NORMAL BLOOD PRESSURE RANGE

- **Normal:** Below 120/80 mm Hg
- **Elevated:** 120–129/<80 mm Hg
- **Hypertension stage 1:** 130–139/80–89 mm Hg
- **Hypertension stage 2**: 140/90 mm Hg or higher
- **Hypertensive crisis:** 180/120 mm Hg or higher

MONITORING BLOOD PRESSURE AT HOME

Home blood pressure measuring device is available for personal use. They come in manual and automatic varieties. Before using you must ensure that you are using the correct cuff size, sit comfortably, keep your arm at heart level, and be still during the measurement. It is useful to monitor blood pressure regularly, especially if you have hypertension or other cardiovascular risk factors. Keep a record of your blood pressure readings, noting the date and time. This information can be helpful for you and your healthcare provider.

LIFESTYLE FACTORS AFFECTING BLOOD PRESSURE

- A diet rich in fruits, vegetables, lean proteins, and low in sodium can help regulate blood pressure.
- Regular exercise is crucial for maintaining a healthy blood pressure.
- Maintaining a healthy weight is important for overall cardiovascular health.
- Excessive alcohol consumption and smoking can contribute to high blood pressure.

RESPIRATION MONITORING

Respiratory monitoring refers to the process of observing, measuring, and assessing various aspects of an individual's respiratory system, including the rate, depth, rhythm, and other characteristics of breathing. This monitoring can be done for various purposes, including healthcare, sports performance analysis, research, and general well-being. The goal is to gain insights into the efficiency and health of the respiratory system. Respiratory monitoring is particularly important in healthcare for patients with respiratory diseases, during surgery, and in intensive care units. The key aspects of respiration monitoring are:

RESPIRATORY RATE

- **Definition:** The number of breaths taken per minute.
- **Monitoring:** Respiratory rate can be monitored visually by counting chest movements or by using sensors and devices.

RESPIRATORY DEPTH

- **Definition:** The amount of air exchanged during each breath, indicating the depth of breathing.
- **Monitoring:** Devices such as respiratory belts or spirometers can measure the depth of breathing.

RESPIRATORY RHYTHM

- **Definition:** The regularity and pattern of breathing cycles.
- **Monitoring:** Observing the regularity of breaths and detecting any irregular patterns.

Capnography

- **Definition:** Measurement of the concentration of carbon dioxide (CO_2) in exhaled breath.
- **Monitoring:** Capnography is often used in medical settings to assess the adequacy of ventilation and respiratory function.

Pulse Oximetry

- **Definition:** Measurement of the oxygen saturation of hemoglobin in the blood.
- **Monitoring:** Pulse oximeters are commonly used to assess how well oxygen is being transported to tissues.

Spirometry

- **Definition:** A lung function test that measures the volume and flow of air during inhalation and exhalation.
- **Monitoring:** Spirometers are used in clinical settings to assess lung function and diagnose respiratory conditions.

Smart Textiles and Wearables

- **Definition:** Clothing or wearable devices embedded with sensors to monitor respiratory parameters.
- **Monitoring:** These devices can continuously track respiratory rate, depth, and other parameters in real-time.

Acoustic Monitoring

- **Definition:** The use of sound-based technologies to monitor breathing patterns.
- **Monitoring:** Microphones or other sound sensors can be employed to detect and analyze respiratory sounds.

Visual Inspection

- **Definition:** Direct observation of chest movements and overall respiratory effort.

- **Monitoring:** This is a basic method often used in emergency situations or as an initial assessment of respiratory function.

Continuous Monitoring

- **Definition:** Monitoring over an extended period, allowing for the detection of trends and changes.
- **Monitoring:** Continuous monitoring is crucial in critical care settings, post-surgery recovery, and for individuals with chronic respiratory conditions.

TYPES OF INJECTION ROUTES

There are several routes for administering medications through injections, each with its own advantages and considerations. The choice of injection route depends on factors such as the medication being administered, the desired rate of absorption, and the patient's condition. Additionally, factors such as the patient's age, medical condition, and the characteristics of the medication also play a role in determining the most appropriate injection route. Some common types of injection routes are explained below:

INTRAMUSCULAR

Intramuscular (IM) injection administers medications into a muscle, typically in the deltoid (upper arm), vastus lateralis (thigh), or ventrogluteal (hip) muscles. The route is commonly used for vaccinations, certain antibiotics, and medications requiring sustained release.

SUBCUTANEOUS

Subcutaneous (SC or SubQ) injection administers medications into the tissue just below the skin. The route is commonly used for insulin, some vaccines, certain hormones, and medications that require slow, sustained absorption.

INTRADERMAL

Intradermal (ID) route is used for injecting medication into the top layer of skin (dermis). It is commonly used for tuberculosis (TB) skin tests, allergy testing.

INTRAVENOUS (IV)

Injection directly into a vein is commonly used for rapid administration of medications, fluids, and blood products.

INTRAOSSEOUS (IO)

Injection into the bone marrow space is commonly used for emergency situations when intravenous access is difficult.

INTRAPERITONEAL (IP)

Injection into the peritoneal cavity, typically through a catheter is used for certain chemotherapy drugs and dialysis.

INTRATHECAL (IT)

Injection into the space around the spinal cord (subarachnoid space) is the choice of route for spinal anesthesia, certain medications for neurological conditions.

EPIDURAL (ED OR EPI)

The route administers the medication into the epidural space, outside the spinal cords protective covering and is the route of choice for pain relief during childbirth, postoperative pain management.

INTRAVENOUS PUSH

Intravenous push (IVP) is the rapid injection of a medication directly into a vein using a syringe. It is commonly used for medications that require rapid administration.

IM INJECTION

"IM" in the context of medical administration typically refers to an intramuscular injection. Intramuscular injections involve the administration of medication directly into a muscle. This route is often used for medications that need to be absorbed more quickly than oral medications.

LOCATION OF INJECTION

The injection is given into a muscle, typically in the upper arm (deltoid muscle), thigh (vastus lateralis muscle), or buttocks (gluteal muscles). The choice of the injection site depends on factors such as the patient's age, the volume of the medication, and the specific medication being administered.

NEEDLE SIZE

The size of the needle depends on various factors, including the patient's size, the specific muscle chosen for injection, and the type of medication. Healthcare providers select an appropriate needle gauge and length to ensure effective delivery of the medication.

Technique

Proper technique is crucial to ensure the medication is delivered safely and effectively. This includes cleaning the injection site, using a quick and steady motion to insert the needle, aspirating to ensure the needle is not in a blood vessel, and slowly injecting the medication.

COMMON MEDICATIONS

Many medications are administered via intramuscular injection, including vaccines, antibiotics, certain hormones, and some pain medications.

Absorption Rate

Intramuscular injections generally allow for a faster absorption of medication compared to oral administration. The muscle's rich blood supply facilitates the rapid uptake of the medication into the bloodstream.

Pain Management

The injection itself may cause some discomfort, but proper technique and the choice of an appropriate injection site can minimize pain. Additionally, some medications can be formulated with additives to reduce injection site pain.

IV INJECTION

"IV" stands for intravenous, and an IV injection involves administering medication or fluids directly into a vein. This method allows for rapid delivery of the substance into the bloodstream, making it an effective route for medications that require quick onset of action or for delivering fluids directly into the circulatory system. Intravenous injections are commonly used in hospitals and clinical settings due to their rapid and efficient delivery of medications and fluids.

LOCATION OF INJECTION

Intravenous injections are typically administered in veins, which are commonly found in the arms, hands, or sometimes other parts of the body depending on the patient's condition and the specific requirements of the treatment.

NEEDLE AND CATHETER

A needle is used to puncture the vein, and a thin, flexible tube called a catheter is inserted through the needle into the vein. Once the catheter is in place, the needle is removed, leaving the catheter in the vein for the duration of treatment.

TYPES OF IV INJECTIONS

Intravenous (IV) injections can take various forms, depending on the specific needs of the patient and the characteristics of the medication or fluid being administered. Some common types of IV injections are:

Bolus or Push

A single, large dose of medication is injected rapidly into the vein.

Infusion

Medication or fluids are delivered continuously over a set period.

IV Drip

Medication or fluids are delivered drop by drop through a gravity-fed system.

IV Pump

An infusion pump is used to control the rate of medication or fluid delivery. IV injections are used for a variety of purposes, including administration of medications (such as antibiotics, pain relievers, and chemotherapy drugs), fluids to maintain hydration, blood transfusions, and nutritional support. Patients receiving intravenous medications or fluids are often monitored closely for any signs of adverse reactions. Healthcare professionals monitor vital signs and the infusion site to ensure the treatment is proceeding as planned. Since IV injections involve puncturing the skin and accessing the bloodstream, there is a risk of infection. Proper aseptic technique is crucial to minimize this risk.

SC INJECTION

"SC" stands for subcutaneous, and a subcutaneous injection involves administering medication into the fatty tissue layer just beneath the skin. This route allows for the gradual absorption of the medication into the bloodstream.

LOCATION OF INJECTION

Subcutaneous injections are typically given into the fatty tissue layer between the skin and the muscle. Common injection sites include the upper outer arm, thigh, abdomen, and buttocks.

The choice of injection site may depend on factors such as the specific medication being administered, the volume of the injection, and patient preference.

NEEDLE SIZE

The needle used for subcutaneous injections is typically shorter and smaller in gauge compared to needles used for intramuscular or intravenous injections.

The size of the needle is selected based on factors such as the patient's size, age, and the specific medication.

Technique

Subcutaneous injections are administered at a 45 to 90-degree angle to the skin surface, depending on the needle length and the amount of subcutaneous tissue.

Pinching the skin at the injection site may be necessary to ensure that the medication is delivered into the fatty tissue.

Common Medications

Many medications can be administered subcutaneously, including insulin for diabetes, certain vaccines, some hormones, and certain types of medications for pain or allergic reactions.

Absorption Rate

Subcutaneous injections provide a slower absorption rate compared to intramuscular injections but are often faster than oral medications. The medication is gradually absorbed into the bloodstream through the capillaries in the fatty tissue.

Pain Management

Subcutaneous injections are generally less painful than intramuscular injections. However, the sensation may vary depending on the individual and the specific medication.

Self-administration

Some patients may be trained to self-administer subcutaneous injections, particularly in the case of chronic conditions like diabetes where regular injections are needed.

OXYGEN THERAPY

Oxygen therapy is a medical treatment that involves the administration of supplemental oxygen to individuals who have difficulty maintaining adequate oxygen levels in their blood.

It is a crucial intervention for people with respiratory or cardiovascular conditions that result in hypoxemia, a condition characterized by low levels of oxygen in the blood. The goal of oxygen therapy is to increase the amount of oxygen available to the body's tissues and organs.

INDICATIONS

- Chronic respiratory conditions such as chronic obstructive pulmonary disease (COPD), emphysema, and interstitial lung disease.
- Acute respiratory conditions like pneumonia, acute respiratory distress syndrome (ARDS), and severe asthma exacerbations.
- Cardiovascular conditions such as heart failure, where oxygen delivery to tissues may be compromised.

DELIVERY SYSTEMS

- **Nasal cannula:** A device with prongs that fit into the nostrils, delivering oxygen to the patient. It is one of the most common and comfortable methods.
- **Oxygen masks:** Covering the nose and mouth, masks can deliver higher concentrations of oxygen compared to nasal cannulas.
- **Venturi mask:** Provides precise control over the oxygen concentration, making it suitable for patients with specific respiratory needs.
- **Non-rebreather mask:** Delivers high concentrations of oxygen and includes a reservoir bag to increase the amount of oxygen available for inhalation.
- **Oxygen tent:** An enclosed environment, often used in pediatrics, where oxygen is supplied to maintain a specific concentration.

Flow Rate

The rate at which oxygen is delivered is measured in liters per minute (L/min). The prescribed flow rate depends on the patient's condition and is adjusted based on their response.

Monitoring

Oxygen saturation levels (SpO_2) are monitored using a pulse oximeter to ensure that the therapy is effective and to avoid over-oxygenation.

Home Oxygen Therapy

Some patients may require oxygen therapy at home, and portable oxygen concentrators or compressed oxygen cylinders may be used. Home oxygen therapy requires proper education and training for patients and caregivers.

Safety Considerations

Oxygen is not flammable, but it supports combustion. Smoking and open flames should be avoided in areas where oxygen is in use. Adequate ventilation is important to prevent oxygen build-up in enclosed spaces.

Titration of Oxygen

Oxygen therapy is often titrated based on the patient's condition and response. The goal is to maintain oxygen levels within a target range.

Oxygen therapy is a critical and life-saving intervention when used appropriately. Healthcare providers determine the appropriate oxygen delivery method, flow rate, and duration based on the patient's condition and specific needs. It is important for patients to follow their healthcare provider's instructions and to use oxygen therapy as prescribed.

NEBULIZATION

Nebulization is a medical process that involves the administration of medication in the form of a mist or aerosol. This method is commonly used for individuals with respiratory conditions to deliver medications directly to the lungs. The device used for nebulization is called a nebulizer, which converts liquid medication into a fine mist that can be inhaled into the respiratory system.

INDICATIONS

Nebulization is often used in the treatment of respiratory conditions, such as asthma exacerbations, chronic obstructive pulmonary disease (COPD) exacerbations, and respiratory infections. It is particularly useful for individuals who have difficulty using inhalers or for young children who may struggle with proper inhaler technique.

NEBULIZER DEVICE

A nebulizer is a small device that converts liquid medication into a fine mist or aerosol. It consists of a compressor, a medication cup, and a mouthpiece or mask. There are different types of nebulizers, including jet nebulizers and ultrasonic nebulizers.

Medications Used

Nebulizers are used to administer a variety of medications, including bronchodilators (to open airways), corticosteroids (to reduce inflammation), and other respiratory medications. Common medications include albuterol, ipratropium, budesonide, and others.

Administration Technique

The liquid medication is placed into the nebulizer's medication cup. The nebulizer is then connected to a source of compressed air or oxygen. When the nebulizer is turned on, it converts the liquid medication into a fine mist, which the patient inhales through a mouthpiece or mask.

Use of Masks

Masks are often used with nebulizers, especially for children or individuals who may have difficulty using a mouthpiece. Masks come in various sizes to ensure a proper fit.

Duration of Treatment

Nebulization treatments typically last for about 10 to 15 minutes, during which the patient inhales the aerosolized medication.

Cleaning and Maintenance

It is important to clean and disinfect the nebulizer regularly to prevent contamination. Proper maintenance ensures the device functions effectively.

Nebulization is an effective way to deliver respiratory medications directly to the lungs. It is important for individuals using nebulizers to receive proper instructions on medication dosage, frequency, and device maintenance from their healthcare provider. Regular follow-ups with healthcare professionals help monitor the effectiveness of the treatment and make any necessary adjustments to the treatment plan.

IV INFUSION (ALSO WITH INFUSION PUMP)

IV infusion, or intravenous infusion, is a medical procedure in which fluids, medications, or nutrients are delivered directly into a patient's bloodstream through a vein. This method allows for the rapid and controlled administration of substances that need to be absorbed quickly and efficiently. Infusions are commonly used in various healthcare settings, including hospitals, clinics, and home care.

INDICATIONS FOR IV INFUSION

- IV fluids are administered to maintain hydration, correct electrolyte imbalances, and restore intravascular volume.
- Many medications, including antibiotics, pain relievers, chemotherapy drugs, and more, are administered via IV infusion.
- Total parenteral nutrition (TPN) or intravenous nutrition is administered to patients who cannot receive adequate nutrition through the digestive system.

IV INFUSION SET-UP

The IV infusion set typically includes a bag or bottle containing the fluid or medication, tubing, and a catheter (cannula or needle) inserted into a vein. The infusion set is connected to a source of gravity (for gravity-driven infusions) or an infusion pump.

Infusion Pump

An infusion pump is a device that delivers fluids or medications at a controlled rate, allowing for precise infusion rates and dosage accuracy. Types of infusion pumps include volumetric pumps, syringe pumps, and ambulatory pumps. Infusion pumps are particularly useful for medications that require a specific rate of administration or for continuous infusions over an extended period.

Administration Rate

The rate of infusion is determined by factors such as the patient's condition, the specific medication or fluid being administered, and the healthcare provider's prescription. The rate may be adjusted based on the patient's response and vital signs.

Monitoring

Patients undergoing IV infusion are closely monitored for any signs of adverse reactions, including changes in vital signs, allergic reactions, or infusion site complications. Regular checks of the infusion site and the IV system are performed to ensure proper functioning.

Site Selection

The choice of the vein for IV infusion depends on factors such as the patient's condition, the duration of treatment, and the type of solution or medication being administered. Common sites include the veins of the hand, forearm, or antecubital fossa.

Complications and Safety

IV infusions come with potential complications, including infection at the insertion site, phlebitis (inflammation of the vein), and infiltration (leakage of fluids into surrounding tissues). Strict aseptic technique is crucial to prevent infections.

Home Infusion

In some cases, patients may receive IV infusion therapy at home. Home infusion may involve the use of portable infusion pumps.

IV infusion is a common and effective way to deliver fluids and medications to patients. The use of infusion pumps enhances the precision and safety of the process, ensuring that patients receive the correct dosage at the prescribed rate.

CARE OF UNCONSCIOUS PATIENT

An unconscious patient is an individual who is not awake, aware, or responsive to their surroundings. Consciousness refers to the state of being aware of and able to respond to one's environment. When a person is unconscious, they lack this awareness and responsiveness. There are various degrees of unconsciousness, ranging from mild confusion or drowsiness to a complete loss of consciousness. The term "unconscious patient" is often used in medical contexts to describe individuals who are in a state of altered consciousness, and it can result from a variety of causes.

COMMON REASONS FOR UNCONSCIOUSNESS

Trauma

Head injuries, severe accidents, or concussions can lead to a loss of consciousness.

Medical Conditions

Certain medical conditions, such as epilepsy, diabetic emergencies, and fainting episodes, can cause temporary unconsciousness.

Stroke

Lack of blood flow to the brain, as seen in a stroke, can result in loss of consciousness.

Cardiac Arrest

A sudden loss of heart function can cause a person to become unconscious.

Severe Infections

Serious infections, sepsis, or other systemic illnesses can affect the brain and lead to unconsciousness.

Overdose or Poisoning

Ingesting toxic substances or overdosing on medications can result in loss of consciousness.

Hypoglycemia

Extremely low blood sugar levels can cause unconsciousness.

Seizures

Seizures, especially if prolonged or repeated, can result in temporary unconsciousness. It is important to note that an unconscious state is a medical emergency that requires prompt evaluation and intervention by healthcare professionals. When caring for an unconscious patient, medical providers will assess the individual's vital signs, conduct diagnostic tests, and initiate appropriate treatment based on the underlying cause of unconsciousness. The level of consciousness is often assessed using tools such as the Glasgow Coma Scale (GCS), which evaluates eye, verbal, and motor responses to stimuli. The goal of medical intervention is to identify and address the underlying cause of unconsciousness, provide supportive care, and optimize the chances of recovery.

The broader guide to the care of an unconscious patient is explained below.

Airway Management

Ensure a clear and open airway. The tongue can fall back and obstruct the airway in an unconscious patient. Use techniques such as the head-tilt, chin-lift manoeuvre or jaw thrust maneuver to open the airway.

Breathing Support

Assess and support breathing. Administer artificial ventilation if necessary, using methods like bag-valve-mask ventilation or mechanical ventilation. Monitor respiratory rate, depth, and pattern.

Circulation Management

Monitor vital signs, including heart rate, blood pressure, and oxygen saturation. Administer intravenous fluids and medications as prescribed to maintain adequate circulation.

Positioning

Position the unconscious patient to maintain a clear airway and prevent aspiration. The recovery position may be used. Regularly change the patient's position to prevent pressure ulcers.

Eye Care

Keep the eyes moist with artificial tears to prevent corneal drying. Protect the eyes from injury by placing a lubricating ointment and covering them with eye patches.

Oral Care

Perform regular oral care to prevent dry mouth and reduce the risk of infections. Moisturize the lips and oral mucosa to maintain oral hygiene.

Skin Care

Turn and reposition the patient regularly to prevent pressure ulcers. Keep the skin clean and dry, using pressure-relieving devices as needed.

Bladder and Bowel Care

Manage urinary elimination with a catheter if necessary. Attend to bowel care by monitoring for constipation and administering appropriate interventions.

Nutrition and Hydration

Administer intravenous fluids or tube feedings as needed. Assess nutritional needs and collaborate with a dietitian to provide appropriate nutrition.

Temperature Control

Maintain a comfortable room temperature to prevent hypothermia. Use blankets or cooling measures as needed to regulate body temperature.

Neurological Monitoring

Assess neurological status regularly, including pupil size and reactivity, motor responses, and Glasgow coma scale (GCS) score. Report any changes in neurological status promptly.

Infection Prevention

Practice proper hygiene to prevent infections, including regular handwashing and use of aseptic techniques. Monitor for signs of infection and implement appropriate interventions.

Psychosocial Support

Provide emotional support to the patient and their family. Communicate effectively with family members, keeping them informed about the patient's condition.

Medication Administration

Administer medications as prescribed and monitor for any adverse reactions. Use pain management strategies if applicable.

Regular Monitoring and Assessment

Conduct frequent assessments to identify any changes in the patient's condition. Collaborate with other healthcare professionals to optimize care.

Caring for an unconscious patient is a collaborative effort involving nurses, physicians, therapists, and other healthcare providers. Effective communication and a systematic approach to care are crucial for ensuring the patient's safety and well-being. Regular assessments help identify any complications or changes in the patient's condition, allowing for timely interventions.

3
CHAPTER

Mechanical Optics, Lenses and Lens Prescription

Ajay Kumar Bhootra, Sumitra Agarwal

A BRIEF HISTORY OF OPHTHALMIC LENSES AND SPECTACLES

HISTORY OF OPHTHALMIC LENSES

The ophthalmic lenses have been used for vision correction for a very long time, although they have evolved from the initial glass reading stone of the 10th century to the current digital lenses with anticipation of further developments.

It was AI-Hazen (996–1038), an Arab physicist, who observed that a segment of glass sphere, in effect a plano convex lens, would magnify images. These primitive single pieces of convex-shaped glass or rock crystals were used as magnifiers for several years.

There is evidence that the renowned Roman Emperor Nero (AD 54) used emerald lenses to view gladiator games. Regardless of whether he could actually see better, his precious gem lenses became an instant, must-have fashion accessory among the upper class.

The early spectacle lenses were made of quartz crystal and were given the name "pebble lenses" in the optical trade. Other early lenses were created from hand-blown glass. As the optical industry grew, hand-blown glass was gradually replaced by more easily-formed lens blanks made from flat sheets of glass. These were called "dropped" lenses because of the process in which flat sheets of glass were heated until they softened enough to drop into cavities that shaped the blanks into a rough curve.

For centuries, the development of spectacle lenses owed more to the development of newer materials for lenses. It was because the focus was more on the transparency of the material. The primary goal was to create clear and transparent materials that could be used to correct vision problems.

The three important properties, i.e., transparency, homogeneity, and dimensional stability, made the glasses the most preferred choice for ophthalmic lenses. In the archives of Venice in 1300 and 1331, edicts appeared forbidding the manufacture of spectacles from any material other than crystal glass. At the end of the 16th century, a German industry was set up at Augsburg, Regensburg, and particularly Nuremberg, where glass was blown and the lenses were thinner, lighter, and cheaper; it was these "Nuremberg glasses" that formed the stock-in-trade of the itinerant Jewish pedlars of the time.

The development of the telescope by Galileo in 1608 gave a marked impetus to the technique of grinding lenses, and the art rapidly spread throughout Europe, particularly in France, Holland, and England. In the middle of the 19th century, Faraday and Stokes in England and Fraunhofer and Guinard in Germany began to improve the quality of glass by adding various oxides in the manufacturing process, and in 1838, the English firm of Chance commenced making a large range of optical glass. Half a century later, developing from the research of Abbe and Schott, the German firm of Zeiss added considerable improvements to the process of manufacturing crown glass (1885 onwards) and rapidly gained what amounted to a world monopoly (von Pflugk, 1913–41), a proud position that is now widely shared. In 1916, World War I started, cutting off America's traditional lens sources in Europe and motivating a team called Bausch and Lomb to launch the first volume factory production of ophthalmic glass in the US.

Spectacle lenses were exclusively made of glass until the introduction of plastic materials. After World War I, advances in polymer technology resulted in new forms of plastics, with the most significant to the optical industry being the invention of polymerized methyl methacrylate (PMMA) in the 1930s.

Around the late 1940s, acrylic lenses were developed in England and introduced on the American market as the first successful attempt by the industry to provide a lightweight substitute for conventionally heavy glass lenses. However, due to acrylic's inherent disadvantages, its popularity was short-lived. The acrylic was just too fragile. It was prone to scratches. However, it served as an impetus for the industry to keep looking for a lightweight alternative to heavy glass lenses.

Another plastic polymer was developed by PPG Industries in the late 1940s and introduced to the market in the early 1950s was CR-39, also known as allyl diglycol carbonate (ADC). It swiftly grew in popularity as a result of being more lightweight, impact-resistant, and easier to produce than conventional glass lenses. They provided greater wearer comfort and greatly decreased the risk of breaking or shattering that was connected with glass lenses. Additionally, the cost of manufacturing CR-39 lenses was lower, increasing the number of people who could purchase eyeglasses. The invention of CR-39 lenses was a crucial turning point in the development of eyewear. It paved the door for additional improvements in lens materials and designs, which had a significant impact on the development of the eyeglass business.

In the 1970s, polycarbonate lenses were developed. When searching for a material with high impact resistance to use in safety eyewear, Dr Daniel Stung and his team at the Foster Grant Company developed these lenses. Because of its safety advantages, polycarbonate lenses soon gained popularity as the best material for safety and sports eyewear. Due to the characteristics of the material, they provided both built-in UV protection and impact resistance. For those looking for both improved safety and vision correction, the advent of polycarbonate lenses was a key development in the eyewear business.

In the 1990s, Mitsui Chemicals unveiled the first in a line of products under the MR™ trademark and a brand-new urethane resin molecule for ophthalmic lens material. It demonstrated exceptional impact resistance, a higher refractive index of 1.60, a higher Abbe value, and low specific gravity, opening the door to a new era of high refractive index lenses. It later debuted MR-7™ in 1991 with an even higher refractive index of 1.67, and MR-174™ in 2000 with a record-breaking refractive index of 1.74. Even with a high lens prescription, these lenses offered unparalleled thinness.

PPG Industries introduced Trivex in the early 2000s. It was designed to provide a combination of features from both polycarbonate and traditional plastic lenses, aiming to offer improved optical quality, lightweight comfort, and impact resistance.

Further advancements led to the development of high-index plastics with superior optical properties. These materials could bend light more efficiently, allowing for thinner and lighter lenses, which were especially beneficial for strong prescriptions.

While materials and transparency were certainly driving forces in the evolution of spectacle lenses, it's also important to acknowledge the concurrent advancements in understanding optical principles, lens design, and the incorporation of new technologies. The combination of these factors has contributed to the intricate and effective spectacle lenses we have today.

The effectiveness of spectacle lenses also rapidly improved. Some of the notable contributions were:
- In 1756, the English optician, John Dollond, first made achromatic lenses by grinding, combining flint and ground glass into a single lens.
- Benjamin Franklin, the great American politician and scientist, designed bifocal lenses for himself probably about 1775.
- John Isaac Hawkins of London introduced trifocal lenses in 1826.

At the same time great advances were made to improve optical forms of lenses, particularly to avoid the astigmatism of oblique rays. The initial meniscus shape suggested by Kepler in his Dioptrice (1611) was greatly improved by the English scientist, WH Wollaston (1804–12), who introduced periscopic lenses, an idea modified to conform with the center of rotation of the eye by A Muller (1889) of Germany and more elaborately by F Ostwald (1898) of France; finally the orthoscopic lenses of Tscherning (1908) corrected distortion and curvature in the periphery in eccentric vision, an idea, however, anticipated by Sir George Biddell Airy (1827). Meantime Allvar Gullstrand (1899–1911) developed his aspherical katral lenses to correct spherical aberration, a problem of considerable importance in the thick lenses used for aphakic patients, and brought forward a solution to the problem of oblique astigmatism in his point focal lenses. Gullstrand's treatment of the subject was further elaborated by Moritz von Rohr (1908–21) and as a result of his work, Zeiss produced thin punktal lenses. H Boegehold (1916–21) was mainly responsible for the theory of astigmatic correction by toric surfaces.

Early in the evolution of ophthalmic lenses, lens producers also looked for ways to develop 'add-on' by simply adding colors to raw glass. In this line, the most elaborate series of experiments was undertaken by Sir Wm. Crookes (1914), who worked on the problem of the protection of glass workers from the development of cataracts. He developed a special color that filtered infrared rays and was named 'Crookes' after the inventor. This cool blue/grey shade was quite effective but unfortunately gave wearers a rather ghastly look, with unattractive shadows beneath the eyes.

Later, American Optical produced a more attractive pink shade called 'Cruxite'. Between the two World Wars, pink lenses became very popular. Bausch and Lomb introduced soft-lite lenses. These lenses provided protection from overbrightness. These lenses have a unique feature for absorbing excess light and preventing glare, which softens the light pleasantly. They have a flesh-like tone, but looking through them, wearers were unconscious of any tint. Color values remain perfectly natural, images are sharp, and vision is acute. The flesh-like hue of 'Soft-lite' lenses closely resembles the natural complexion, making them the least conspicuous of all eyeglasses available. Bausch and Lomb developed Ray-Ban and G-15 proprietary sunglass lenses. The addition of specific oxides to the glass mixture produced a solid tint. In high-lens prescription, these solid tints produced an uneven color, which was later resolved by using a vacuum coating process and a dye bath on plastic lenses. The dye was then absorbed into the lens surface, allowing for uniform tint density.

Photochromatic tints were also developed that darken when exposed to sunlight and fade back indoors. The first photochromic technology was offered for glass lenses in 1966 by Corning. Silver halide crystals added to the molten glass would cause the finished lenses to darken in reaction to UV in just a few minutes and would achieve maximum darkness after about 15 minutes. The more intense the UV exposure, the deeper the darkness, so the lenses could provide constantly adjusting comfort in a variety of light conditions. These lenses also protect the eyes from UV exposure. Early lenses would return to 65 percent transmittance in about 10 minutes after the UV exposure was terminated and reach 85 percent transmittance after an hour.

The first commercial plastic photochromatic lens was introduced in 1982. The organic photochromic material used in plastic lenses may include spiropyrans, spirooxazines, and naphthopyrans. High refractive index plastic materials were not readily responsive to standard photochromatic dyes until a process was developed in which spiroindoline photochromatic dye was inserted between several coatings of polyurethane on the surface of polycarbonate lenses, allowing for uniform tint density across the lens.

The initial light-responsive lenses were slow to darken and fade back to their clearest state. But further development improved them a lot, and today's best photochromic lenses can change from clear to dark in less than 15 seconds and then fade back to the clearest state in 2-20 minutes, depending on the manufacturer and temperature.

Plastic lenses were prone to scratches; therefore, a scratch-resistant coating was recommended. It was achieved by vacuum depositing a layer of silicone dioxide or using a dip- or spin-coat process on the lens surface. While the concept of anti-reflective lens coating was initially proposed in 1880, it was British physicist John William Strutt and 3rd Baron Rayleigh, who was awarded the Nobel Prize in Physics in 1904, who made significant contributions to the study of optics. In 1886, he discovered the first practical and simplest type of anti-reflective coating, often referred to as the Rayleigh or Rayleigh-Rice coating. This coating reduced the reflection of light from glass surfaces, improving the clarity of lenses and optical instruments. Lord Rayleigh's work laid the foundation for the development of modern anti-reflective coatings used in eyeglasses and optical devices today.

In 1935, Carl Zeiss indeed produced one of the earliest interference-based AR coatings for eyeglass lenses. This type of AR coating involves applying a thin film of a transparent material, typically magnesium fluoride, to both surfaces of the crown glass lens. The thickness of this coating is designed to be one-quarter (1/4th) the wavelength of the incident light, and the material used should have a lower refractive index than the lens substrate. This interferes with and reduces surface reflections, enhancing optical clarity.

When plastic materials were introduced there were initial challenges in the application of ARC on plastic lenses which were overcome with the use of a double layer coating. Currently, multiple layers are applied on each lens surface, using physical vapor deposition technique, consisting of four layer coatings of alternating high (either titanium oxide or zirconium dioxide) and low index (silicone dioxide) dielectric materials.

Recently, multi-stack layer surface coatings were adopted. These comprise a primer coating that improves the impact resistance of the lens, a hard coating, multiple layer anti-reflective stack and a top coat. The top coat provides a hydrophobic property by electrostatically repelling water molecules, and an oleophobic function that prevents grease deposit formation on the lens surface.

The Future

Many concepts and technologies using prototype materials have been proposed to aid in vision correction. These innovations aim to improve the quality of life for people who need vision correction.

Adaptive lenses seem to have promises for future lenses. These lenses correct refractive error by reversibly altering either the refractive index or lens curvature. Liquid crystal (LC) designs combine the properties of both crystalline solids and liquids and have received much attention, especially in the correction of presbyopia. In their solid state, the liquid crystal molecules are in regular order and held in fixed positions. Upon application of a controlled electrical current, the liquid crystal molecules rotate into a liquid formation, thus changing the refractive index and therefore the focal length. Switching from distance to near vision requires external electronics, possibly wireless technology, using blink detection or proximity sensors that track eye convergence or a change in pupil size during convergence as possible approaches for inducing the change in the refractive power.

Recently, a 3D printing platform has been introduced into an ophthalmic laboratory setting. The custom-designed lenses are printed on demand, requiring a few hours for the finished product, negating the need for stock-on-hand while reducing waste, water, and energy consumption.

HISTORY OF SPECTACLES

Spectacles were regarded as one of the wonders of the age in literature. Unfortunately, the exact origin of spectacles is not definitely known, and there are several conjectures and theories regarding their development. The information about the early development of spectacles is mostly derived from their mention in literature and the forms they took in mediaeval art. The approach allows for a more reasonable understanding of the development and use of spectacles throughout history.

Greeff (1921) has examined a great mass of data about the invention of spectacles. He points out that it is not right to neglect the evidence as shown in ancient arts, but it would be naive to conclude that any spectacles shown were of the epoch the picture represents. Throughout history, artists have often incorporated spectacles into their depictions of characters engaged in deep study or meditation, even in scenes set in ancient times. While this artistic choice can enhance the sense of authenticity and realism, it is important to note that there are instances where the presence of spectacles may appear out of place within the historical context. Still, it may be accepted as evidence that the use of spectacles dates from about the 13th century, as the earliest historical figure documented wearing eyewear was Bishop Ugone da Provenza **(Fig. 3.1)**. This Dominican priest was portrayed in a painting by Tomaso da Modena in the year 1252. His glasses were really nothing more than simple magnifying lenses with two monocles riveted together so they could perch on his nose. The spectacles worn by the Cardinal were so riveted together that they could have been stable on a prominent nose.

Another extensive study by a group of researchers concluded after examining mass data concerning the invention of spectacles that AD 1280 was the probable time of the invention and it was Salvino d'Armati of Florence who was considered the probable inventor, as this fact is inscribed on his tombstone. Early iterations of spectacles typically comprised two separate monocles, each housing quartz crystal lenses, and were attached to a frame worn low on the forehead.

Some theories suggest that ancient Chinese and Arabian civilizations might have had some form of basic magnification device or lens that could have been used to aid vision. Ancient Chinese texts describe the use of crystal lenses for magnification, and the Arab scholar Alhazen wrote about the properties of light and lenses.

Laufer's assertion from his study in 1907 suggests that spectacles may have originated in India during the Mongolian dynasty in early 14th century, and then made their way to

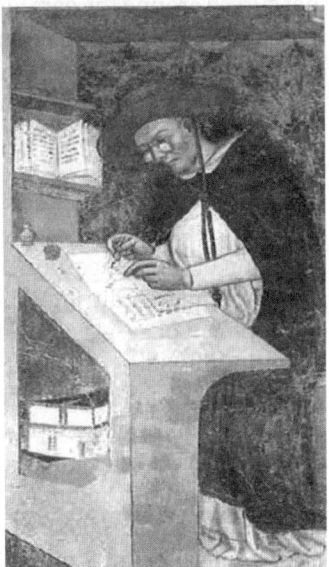

Fig. 3.1: Bishop Ugone da Provenza, shown in this 13th century painting is the first historical figure known to wear eye wear.

China through Turkistan. However, it is worth noting that the exact origins and diffusion of spectacles remain a topic of ongoing scholarly debate, with various theories and evidence contributing to our understanding of their history.

It is true that the widespread use of spectacles became more common after Johannes Gutenberg's invention of the printing press in the mid-15th century. Gutenberg's invention revolutionized the production of books and printed materials, leading to an increase in literacy and the availability of printed materials for a broader population. This, in turn, contributed to a greater need for vision correction. The event marked the real beginning of the need to correct vision with spectacles. Lenses used were biconvex in form and used primarily to correct presbyopia. During this period, it was also thought that biconcave lenses would help nearsighted persons see more clearly in distance vision. Johanes Kepler was the person who introduced the concept of lens grading by their focal power. Until then lens power were defined by the age of the person wearing them.

By this time, Venice became the hub for eyeglass production, with skilled artisans crafting spectacles with metal or bone frames. These early spectacles were rudimentary, featuring lenses that were not necessarily tailored to individual prescriptions. As the demand increased, new spectacles-making centers were opened up in Holland and Germany. At the end of the 15th century bow spectacles were made, which used elastic pressure to hold them in position. Steel was used as the spring and also to hold the lenses in mounting.

In 1560, a painting by J Van Straet depicts a man walking and holding a single glass to his eye, and it was recorded that during 1583 single glasses in horn, leather or metal mountings were sold in great quantities at Nuremberg in Germany. The 16th century saw the development of concave lenses to correct nearsightedness. By the 17th century, Benjamin Franklin's invention of bifocal lenses further expanded the functionality of eyeglasses. The 17th century also brought changes to frame design, with a shift from the rivet style to "temple spectacles," which had arms that curved around the ears for a more secure fit. Frames made from materials like tortoiseshell, ivory, and metal became popular among the wealthy. These temple spectacle frames replaced all other forms including folding spectacles.

In the 18th century, advancements in lens grinding techniques improved the precision of eyeglasses. The use of gold, silver, and tortoiseshell for frames added aesthetic value to the eyewear.

The 19th century marked a period of rapid progress in eyewear technology. The invention of the adjustable nose bridge in the early 1800s allowed for a more customized fit. The invention of the "pince-nez" style, which rested on the bridge of the nose without earpieces, gained popularity during this era. Manufacturing techniques continued to evolve, with the development of eyeglass frames made from various materials such as steel and celluloid.

During this period, most glasses were sold in hardware stores. Gradually, gold and silver were used as frame materials, and jewellers became the logical successors to hardware merchants. Merchants selling glasses purchased them as ready-made glasses, usually one dozen per box, and sold them under an "inch-number" system. Away from large cities, itinerant eyeglass peddlers were the primary method of eyeglass distribution. Most of their wares were produced by European sources. People who thought that they needed glasses would try on ready-made glasses, one after another, until they found a pair that helped. The lenses in this factory-made eyewear were always the same power for each eye.

The early 20th century saw the rise of mass production techniques for eyeglasses, making them more affordable and accessible to a wider population. The introduction of plastic frames in the 1950s brought about new possibilities for design and comfort. Transition lenses, which darken in response to sunlight, were introduced in the 1960s.

The 21st century has seen significant advancements in eyewear technology, including the development of progressive lenses that correct multiple vision problems in one lens. The integration of smart technology has led to the creation of smart glasses, which can display information, take pictures, and perform other functions.

Throughout its history, the evolution of spectacles has been driven by a combination of scientific understanding, technological innovation, and changing fashion trends. Today, eyeglasses continue to be an essential tool for correcting vision and a fashion statement for many.

TERMS USED IN LENS WORKSHOP

The purpose of workshop process is to give the product a desired shape so that it can be put to the desired use by the consumer. The onus is the efficient utilization of equipment and tools to work with the raw materials in a most effective manner to manufacture the finished products. While working in the workshop the workers and other individuals engaged in the task execution uses industry relevant jargon and various terms to describe and communicate. An understanding of these specific terms is critical to success. Similarly in a lens work shop, while manufacturing spectacle lenses various terms and jargon are used to describe different aspects of eyeglass lenses, their manufacturing processes, and related equipment. Some of the common terms are listed down:

LENS BLANK

A lens blank is a semi-finished lens that has the basic lens shape and curvature but has not yet been finished to an individual's lens prescription. Lens blanks come in various materials, designs, and sizes. Lens blanks are also known as moulding or pressing.

LENS SURFACING

Lens surfacing refers to the process of grinding and polishing the lens blank to achieve the specific lens prescription of an individual job order. This process involves shaping the lens to the correct curvature and thickness. The process converts a blank into a transparent lens. The complete surfacing process starts with generation of curvature and finishes with polishing.

LENS PRESCRIPTION

A prescription is a written order from an eye care professional (optometrist or ophthalmologist) specifying the exact corrective lens power sphere, cylinder, axis, and other parameters needed to correct a person's vision.

LENS DIAMETER

The lens diameter refers to the measurement of the width of a lens, typically measured across the widest part of the lens. It is an important dimension when selecting eyeglasses, sunglasses, or other eyewear because it affects the overall size and fit of the glasses on your face.

EFFECTIVE DIAMETER

While the diameter refers to the measurement of the widest width of the lens, effective diameter represents the size of the lens needed to ensure that the major reference point of the lens aligns correctly within the lens aperture of the frame. This alignment is essential for achieving optimal optical performance and clear vision when wearing eyeglasses. Effective diameter takes into consideration both the physical size of the lens and the placement of the major reference points within that lens. In spectacle dispensing, the major reference point is typically the optical center of the lens or the fitting cross position of the progressive lens which should align with the wearer's pupil when looking straight ahead. Effective diameter is measured as follows:

- Mark the positions of the monocular interpupillary distance (IPD) or fitting cross on the lens insert.
- Now measure the distance from the marked position on the lens insert to the apex of the lens bevel farthest from it.
- Multiply it by 2.
- Add 1 or 2 mm for the depth of the groove.
- The result is effective diameter of the lens in millimeter needed for appropriate dispensing.

REFRACTION INDEX

The refractive index is the measure of light bending ability of the lens material, i.e., how much a lens material can bend or refract light. Materials with a higher refractive index, i.e., high-index lenses can produce thinner lenses for a given prescription.

ABBE NUMBER

A numerical expression of how prone a lens material is to causing chromatic aberration. It is also referred to as constringence. It is an important number for the calculation of chromatic aberration. The higher the number, smaller will be the light dispersion and chromatic aberration through the lens material.

CROWN

In ophthalmic optics, glass with a refractive index of 1.523 is known as crown. In scientific optics, the term is used to denote a lens material which is low in index and high in constringence when combined with higher index glass, i.e., flint produces achromatic lenses.

CR-39

CR-39 denotes a type of plastic lens material derived from allyl diglycol carbonate. It was developed by the PPG Industries in the late 1940s and became widely used for eyeglass lenses due to its excellent optical properties. CR 39 has a refractive index of 1.498.

SPHERICAL

In a lens workshop, the term "spherical" is used to mean two different understandings. In the context of lens, the term "spherical" refers to a specific type of lens curvature or denotes the shape of lens surface. Spherical curve implies that the lens surface has a uniform curve across its entire surface, much like a section of a sphere. This curvature is consistent in all meridians.

The term "spherical" is also used as a part of lens prescription in the job order which is used to describe the primary component of a lens prescription that corrects basic refractive errors, indicating the degree of refractive correction. It is prefixed with either plus or minus sign. Plus spherical will result in converging lens and minus spherical lens will result in diverging lens.

CYLINDER

Like spherical the term "cylinder" is used to mean two different understandings. In the context of lens the term "cylinder" refers to lens that has a power meridian which is paired with-plano

Chapter 3: Mechanical Optics, Lenses and Lens Prescription

meridian. In its most basic form, it is the sub-section of a solid cylinder glass or plastic. Cylinder lens differs from spherical lens because of their geometrical shape.

The term "cylinder" is also used as a part of lens prescription in the job order which is used to describe one of the components of a lens prescription that corrects astigmatism. The lens power is only in one dimension and will not affect the light in the perpendicular dimension. Like spherical cylinder can also be prefixed with either plus sign or minus sign.

AXIS

The axis specifies the orientation of the cylinder correction. The cylinder axis is a crucial component of a lens prescription. It is one of the three main elements in an astigmatic prescription, alongside the sphere and cylinder values. It can be defined as:
- A line of zero curvature on a cylindrical surface.
- The principal meridian of a plano cylinder in which the power is zero.
- More generally, that principal meridian of an astigmatic lens in which the focal power is that of the spherical element only of the lens prescription.

The axis value ranges from 0 to 180 degrees, with 90 degrees representing the vertical meridian of the eye and 180 degrees representing the horizontal meridian.

The cylinder axis is crucial for ensuring that the astigmatic correction is precisely aligned with the eye's astigmatism, allowing for clear and focused vision. Properly oriented cylindrical corrections can significantly improve visual acuity and reduce the blurriness associated with astigmatism.

MERIDIAN

A meridian is an imaginary line that crosses the optical center of the lens. The power of a correcting lens may vary in different meridians, from minimum power along one meridian, gradually increasing to a maximum power along another meridian at right angle to the first meridian. The minimum and maximum meridians are known as the principal meridians of the lens that lie perpendicular to each other and meet at the optical center of the lens. The rays of light passing through this meeting point travel undeviated. When these two meridians carry same power, the lens is known as spherical lens and when these two meridians carry different power, the lens is known as sphero-cylinder lens. In case of plano-cylinder lens, one meridian has no power and other carries the lens power.

OPTICAL CROSS

An optical cross is a diagrammatic representation of the orientation of the two principal meridians of an ophthalmic lens that shows the dioptric strength of the lens along the respective meridians. The two principal meridians are perpendicular to each other, for example, if one principal meridian is at 90 degree, other would be at 180 degree and so on. The two principal meridians are commonly known as axis meridian and power meridian. Axis meridian has the minimum lens power and power meridian has the maximum lens power as shown in **Table 3.1**.

Table 3.1: Comparison of axis meridian and power meridian in reference to lens-power.

Lens power	Axis meridian	Power meridian
Spherical	Amount of spherical	Same as axis meridian
Plano cylinder	Plano	Cylinder element
Sphero-cylinder	Spherical element	Summation of both spherical and cylinder

NEAR ADD

"Near add" is a term used in lens prescription to indicate the additional spherical power needed for near vision correction. It is typically prescribed as an additional power, measured in diopters (D), and is added to the main spherical element of distance vision correction. Near add is also known as the "addition" or "reading addition."

PRISM

Prism is also an important component of lens prescription. A prism is used to correct eye alignment issues. It is measured in prism diopters and is specified in the prescription when needed.

In the context of a lens workshop, a prism refers to a wedge-shaped lens that has the ability to deviate light as it passes through.

Prism power is measured in prism diopter (Δ). Prism diopter indicate the amount of deviation or displacement of light that occurs as it passes through the prism. Prism power can be specified in either horizontal (base in or base out) or vertical (base up or base down) directions. For example, a prescription may include a prism correction of 2.00Δ base out.

DECENTRATION

Decentration refers to the displacement of optical center of the lens either horizontal or vertically or both from the standard optical center position.

BASE CURVE

The base curve determines how steep or flat the lens appears when viewed from the side. It is typically measured in dioptres (D) and represents the degree of curvature of the lens. A steeper base curve means a more curved or "bowl-shaped" lens, while a flatter base curve results in a less curved or more "plate-like" lens.

In the context of spectacle lenses, the base curve refers to the curvature of the front surface of the lens. The selection of the base curve is crucial first step in ensuring that the prescription lenses match the curvature as appropriate for the given lens prescription. A properly matched base curve helps in achieving the best form lens that provides best visual clarity and minimizing distortions and also ensures best cosmetic appeal.

OCULAR CURVE

The "ocular curve" refers to the curvature of the back surface of a spectacle lens which is the result of the selection of the base curve. Ocular curve is one of the important determinants for the vertex distance of the spectacle lens.

CROSS CURVE

In the context of eyeglass prescriptions, the "cross curve" refers to the combined curvature of the base curve and the cylinder component of a prescription lens. It is the sum of the base curve and the cylinder, defining the overall curvature of the lens surface when astigmatism correction is incorporated. It accounts for both the spherical correction (base curve) and the cylindrical correction, ensuring that the lens surface provides the appropriate refractive correction for the patient's vision needs.

Most sphero-cylinder lenses have the cylinder power on the back surface of the lens. They are ground using lap tools having two curves. The first and weaker curve gives the spherical power and is called the back base curve. The second, more minus curve is called the cross curve and includes added value necessary to create cylinder power. The tool value is denoted as back base curve/cross curve. In other words, the surface power in the meridian at right angle to that of the base curve of the toroidal surface.

SURFACE POWER

The ability of a surface of the lens to alter the vergence of incident light is called its surface power. A lens has two surfaces, either of which may be positive or negative or zero, separated by a thickness of lens material. Each surface of a lens will have a converging or diverging effect of its own which depends upon the radius of curvature of the surface and the refractive index of the material.

SURFACE CURVATURE

Surface curvature is the geometrical property of the surface of the lens. In case of simple spherical surface, it depends only on radius of curvature of the surface, not in any way on the material of the surface. Surface curvature is the angle through which the surface turns in unit length of arc.

CORRIDOR LENGTH

Corridor length of the progressive addition lens defines the section on the umbilical line that features gradual change in base curve from a minimum value to value that is 85% of the maximum value. The top end of the corridor length is at the center of fitting cross and the bottom end of the corridor length is at the point where 85% of the near addition is achieved. This is usually achieved at the top edge of the near power circle depending upon lens design. A shorter corridor length implies that the optics of lens design is compressed, due to mathematical constraints of progressive lens design that increases the rate of change in unwanted cylinder across the lens design, leading to narrower central viewing zone and reduced intermediate utility.

FREE-FORM TECHNOLOGY

Free-form technology, also known as free-form lens design or digital lens surfacing, is an advanced method of manufacturing eyeglass lenses that provides highly customized and precise vision correction. Unlike traditional lens manufacturing, which involves grinding the prescription onto the front surface of a lens blank, free-form technology uses computer-controlled equipment to create lenses with complex, customized surfaces on one or both the front and back sides of the lens.

LACQUER

Lacquer is used in lens workshop for the purpose of applying scratch resistant coating to the lens surface of plastic lenses, which help protect the lenses from everyday wear and tear, including minor scratches and abrasions. Some lenses are coated with a lacquer containing UV-blocking properties to provide additional protection against harmful ultraviolet (UV) rays from the sun. Lacquer is also used as a coat of primer before applying anti-reflective coating on polycarbonate lenses. Lacquer comes in different refractive indices for different indices of lens material.

ETCHING

Etching is the process applied to prepare the lens surface for various coatings and improve their adhesion and longevity.

Before applying scratch-resistant coatings to lenses, lens laboratories often use an etching process to clean and prepare the lens surface. This preparation involves removing any contaminants and creating a surface that promotes better adhesion for the scratch-resistant coating. Etching can be achieved using warm sodium hydroxide (NaOH) solutions in ultrasonic baths. This process helps increase the lifespan of the scratch-resistant coating by ensuring it adheres well to the lens surface.

Similarly, before applying anti-reflective (AR) coatings to lenses, lens laboratories may use a different type of etching process. Instead of a chemical etching process, an ion gun is often used to etch the lens surface. This ion-assisted etching creates a clean, microscopically rough surface that enhances the adhesion of the anti-reflective coating. It also helps in reducing reflections and glare, improving optical clarity.

GENERATOR

Generators are the important equipment for lens workshop. They are used to generate concave, convex, spherical and cylinder curves on lens blanks. There are generators for only glass lenses and there are generators for only plastic lenses and there are generators that can be used for both materials. Lens laboratories often use automated machines for this purpose.

LENS SURFACING

Lens surfacing is the process of generating, shaping and polishing the surfaces of eyeglass lenses to achieve the desired prescription and optical properties.

LENS POLISHING

Lens polishing is the ultimate step in the lens surfacing procedure, yielding specular reflection rather than diffuse reflection and consistent transmission instead of random transmission.

CHILLER

Chiller is the equipment used for cooling lens and various components involved in the lens manufacturing and surfacing lenses.

VARNISH

Varnish is the scratch-resistant coating applied on the lens surface to protect the lens surfaces from minor scratches and abrasions. This helps extend the lifespan of eyeglasses and maintain optical clarity.

EDGING

Grinding the edges of a lens to the finished shape and size as required and at the same time imparting the desired edge form, such as flat, bevelled, etc., is known as edging of lenses.

GLAZING

Strictly, the fitting of lenses to a frame or mount, but often used to include the cutting and edging processes.

BEVEL

Bevel refers to a specific cut or angled edge that is applied to the perimeter of a lens while finishing the lens edging. Beveling is an essential step in the lens finishing process, and it makes it easier to insert the lenses into the eyeglass frames lens grooves. The beveled edges allow the lenses to slide into place without catching or causing damage to the frame remains stable. Beveling is tailored to match the specific frame design and lens groove shape, ensuring compatibility and a seamless fit.

LENS GROOVING

Lens grooving is a process in eyeglass lens manufacturing and edging where a groove or channel is created on the edge of a lens. This groove is typically made to accommodate a nylon or plastic cord that holds the lens securely in the eyeglass frame.

EMERY

Emery is granular rock consisting of a mixture of the mineral corundum and iron oxides used as an abrasive or polishing material during lens surfacing.

ABRASIVES

Abrasives are materials used for grinding, smoothing, shaping, and polishing eyeglass lenses during the lens manufacturing and surfacing processes. The choice of abrasive material and grit size depends on the specific lens finishing tasks and the type of lens material being processed.

CHUCK

Chuck typically refers to a specialized tool or device used to hold and secure eyeglass lens blanks during various stages of the lens surfacing process.

NEWTON'S RING

Newton's ring is an interference pattern that arises due to variations in the optical path length between two interacting surfaces.

TEST PLATE

A "test plate" is a finely polished plate or lens with a highly accurate and well-shaped surface, used for examining and evaluating the surface quality of another lens with a curvature opposite to its own by observing Newton's rings. This technique helps assess the quality and correctness of the lens under examination based on the interference pattern created by the interaction of light between the two surfaces.

BUTTON

Buttons are used to manufacture glass bifocal blanks. Bifocal lenses have two distinct optical powers in a single lens, typically with the upper portion for distance vision and the lower portion for near vision. Buttons serve the purpose of near segment in the context of glass bifocal lenses.

DEPRESSION CURVE

The power of the surface worked on the main lens to receive the button.

CRIBBING

Cribbing in the context you provided typically refers to the process of removing excess material from a lens to achieve the desired shape and size. It is a machining or finishing operation commonly used in lens manufacturing to ensure that the final lens conforms to the precise specifications and dimensions required for its intended optical function.

SHANKING

Shanking refers to the process of roughly trimming the edges of a lens to achieve the desired size and shape by using special pliers to crumble or break away the excess material. This procedure is often a preliminary step in lens manufacturing, helping to bring the lens closer to its final dimensions before more precise finishing operations are performed.

TREPANNING TOOL

Some ophthalmic lenses, especially rimless or semi-rimless frames, require holes for mounting. Trepanning tools can be used to drill precise holes in the lenses for screws or other mounting hardware.

LENS FORM

Lens form typically refers to the specific curvature, shape, and design of a lens. It describes how the lens is ground, shaped, and curved to correct vision problems or meet particular optical requirements.

LENS MARKING

The marking of lens blank for control of centration, axis direction, segment setting, etc.

SURFACE POWER

The power in diopter of a single surface, numerically equal to $(n_2 - n_1)/r$, where n_1 and n_2 are the refractive indices of two lenses and r is the radius of curvature in meters.

TRANSVERSE TEST

Transverse test is a method of estimating focal power of lens by observation of 'against' or 'with' movements.

VERTEX

Vertex in the context refers to the point of intersection of the optical axis with a surface of a lens.

C-SIZER

A tool used to measure the circumference of a cut lens.

CALIPER

The tool used to measure the thickness of a lens.

COLMASCOPE

A tool used to test the stress a lens is under. It will reveal a lens that is too tight in an eyewire or a glass lens that has been properly treated for impact resistance.

CRAZING

Crazing refers to a lens that has cracked or has a web-like pattern of splits cross the entire lens surface. Crazing is caused by chemical reaction.

EDGER VOMIT

Edger vomit refers to the mix of water and swarf that collects under a wet cut edger.

EQUITHIN

Equithin is a laboratory process used on progressives to thin the lens. The process creates prism in the lenses but the prism is balanced in such a way that it is unnoticed by the wearer.

GROOVER

The lab tool that cuts the slot on the lens edge that catches the nylon cord in semi-rimless frames.

HIDE-A-BEVEL

A generic term for a bevel placed in the best position to hide the edge thickness of a lens.

HYDRO-PHOBIC

A lens coating that resists water build-up, sheds rain drops and prevents fogging.

IMAGE JUMP

Image jump refers to the shift of image that an individual person may experience when changing the gaze from the distance portion of a lens to the magnifying segment area in a lined bifocal.

IMPACT RESISTANCE

A way of expressing how much force a lens can take before breaking.

SEGMENT INSET

Segment inset refers to how much the reading area of a lens is moved inward nasally to match patient convergence. It is equal to the far pupillary distance minus the near pupillary distance.

LAMINATED

A lens that is multi-layered. The term is used in explain the features of polarized lenses.

LAP

The tool that holds the pads and polishes the lenses during surfacing is called lap.

LENS CLOCK

A tool that reads curvature of the lens surface is called lens clock. It is capable of reading both plus and minus curvature and can be used to accurately read a prescription without the use of a lensometer.

LENS WASHER

A thin strip of plastic used to increase the circumference of a lens that has been cut too small for an eyewire.

SAFETY BEVEL

The smoothing out of the leading edge of a lens so that it is not sharp.

SWARF

The debris left over from lens processing in surfacing and finishing.

OPHTHALMIC LENS MATERIAL

All the ophthalmic lenses currently available in the ophthalmic industry can be classified into two broad categories as shown in **Flowchart 3.1**.

GLASS LENS

Glass lenses are made of natural minerals. There are some intrinsic qualities of mineral glass material which make it unique. These qualities are listed below:
- Transparency
- Dimensional stability
- Chemical stability
- Hardness
- Suitability for forming and machining
- Heat resistant

Flowchart 3.1: Two types of lens material.

The glasses are incredibly stable even at all temperature, exhibiting no signs of fatigue. Despite their fragility, they prove highly resistant to scratches. The components used for glasses for spectacle lenses are vitrifiable mixture which is put into the melting tank in the form of extremely pure raw materials so as to obtain perfect quality glass. The basic components such as silica and alumina are introduced in the respective forms of iron-free sand and feldspar. The alkaline oxides, i.e., sodium or potassium are generally added in the form of carbonates or nitrates. Lime and magnesia are sometimes replaced by limestone and dolomite. These basic components are accompanied by numerous other ingredients such as rare earths. Natural glass has a clear advantage here as its refractive index range extends from 1.5 to 1.9. Natural glass also has a greater density than plastic. The result-even when the refraction index is the same, lenses made of glass are always thinner than those made of plastic, but they are substantially heavier.

RESIN LENS

Resin or plastic lenses are made of organic materials, offering a versatile and accessible alternative to traditional glass lenses. Organic compounds, which are particularly light in weight, generally offer the advantages and drawbacks of a structure which has been formed at a low temperature. They are considerable less stable than mineral glasses and scratches much more easily. Plastic spectacle lenses have revolutionized the eyewear industry. Their popularity stems from a combination of factors, including durability, lightweight design, and affordability.

Chapter 3: Mechanical Optics, Lenses and Lens Prescription

Plastic spectacle lenses are typically made from various types of polymers, with CR-39, polycarbonate and high-index plastics being among the most common choices. These materials share several key characteristics:

* Plastic lenses are significantly lighter than traditional glass lenses, making them more comfortable for extended wear.
* Polycarbonate lenses, in particular, are known for their exceptional impact resistance.
* Plastic spectacle lenses are less prone to shattering than glass, reducing the risk of injury in case of accidental drops or impacts.
* Plastic lenses are generally more affordable than glass lenses, making them an accessible option for a wide range of individuals.
* Plastic lenses are also available in several high indices to make the lens thinner and more aesthetic.
* Many plastic lenses can be coated to provide UV protection, safeguarding the eyes from harmful ultraviolet rays.

For an individual person ophthalmic lens material is selected based on its optical properties, durability, weight, and compatibility with various lens treatments and the desired performance of the finished lens in terms of three factors as shown in **Flowchart 3.2**.

While vision is the function of optical properties of lens material, comfort and safety are more associated with the physical properties of the lens material. Cosmetic factors in eyeglasses and other optical devices often depend on the optical properties of the lens material and any additives or coatings that are applied to modify these properties.

There are three principal optical factors that govern the selection of appropriate lens material. These are shown in **Flowchart 3.3**.

Refractive Index

The refractive index of a lens material is the ratio between the velocity of the monochromatic light in air to the velocity of light in the given lens material and is denoted by 'n'.

$$n = \frac{\text{The velocity of light in air}}{\text{Velocity of light in lens material}}$$

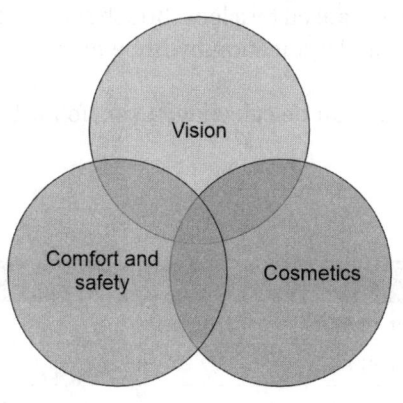

Flowchart 3.2: The three important factors that drive lens material selection.

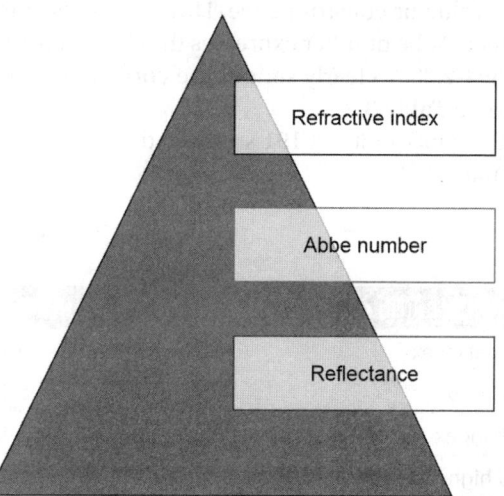

Flowchart 3.3: Three important optical factors.

The reference wavelengths used for the determination of refractive index are as follows:
- Mercury e-line λe = 546.07 nm
- Helium-d line λd = 587.56 nm

These lines are used out of convention because they are close to the middle of the visible spectrum. Historically, different countries have their own preference between the two. However, in real terms it makes very little difference. For example, for CR_{39}, nd = 1.498 and ne = 1.501, both of which round to 1.50 at two decimal places.

This is a number, which has no unit and is always greater than 1. When the light passes from air to, say glass, i.e., rare medium to denser medium, the speed of their propagation slows down.

The refractive index defines the velocity of light with which it travels in the respective material. Thus, it describes the ability the lens material to bend light. The velocity of light in a vacuum is approximately 186,000 miles or 300,000 kilometers per second. Its velocity through differing lens materials varies as some materials offer more resistance than others, the higher the refractive index the greater its resistance or slower its speed. A higher index of refraction results in a lower angle of refraction which means the bent light ray comes closer to the normal (perpendicular) line. In other words, for a given angle of incidence, the higher the index, the more light is bent. That is why "high index" lenses can be thinner for a given prescription compared to the lower index lenses. **Table 3.2** gives the classification of refractive index within BS 7394-2-2007 from normal to very high index.

It is important to know that two lens materials of the same index will have similar center substance. For example, glass lenses are more rigid, whereas plastic lens material is not as hard as glass. It may be that a plastic lens of the same refractive index requires a thicker center substance in order to have sufficient mechanical strength to avoid it buckling under the tension imposed during glazing the lens to a frame.

With plus lenses, differing edge thicknesses is possible due to the lens size as an aspheric lens with normal index may show thinner edge profile the spherical lens design. Patients are most frequently disappointed when they are dispensed higher refractive index lenses from stock when they have previously had a lower index lens surfaced to minimum size uncut. **Figure 3.2** shows the edge thickness of minus lenses as dispensed.

Abbe Number

The Abbe number, denoted by the lower case the Greek letter "nu" (v), is often referred to as the V-value or constringence. However, these terms are now superseded by the term Abbe number. Abbe number expresses the chromatic dispersion caused by a lens. British standards BS 7394-2:2007 clearly set out the correct terminology for classification by Abbe number as shown in **Table 3.3**.

BS EN ISO 13666:20191 suggests that the Abbe Number can be calculated using following formula:

$$v_d = \frac{(n_d - 1)}{(n_F - n_c)}$$

Table 3.2: British standard classification of refractive index.	
Normal index	≥ 1.48 but <1.54
Mid index	≥ 1.54 but <1.64
High index	≥ 1.64 but <1.74
Very high index	≥ 1.74

Chapter 3: Mechanical Optics, Lenses and Lens Prescription

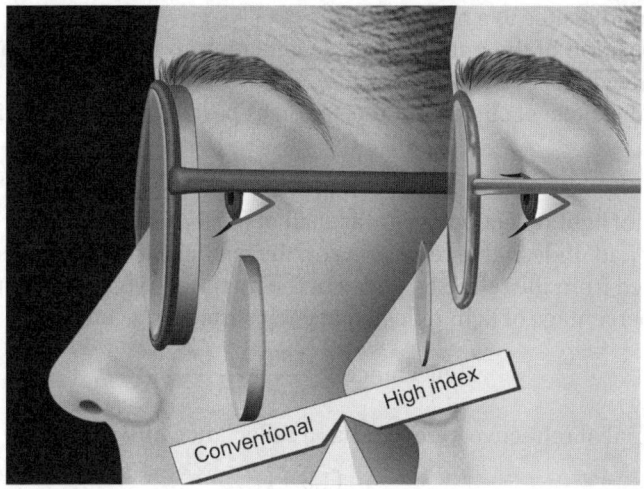

Fig. 3.2: Thinner edge profile of minus lenses.

Table 3.3: Abbe number as classified by British standard.	
Low dispersion	≥ 45
Medium dispersion	≥ 39 but <45
High dispersion	<39

Where,
- v_d **is the Abbe number**
- n_d **is the refractive index of lens material at "D"** spectral line (approx. 587.6 nm)
- n_f **is the refractive index of lens material at "F"** spectral line (approx. 486.1 nm)
- n_c **is the refractive index of lens material at "C"** spectral line (approx. 656.3 nm)

Abbe number is the reciprocal of the dispersive power (ω), therefore:

$$\text{Abbe number} = \frac{1}{\omega}$$

Abbe value is the number that is the measure of the degree to which light is dispersed when entering a lens material. The light passing through the lens periphery disperses due to prismatic effect and causes chromatic aberration as different wavelengths of light are refracted at varying degrees, resulting in color fringes or blurriness. The effect can be more pronounced in higher lens power and also with the lower the abbe number of the lens material. Abbe number of 60 is considered to have the least chromatic aberrations and Abbe number of 30 is for the most chromatic aberrations. Thus, chromatic aberration is inversely proportional to the Abbe number. Transverse chromatic aberration (TCA) is more important for spectacle lens design and is expressed in prism dioptres (Δ).

Abbe value is the property of the lens material and cannot be affected by any surface technique. However, the effect of dispersion can be minimized by important dispensing factors:
- Always use monocular pupillary distances
- Consider modifying pantoscopic angle

- Keep back vertex distance to a minimum
- Consider the position of the optical centers in relation to horizontal center line and edge thickness differences

Figure 3.3 shows the effect of chromatic aberration as perceived by an individual.

Reflectance

The phenomenon of light reflection occurs at each of the lens surfaces. The result is the loss of lens transparency and undesirable reflections on the lens surfaces. The reflectance of the lens surface is calculated from the refractive index of the material. When the light is normal on the lens surface, the percentage of light reflected at each surface is given by:

$$\text{Reflectance} = \frac{100\,(n-1)^2}{(n+1)^2}\%$$

Therefore, a material of refractive index 1.5 has a reflectance of:

$$100\,\frac{(1.5-1)^2}{(1.5+1)^2}$$

$$\text{Or, } 100\,\frac{(0.5)^2}{(2.5)^2}$$

$$\text{Or, } 100 \times \left(\frac{0.5}{2.5}\right)$$

Or, 3.9% per surface.

From the above, it can easily be said that as the refractive index increases, reflectance also increases. The higher the refractive index, the greater the proportion of light reflected from the surfaces. The unwanted reflection can be almost completely eliminated by applying an efficient anti-reflection coating, the need of which is more in higher index material. **Table 3.4** gives the percentage of light lost due to surface reflectance.

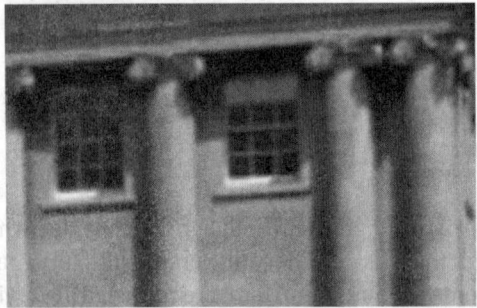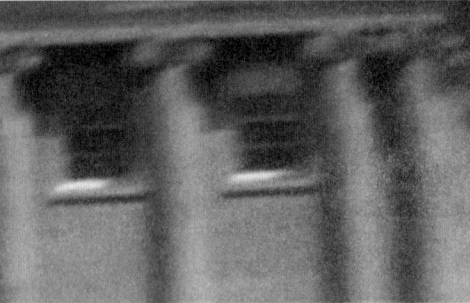

Fig. 3.3: Chromatic aberration as perceived by an individual.

Table 3.4: Loss of light due to surface reflectance.

Refractive index	% of light reflected
1.5	7.8%
1.6	10.4%
1.7	12.3%
1.8	15.7%
1.9	18.3%

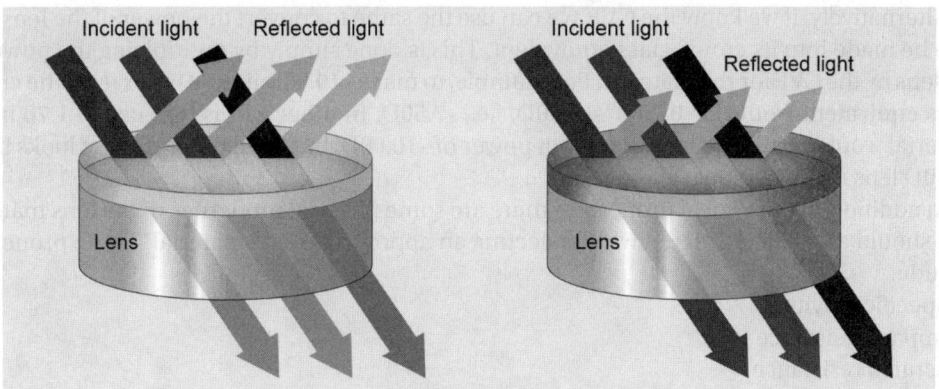

Fig. 3.4: Loss of light because of surface reflection.

Figure 3.4 shows the effect of surface reflection as light transmitted through the lens reduces.

Absorption

The amount of light which goes through a lens can be reduced because of absorption by the lens material. This is negligible in case of a non-tinted lens, but constitutes an intrinsic function of a tinted or photo chromatic lens. Absorption of an ophthalmic lens generally refers to its internal absorption, i.e., to the percentage of light absorbed between the front and the rear lens surfaces. Lens absorption occurs according to Lambert's law and varies exponentially as a function of lens thickness.

CURVE VARIATION FACTOR

Curve variation factor shows the variation in surface power when the lens material is other than crown glass, so providing an indication of the change in thickness. It can also be used in tool power calculation. It is useful to know the likely change in the volume and thickness which will be obtained when another material is compared with the standard crown glass. This information enables a direct comparison in the thickness to be obtained. For example, 1.70 index materials have a CVF of 0.75D, which will be about 25%, if this material is substituted for crown glass. For a given refractive and a standard index, the CVF is given by:

$$CVF = \frac{Ns - 1}{Nr - 1}$$

Where,
Ns = Refractive index of standard lens material.
Nr = Refractive index of substituting lens material.

CVF in above example would be:

$$CVF = \frac{1.523 - 1}{1.70 - 1}$$

$$= \frac{0.523}{0.700}$$

$$= 0.747 \text{ D}$$

$$= 0.75 \text{ D approx.}$$

Alternatively, if we know the CVF, we can use the same to convert the power of the lens that is to be made into its crown glass equivalent. This is done simply by multiplying the power of the lens by the CVF for the material. For example, to make –10.00D in 1.70 index lens, the crown glass equivalent would be 0.75 × –10.00D, i.e., -7.50D. In other words, the use of 1.70 index material would result in a lens that has a power of –10.00D, but in all other respect looks like a –7.50D lens made in crown glass.

In addition to the optical properties, there are some physical properties of the lens material that should also be considered while selecting an appropriate lens material. These properties include:

- Specific gravity
- Impact resistance
- Scratch resistance

Specific Gravity

Specific gravity is the measurement of physical density or weight of the material in grams per cubic centimeter. In deciding the weight of lens material, a lens material with low specific gravity will produce a lighter lens. Reduction of weight improves wearing comfort, and eliminates the indentations from nose pads that are produced by wearing heavy glasses. However, low density does not always mean a lighter lens—the amount of material depends on the refractive index and the minimum thickness. But low specific gravity is very important for prescriptions that require high powered plus or minus lenses. Patients with high power prescriptions are usually advised to use higher index glasses. Although they offer thinner lenses, they are not necessarily more comfortable to wear because of their high specific gravity. **Table 3.5** shows the specific gravity of various lens materials:

Impact Resistance

In 1971, the Food and Drug Administration (FDA) adopted a procedure to ensure the level of protection provided to the consumer for "street wear". More stringent standards are applied for industrial protection. The standard involves dropping a 5/8″ steel ball from a height of 50″ onto the lens and the lenses that survive this test are deemed impact resistant **(Fig. 3.5)**. The implementation of this standard in the USA led to increased use of hard resin lenses. Only a sample of hard resin lenses is needed to be tested for impact resistance, whereas every glass lens is needed to be tested. This accelerated the shift towards the plastic lenses.

Scratch Resistance

One of the great advantages of glass lenses is abrasion resistance. Plastic lenses need to be coated with an additional resin to match the scratch resistance of glass material. These resin coatings can be applied in a number of ways. Lenses may be dipped, or a thin layer of resin may be spun onto the lens surface. These coating layers are usually 5 micron thick.

Table 3.5: Specific gravity of different lens material.

Material	Refractive index	Specific gravity
Polycarbonate	1.590	1.20 g/cc
CR-39	1.498	1.32 g/cc
Crown glass	1.523	2.54 g/cc
High index glass	1.60	2.63 g/cc

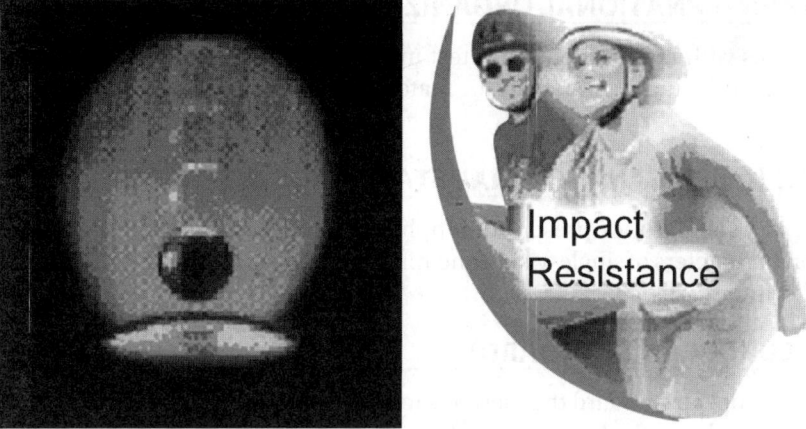

Fig. 3.5: Drop ball test for impact resistance.

While abrasion resistance is an important property for spectacle lenses, it is not crucial to the normal use of the product. Appropriate education of patients can assist them in avoiding situations where abrasion resistance becomes important, especially since the majority of scratches are put into the lenses by wearers themselves.

LENS STANDARDS

There are various standards and regulations related to spectacle lenses that ensure their quality, safety, and performance. These standards are set by international organizations and national bodies to ensure that eyeglasses provide accurate vision correction and maintain acceptable levels of quality. However, the standards can evolve over time, so it is possible that there may be changes from time to time. It is also possible that the different countries may adopt their own variations or equivalents. Eyewear manufacturers and optical laboratories typically adhere to these standards to ensure the quality and safety of the products they produce.

ISO 8980 (INTERNATIONAL ORGANIZATION FOR STANDARDIZATION)

ISO 8980 consists of several parts that deal with different aspects of ophthalmic optics and instruments. Part 1 of this standard covers terminology, part 2 addresses test methods for determining optical properties, and part 3 specifies tolerances for optical properties of lenses.

ISO 12870 (INTERNATIONAL ORGANIZATION FOR STANDARDIZATION)

ISO 12870 is a standard that focuses on prescription swimming goggles. It outlines requirements for prescription goggles, including optical properties, materials, and impact resistance.

ISO 14889 (INTERNATIONAL ORGANIZATION FOR STANDARDIZATION)

ISO 14889 is a standard that addresses the mechanical properties of spectacle frames and sunglasses. It includes tests for frame strength, durability, and resistance to corrosion.

ISO 16034 (INTERNATIONAL ORGANIZATION FOR STANDARDIZATION)

ISO 16034 specifies requirements for ready-to-wear spectacles frames. It covers aspects such as dimensions, materials, and labeling.

ISO 21987 (INTERNATIONAL ORGANIZATION FOR STANDARDIZATION)

ISO 21987 deals with requirements and test methods for non-prescription spectacle frames and sunglasses. It includes guidelines for materials, construction, and performance of these products.

ANSI Z80.1 (AMERICAN NATIONAL STANDARDS INSTITUTE)

ANSI Z80.1 is a standard for prescription ophthalmic lenses. It provides guidelines for the prescription parameters of single-vision and multifocal lenses, including tolerances for power, prism, and cylinder axes.

EN 1836 (EUROPEAN STANDARD)

EN 1836 is a European standard that pertains to sunglasses and sunglass lenses. It outlines the requirements for the optical properties of sunglasses, including transmission factors, color perception, and impact resistance.

AS/NZS 1067 (AUSTRALIA/NEW ZEALAND STANDARD)

This standard covers sunglasses and fashion spectacles. It provides guidelines for the labeling, testing, and categorization of sunglasses based on their level of protection against solar radiation.

India also has its own standards and regulations related to spectacle lenses and eyewear. The Bureau of Indian Standards (BIS), which is the national standards body of India, sets standards for various products, including ophthalmic optics. Some relevant Indian standards for spectacle lenses are listed below:

IS 14889: 2019—Ready-to-Wear Spectacle Frames

This Indian Standard specifies requirements for ready-to-wear spectacle frames, including dimensions, materials, design, construction, and labeling.

IS 12609 (Part 1): 2015—Prescription Ophthalmic Lenses

Part 1 of this standard deals with the specification for uncut finished prescription ophthalmic lenses. It covers aspects such as optical and geometrical properties, mechanical properties, marking, and labeling.

IS 12609 (Part 2): 2015—Prescription Ophthalmic Lenses

Part 2 of this standard focuses on test methods for prescription ophthalmic lenses. It provides procedures for testing optical and geometrical properties, as well as impact resistance and mechanical properties.

IS 12609 (Part 3): 2015—Prescription Ophthalmic Lenses

Part 3 of this standard specifies tolerances for prescription ophthalmic lenses. It outlines allowable deviations from the prescribed values for power, prism, and cylinder axes.

IS 12609 (Part 4): 2015—Prescription Ophthalmic Lenses

Part 4 of this standard addresses the specification and test methods for progressive addition lenses.

Chapter 3: Mechanical Optics, Lenses and Lens Prescription

These Indian standards help ensure the quality, safety, and performance of spectacle lenses and eyewear products sold within the country. Manufacturers and suppliers in India should adhere to these standards to meet regulatory requirements and provide consumers with reliable and high-quality eyewear.

ANSI Z80.1-2005 of American National Standard Institute provides recommendations for prescription ophthalmic lenses, and also contains the tolerance on refractive power.

		ANSI Z80.1–2005 Power/sphere-cylinder Single vision and multifocal lenses			
Meridian of most power	Tolerance each meridian	Tolerance 0.00 0.75	On nominal >0.75 4.00	Value of >4.00 6.00	Cylinder >6.00
0.00–3.00	+/–0.12	+/–0.09	+/–0.12	+/–0.18	+/–0.25
3.00–6.00	+/–0.12	+/–0.12	+/–0.12	+/–0.18	+/–0.25
6.00–9.00	+/–0.18	+/–0.12	+/–0.18	+/–0.18	+/–0.25
9.00–12.00	+/–0.18	+/–0.12	+/–0.18	+/–0.25	+/–0.25
12.00–20.00	+/–0.25	+/–0.18	+/–0.25	+/–0.25	+/–0.25
20	+/–0.37	+/–0.25	+/–0.25	+/–0.37	+/–0.37

		ANSI Z80.1–2005 Power/sphere-cylinder Progressive and aspheric lens			
Meridian of most power	Tolerance each meridian	Tolerance 0.00 0.75	On nominal >0.75 4.00	Value of >4.00 6.00	Cylinder >6.00
0.00–3.00	+/–0.12	+/–0.12	+/–0.18	+/–0.18	+/–0.25
3.00–6.00	+/–0.12	+/–0.12	+/–0.18	+/–0.18	+/–0.25
6.00–9.00	+/–0.18	+/–0.18	+/–0.25	+/–0.25	+/–0.25
9.00–12.00	+/–0.18	+/–0.18	+/–0.25	+/–0.25	+/–0.25
12.00–20.00	+/–0.25	+/–0.18	+/–0.25	+/–0.25	+/–0.25
20	+/–0.37	+/–0.25	+/–0.25	+/–0.37	+/–0.37

	ANSI Z80.1–2005 Cylinder axis tolerance			
Cylinder power	To 0.37	>0.37 0.75	>0.75 1.50	>1.50
Degrees of tolerance	+/–7	+/–5	+/–3	+/–2

	ANSI Z80.1–2005 Multifocal progressive add power	
Nominal add power	Up to 4.00	>4.00
Add power tolerance	+/–0.12	+/–0.18

ANSI Z80.1–2005 Precribed prism tolerance	
Prismatic power	*Tolerance*
0.00 to 2.00	+/−0.25
Over 2.00 Up to 10.00	+/−0.37
Over 10.00	+/-0.50

Base curves ANSI Z80.1 95
± 0.75 Diopters

OPHTHALMIC LENS BLANK MANUFACTURE—GLASS AND PLASTIC

GLASS LENS BLANK MANUFACTURING

Optical glass blank is manufactured in a multi-step process that begins with the selection of appropriate raw material that will be measured and combined to create the glass formulation. The process may vary somewhat based on the specific type of optical glass being manufactured and its intended application. However, before discussing the process of manufacturing it would be useful to understand the intrinsic qualities of mineral glass which make it such a unique material. Among these considerations, the fundamental elements are mentioned in **Table 3.6**.

The ophthalmic industry is a sector where mineral glass has long played a major role due to its fundamental properties, affording the production of all types of corrective lenses, from simplest to the most complex, as well as for sun and industrial protection glasses.

The step-by-step manufacturing process of ophthalmic glass blanks is shown in **Flowchart 3.4**. **Figure 3.6** shows the schematic representation of typical end to end production line of the ophthalmic glass blank manufacturing unit.

Table 3.6: Elements that makes the glass a unique material.

Elements	*Implications*
Transparent	Depends on the degree of control of impurities to the glass formulations
Homogeneity	Process dependent, requires proper mixing and slow cooling to achieve minimal birefringence
Hardness	Hardness provides for robustness and durability, also makes it suitable for forming and machining
Dimensional stability	Important for lens to retain its curvature, shape and form
Chemical stability	Ability to resist chemical reaction when exposed to chemicals, environment or potentially damaging substances
Melting point	Retains its structural integrity and functional properties even when exposed to extreme heat

Chapter 3: Mechanical Optics, Lenses and Lens Prescription

Flowchart 3.4: Step-by-step manufacturing process of ophthalmic glass lens blanks.

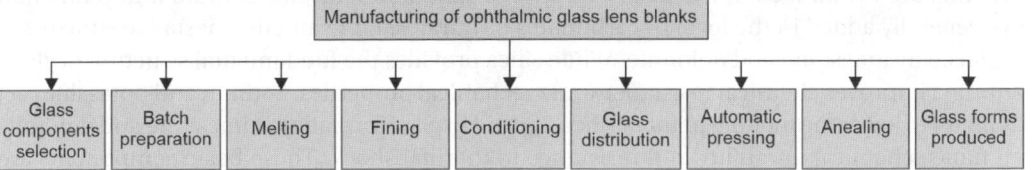

1. Raw materials
2. Batch preparation
3. Melting
4. Fining
5. Conditioning
6. Automatic pressing
7. Heat treatment
8. Packing
9. Quality control
10. Laboratory measuring

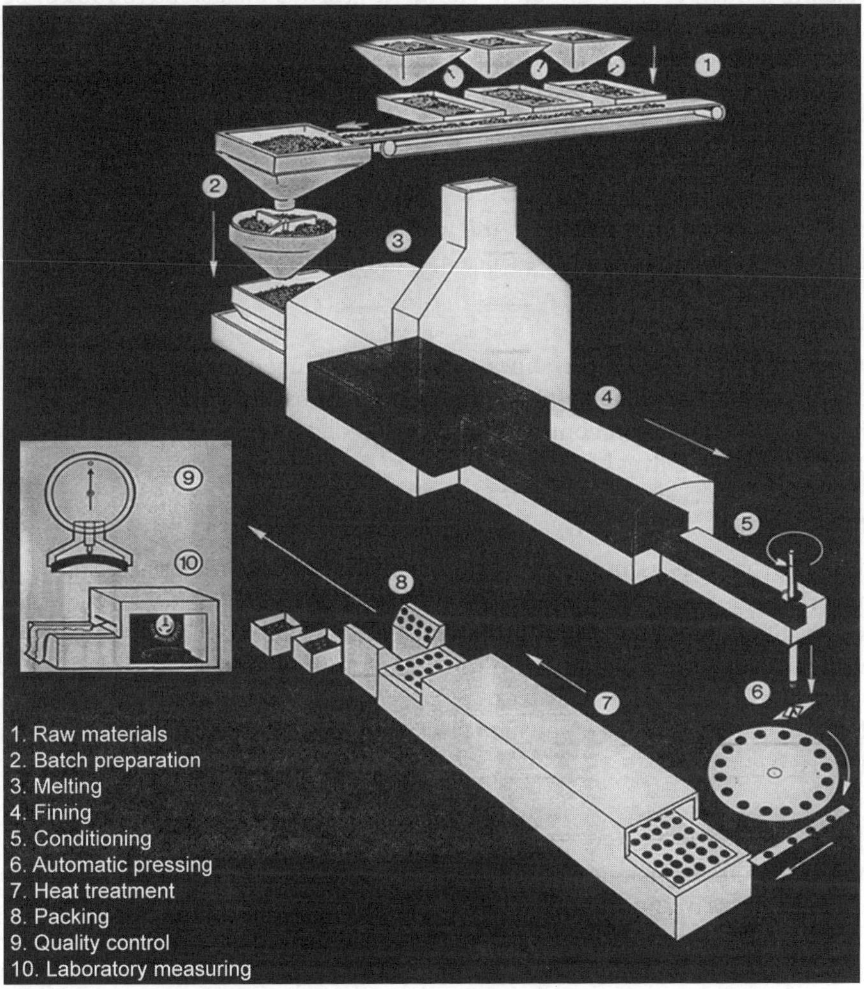

Fig. 3.6: Schematic representation of production line for spectacle glass blanks.

Glass Components Selection

The process begins with selecting the appropriate glass material. Ophthalmic lenses are made from various types of glass, each with specific optical properties, refractive indices, and characteristics. The components of ophthalmic glass are vitrifiable mixture or composition which is put into the melting tank in the form of extremely pure raw materials so as to obtain perfect quality glass.

The basic components are silica, alumina, sodium, potassium, lime, magnesia. Silica and alumina are introduced in the form of iron free sand and feldspar. Sodium and potassium are generally added in the form of carbonates or nitrates. Lime and magnesia are sometimes replaced by limestone and dolomite. While silica provides the fundamental structure of glass, alumina improves chemical resistance and mechanical properties. Sodium and potassium act as fluxes to lower the melting point of silica and aid in glass formation. Limestone and dolomite en hance chemical durability and resistance to thermal shock. These basic components are accompanied by numerous other ingredients such as rare earths. Some refiners like antimony oxide, alkaline nitrate, etc., are added to eliminate gaseous inclusions (bubbles) in molten glass. Colorants may be added to determine the tint. For example, inclusion of ferrous oxide gives blue tint and provides absorption in red and infra red end of spectrum, ferric oxide gives a greenish yellow tint, nickel oxides for brown tint. Various rare earths like neodyme, erbium, etc., are also used.

Crown

The composition of crown is similar to the window glass with high silica, lime and sodium content. The extra white crown is pure silica based which is extremely transparent.

Photochromatic Lens

The composition is much more elaborate owing to the need for the glass to have special properties of reaction to certain light radiation. The vitreous structure is extremely stable, viz, a borosilicate with high boron content to which is added a series of elements introduced to develop micro crystal of silver halide.

High Index Glass

To produce high index glass, traditionally contained lead oxide to increase the refractive index of the material. This produces 'flint' glass. Today for high index single vision lens lead oxide is replaced by titanium oxide thus preserving high index while reducing glass density. Certain other elements such as niobium, zirconium and strontium are also included for adjusting optical properties.

To obtain an improved range of segment glasses for fused multifocals, lead oxide is replaced by barium oxide.

Batch Preparation

Batch preparation is an operation of the utmost importance and is vital for the homogeneity and refractive index of the finished glass product. It consists of the preparing and close blending of the raw materials so as to obtain the proper composition from the furnace. Batching involves combining the mixed raw materials in the appropriate proportions based on the glass recipe. The exact formula will depend on the type of glass being produced and the desired optical characteristics.

Components are precisely weighted to obtain the exact amounts of materials as required on the glass weighing sheet. In scenarios where even a small ingredient can significantly impact specific glass properties, the level of weighing precision can be as fine as 1 in 10,000. Accurate measurement of raw materials is crucial to achieve the desired glass properties. Each raw material is weighed according to the specific formula for the glass composition. The weighing process may involve the use of electronic scales and sophisticated weighing systems to ensure precision.

The weighed raw materials are mixed thoroughly to achieve uniform distribution. Proper mixing ensures that the final glass composition is consistent throughout the batch. The blending of all of the various materials is performed in a mixer. A predetermined mixing time must be respected for each glass type. The batch is then transferred to the furnace area for melting.

Melting

The melting of an ophthalmic glass batch is a critical step in the production process, as it involves transforming the raw materials into a homogeneous molten state that can be further processed to create high-quality lenses. The melting process requires careful control of temperature, time, and conditions to ensure that the glass composition remains consistent and free from defects.

The batch is put into the part of the furnace where the melting operation actually takes place, usually mixed with cullet. Cullet is in fact glass of the same composition collected from previous manufacturing cycles and then crushed. A certain amount of cullet is useful in melting operation.

To melt the batch and produce a homogeneous product, the temperature of the furnace must be sufficient for the glass batch to reach a liquid state which may gradually be increased up to 1500 degree celsius, depending upon the glass type. As the temperature increases, the raw materials will begin to melt and form a molten glass mixture. It is crucial to maintain a consistent temperature within the furnace to ensure that all components of the batch melt evenly and thoroughly.

Depending on the furnace design, stirring mechanisms may be employed to promote mixing and homogenization of the molten glass. Stirring helps distribute the components evenly and reduce the formation of localized variations in composition.

During the melting process, volatile components and gases may be released from the batch. These gases can lead to defects such as bubbles in the final glass. Some furnace designs include degassing mechanisms to remove these gases from the molten glass. Precise temperature control is essential during the melting process. Deviations from the target temperature can affect the glass's composition and properties.

Refining agents may be added to the molten glass to remove impurities and trapped bubbles. These agents help improve the optical quality and overall purity of the glass.

Throughout the melting process, the molten glass is monitored for its composition, temperature, and visual appearance. Quality control checks can identify any variations or defects that need correction.

Fining

The fining stage of production consists of raising the glass temperature for greater liquidity so as to permit the escape of gases which are still present in the melt. This operation is carried out in a second part of the furnace which is called the fining chamber.

Given the temperature attained up to 1600°C; standard refractory material cannot be employed, simply because they would be adversely affected by the heat and consequently contaminate the glass with impurities such as coloring.

This is why platinum is used, a refractory material which is virtually unaffected by hot glass.

Conditioning

In the fining stage, the glass is at too high a temperature to be used for forming. It is too fluid and insufficiently homogeneous. This is why glass temperature must be reduced as soon as it leaves the fining stage. The aim is for the glass to reach the forming stage in a more viscous state and with a uniform mass temperature.

Also, to reach optical quality standards, i.e., perfect homogeneity, the glass must undergo constant blending using a stirring process. After the blending and homogeneous temperature reduction operation, the glass leaves the delivery tubes at working viscosities which vary between 1000 and 10000 poises, according to the type of glass.

Glass Distribution

The purpose of this operation is to feed the presses with constant weight quantities of glass. To do this, the glass which comes out of each delivery tube at a stable flow rate is cut by shears made from special steel. The operating cycle of the shears is synchronized with that of the press.

The constant weight glass quantities are called parisons, i.e., a rounded mass of molten glass formed by rolling the substance immediately after removal from the furnace.

Automatic Pressing

Properly produced parisons at the required viscosity level are essential for obtaining good quality mouldings. They serve as the starting material for creating the blanks. Each press position corresponds to a precise work phase—loading, pressing, cooling and takeout.

The system of continuous pressing is responsible for production rates of several thousand mouldings per hour.

The press tooling determines the dimensional features of the moulding. It comprises four basic parts:
1. The mould provides the peripheral size and shape
2. The valve shapes the convex face of the moulding
3. The plunger compresses the mass of glass and forms the concave surface
4. The ring closes the whole assembly and determines the shape of the moulding edge nearest to the plunger.

Different types of presses are used according to moulding shapes and to the physical characteristics of the glass.

Annealing

When the moulding leaves the press, it passes by conveyer belt into an annealing lehr. Annealing is an operation of heating the mouldings to a reduced and controlled temperature, the aim of which is to reduce considerably thermal internal stresses or strain and improve its structural integrity and optical properties. Annealing helps enhance the optical clarity of the glass by minimizing birefringence (double refraction) and other optical distortions. It also improves the mechanical strength of glass lenses. Annealing temperature is set slightly below the glass melting temperature. The molten material is held at the annealing temperature for a specific period of time. This duration allows the internal stresses within the molten glass to relax and gradually dissipate. The hold time varies based on the glass composition and thickness of the glass objects being annealed.

The moulding is heated to a temperature ranging from 550 to 770°C according to the nature of the glass and then cooled at a controlled rate. The reduction of stresses within the moulding facilitates the surfacing operation without the risk of breakage.

Glass Forms Produced

Glass blanks are produced and are delivered in varying forms according to processing required for transforming them into ophthalmic lenses with specific optical properties **(Fig. 3.7)**.

Chapter 3: Mechanical Optics, Lenses and Lens Prescription

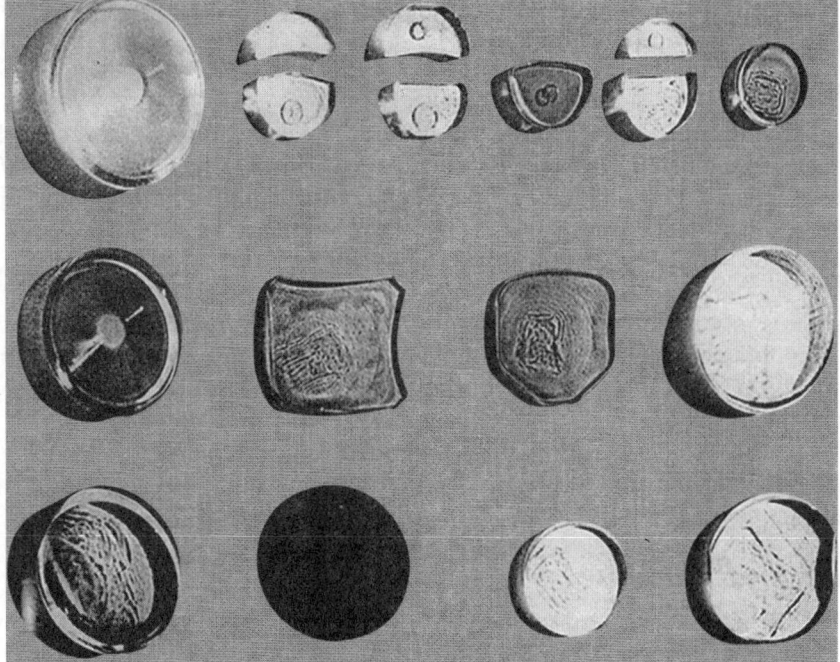

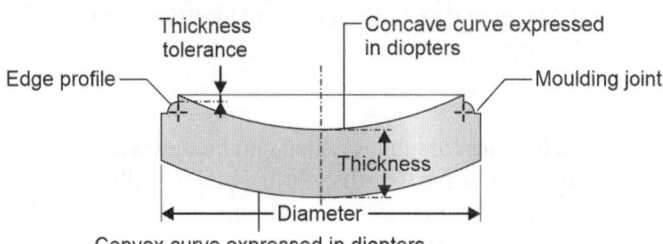

Fig. 3.7: Range of formed blanks.

The blanks so formed are defined by combination of curves expressed in diopter on the basis of refractive index and their shape and size.

Controls

Not only is the glass mouldings inspected after the final stage of production, but also the whole production line is subjected to inspection controls from raw material acceptance, tooling, annealing and product shape and appearance down to their chemical and physical characteristics. This is known as quality assurance.

The main controls carried out on the production lines are:
- Quality control
- Laboratory measuring

Quality Control

The purpose of quality control is to be absolutely sure about dimensional characteristics and product appearance.

On the manufacturing, line there are two types of quality control which are carried out several times during the production:

Controls at the press

These controls give initial information as to product quality with respect to compliance of dimensional characteristics like thickness, curves and weight, glass quality, visible defects that include folds, checks. People in charge of manufacturing can then immediately correct any process deviation, be it at the production stage or pressing stage.

Controls at the end of annealing lehr

The purpose is to guarantee predetermined quality for customers. Following the laws of statistics, a certain amount of product (sampling) is selected and according to the guaranteed level of quality, an acceptance or rejection system is put into use. To offer the best possible guarantees, all dimensional glass quality and appearance controls are carried out.

When a lot is accepted it is put into the warehouse to await shipment.

When a lot is rejected, and level of quality permitting, each piece of the lot is inspected individually.

Laboratory Measurements

Controlling dimensional and visual quality is not enough to guarantee the product's characteristics. Consequently, several blanks are taken several times a day and send to laboratory to be measured:

- Refractive indices at different state of annealing and at different wave-lengths
- Constringencies or Abbe number at the same wave lengths
- Thermal expansion
- Density
- Chemtempering characteristics for lenses which can be tempered
- Light transmission at different wave lengths in ultra-violet, visible and infra red ranges
- Color by determination of trichromatic coordinates in the international CIR system

Other measurements are also taken but with less frequency: Chemical durability, thermoviscous characteristics and chemical composition.

However, in case of photochromatic glasses special instruments are used for measuring transmittance and colors (trichromatic coordinates) under different state of illumination:

- Virgin color (first exposure to illumination)
- State after varying times of controlled illumination
- State after varying times of fading

Taking account of the manufacturing process and the composition of these glasses, their chemical analysis is carried out by physical analytical methods every hour. Computer processing of this data helps to ascertain very quickly the photochromatic properties of the production in progress.

PLASTIC LENS BLANK MANUFACTURING

Plastics lenses are made of polymers, derived from synthetic materials obtained through organic chemistry. Polymers are large molecules composed of repeating units called monomers. Polymers are formed through a process called polymerization, where monomers undergo chemical reactions to link together and form the polymer chain.

Polymers can indeed be categorized into two broad types based on their behavior when heated:

Thermoplastics

These polymers can be melted and reshaped multiple times without undergoing a chemical change. They soften when heated and solidify when cooled. Common examples include polyethylene, polypropylene, and PVC.

Thermosetting

These polymers undergo a chemical cross-linking reaction when heated, which permanently sets their structure. Once they are formed, they cannot be melted and reshaped. Common examples include epoxy resin and phenolic resin.

The most common polymers used to manufacture ophthalmic plastic lenses are CR-39, polycarbonate and various hi-index plastic materials. Allyl Diglycol Carbonate, Bisphenol A, and Urethane are common monomers respectively.

The history of development of plastic material for ophthalmic lenses has long story of development of most suitable monomer which can be used for ophthalmic lenses consistently and can also serve desired objective. Two motivated factors for a plastic lens material were the safety issue (greater resistance to impact) and comfort (lighter weight lenses). A company called Columbia Southern Chemical Company in Barberton, Ohio which was the subsidiary company of Pittsburgh Plate Glass Co discovered the compound Allyl Diglycol Carbonate monomer around 1940 which they marketed under batch name "CR 39". Polycarbonate was developed in the 1970s for aerospace applications. Lenses made of polycarbonate were introduced in the early 1980s in response to a demand for lightweight and impact-resistant lenses. In chemical terms, polycarbonate is a linear polymer thermoplastic with amorphous structure. Its carbonate skeleton is made of succession of carbonate radicals and phenol. Bisphenol A is common monomer. In 2001, PPG Industries introduced a material called Trivex. Trivex lenses are composed of a urethane-based monomer and are made from a cast moulding process similar to CR-39 are made.

Manufacturing of Thermosetting (CR-39)

Preparation of Monomer

CR-39 monomer is supplied in liquid form by industrial chemical supplier. It has to undergo filtering, degassing and addition of catalyst. Two alternate catalysts may used in the form of pure dry benzoyl peroxide or iso-propyl percarbonate in the proportion of 3 to 3.3% by weight. Large drums of monomer must be stored at a temp of less than 4 deg celsius.

Mould Assembly

Mold consists of two glass or metal parts, assembled either by pressing against a circular ring (gasket) or tightening with clip, or by using adhesive tape.

Filling

The empty space created between the two parts of the mould is filled with liquid monomer.

Polymerization

The filled mould is placed in an oven where it undergoes a heat cycle for several hours, or for certain material are exposed to UV radiation for a few minutes to provoke gradual hardening of the resin. CR-39 shrinks by about 14% in all directions during polymerization.

De-moulding

The clips or tapes are removed and moulds are separated to release the lenses. The lens is then inspected and treated as necessary.

The aforesaid procedure is applicable to both semi-finished and finished lenses. The hard coating may be applied in the form of polysiloxane lacquer to lens surface or by applying quartz-like layers to each surface.

Manufacturing of Thermoplastic (Polycarbonate)

Preparation of Material

Raw material, made of transparent granules is dried up with hot air and loaded into position on the press.

Setting the Press

The moulds are positioned, setting the pressure, mould temperature, injection and cooling time and heating of the material (About 300°C).

Injection

The molten material is injected under pressure into moulds.

Cooling

The material is solidified by conduction through the mould.

De-moulding

The press and the mould support block are opened and the lenses are released. The lens is taken out and then sent for varnishing.

The technology allows lenses of any design to be manufactured simply by filling different moulds in the press. These lenses may be either finished or semi-finished which require subsequent surfacing of back surface.

OPHTHALMIC PRESCRIPTION LENS MAKING

INTRODUCTION

A semi-finished lens has to undergo surfacing process so that it can be used as ophthalmic lens by the wearer. During the surfacing process, a specific lens surface curvature is generated and the difference of curvature between the front surface and back surface gives us the required dioptrical value. The required curvature is attained by a series of operations and the blank is held against a tool of opposite curvature. A wide range of tools, calibrated for a specific curvature of the lens and are made of cast iron are used in the process. The front surface known as '+' side of the lens is surfaced on the concave tools to make required curvature and the back surface is surfaced on the convex tools (**Fig. 3.8**). These cast iron tools must be checked frequently by means of a brass template or gauge of opposite curvature and if required the tools may be trued by means of tool truing device to rectify the curvature. **Flowchart 3.5** shows the sequential processes needed for lens surfacing.

Chapter 3: Mechanical Optics, Lenses and Lens Prescription

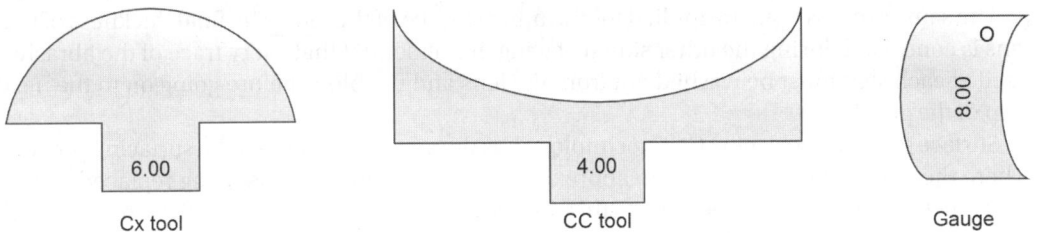

Fig. 3.8: Tools used in lens prescription laboratory.

Flowchart 3.5: Sequential process for lens surfacing.

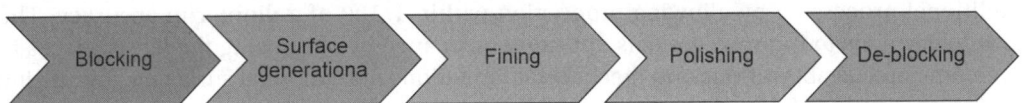

Step 1

The blank is attached to a cast iron or metal block with the help of pitch or lac or soft metal alloy. The metal block provides a support for holding blank throughout the grinding operation.

Step 2

Now, the assembly is put to the roughing process. Roughing implies generating the desired curvature. The surface of the blank is brought to its approximate curvature by rotating the blank against the tool of desired curvature. During this process, a course abrasive powder is used. Carborundum/sand is the commonly used abrasive powder. We obtain rough surface of the lens.

Step 3

After the roughing is completed the blank is now ground on the proper tool as required by the specific lens power with the help of finer grain abrasive like aluminous oxide. Two grades of abrasive are used which are commonly expressed as 302 and 303. The surface of the blank is trued with the help of grade 302 and then it is finished by smoothing with the grade 303. The correct surface curvature is now obtained and the lens is ready for the final polish.

Step 4

Now the lens is ready by polishing. A soft pad either felt cloth or wool cloth or specially designed polishing pads are attached to the tool and rouge (iron oxide) commonly known as 309 or cerium oxide is applied to polish the lens. The rouge is mixed with the water and is applied to the attached pad to polish the lens surface.

Step 5

The polished lens surface is to be inspected by putting it under an incandescent bulb and if found satisfactory, the lens is de-blocked from the metal block. The lens and the block are immersed in the cold water and the block is tapped by a wooden mallet. Ice cubes may also be used to facilitate the de-blocking process. The thermal change causes the lens to come out from the block and also from pitch. If any particles of the pitch are still found on the surface, it is being cleaned by using thinner.

The same process is again applied for the other surface of the lens. The final thickness of the lens is controlled during the other side surfacing. It is essential that every trace of the abrasive used at each step must be washed out from the lens and the block before going on to the next step of the grinding.

Surface generation by new CNC technology has dramatically changed the surfacing process where the lens surface is brought to approximately correct curvature is being replaced by the faster method of surface generating. In this process, the required curvature of the lens is formed simply by tilting the specially designed tools on the blanks at a predetermined angle.

The most latest is free form technology that involves a highly sophisticated proprietary software and CNC multi-axis surfacing technology systems to produce the complex lens surfaces precisely. This new surfacing technology creates a significant improvement over traditional processing by allowing production within 1/100 of a diopter in accuracy. The technology aims to improve the lens optical performance by optimizing the lens surfaces to overcome optical aberrations and mechanical limitations of traditional surfacing, framitizing the lenses to specific frame fitting and adjustment characteristics, and personalizing the lenses to an individual prescription and individual viewing habits of the user.

LENS DEFECTS

Lens defects refer to imperfections or abnormalities in optical lenses that can adversely affect their performance in terms of image quality, clarity, and functionality. Lens defects can be because of limitations of optics or material intrinsic or they can result from manufacturing errors, design flaws, or physical damage. **Flowchart 3.6** shows the different groups of lens defects.

OPTICAL ABERRATIONS

Optical aberrations are primarily due to the inherent limitations of optics and the way light behaves as it passes through lenses. These aberrations result from deviations from ideal optical behavior and can affect the quality and accuracy of images formed by lens. These are deviations from ideal optical behavior in which the lens fails to focus light perfectly. There are two broad types of optical aberrations as shown in **Flowchart 3.7**.

Flowchart 3.6: Different types of lens defects.

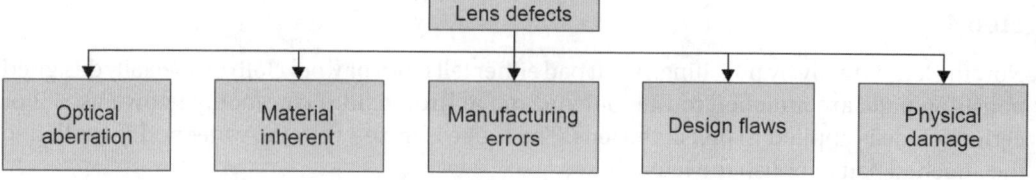

Flowchart 3.7: Types of optical aberrations.

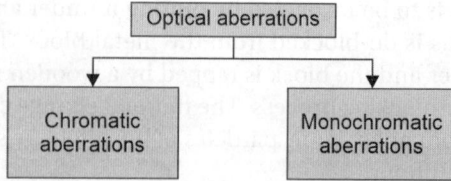

Chromatic Aberrations

Chromatic aberration occurs when the different wavelengths of light **(Fig. 3.9)** are not brought to the focus at the same point. Blue wavelength is refracted more than the red wavelength of light when it passes through a lens. The result is out of focus image. The wearer complains of peripheral color fringes around the object which is more pronounced off-axis. The higher the power of the lens—the greater is the chromatic aberration.

Chromatic aberration depends upon the material of the lens. Since the lens materials have a different refractive index for different wavelengths of light—the lens will have a different focal length for each wavelength. The refractive index is higher for shorter wavelength than the longer wavelength light, so focal length is less for shorter wavelength than that of the longer wavelength of light.

Since chromatic aberration occurs because the refractive index of the lens material varies with the wavelength of the incident light, it gives rise to what is called the Abbe value of the lens material which is denoted by V-value. Higher Abbe value implies low chromatic aberrations and vice- versa. So polycarbonate lens with Abbe value of 30 causes more chromatic aberration than CR 39 lens with Abbe value of 58.

Monochromatic Aberrations

Monochromatic aberrations primarily result from deviations in the shape or surface quality of lenses. These aberrations can indeed be influenced and minimized through careful lens design and control of lens size and shape.

Lens Design

Optical engineers use sophisticated design techniques to minimize monochromatic aberrations during the lens design process. This involves selecting appropriate lens shapes, curvatures, and materials to reduce or eliminate specific aberrations like spherical aberration, coma, oblique astigmatism, and distortion. Aspheric lens surfaces, which deviate from a simple spherical shape, are often employed to reduce spherical aberration and effect oblique astigmatism.

Lens Size and Aperture

The size of the lens elements, particularly the aperture size, can impact the correction of aberrations. Larger aperture lenses capture more peripheral light and potentially increase peripheral aberrations, although they can also introduce other challenges like increased weight and complexity.

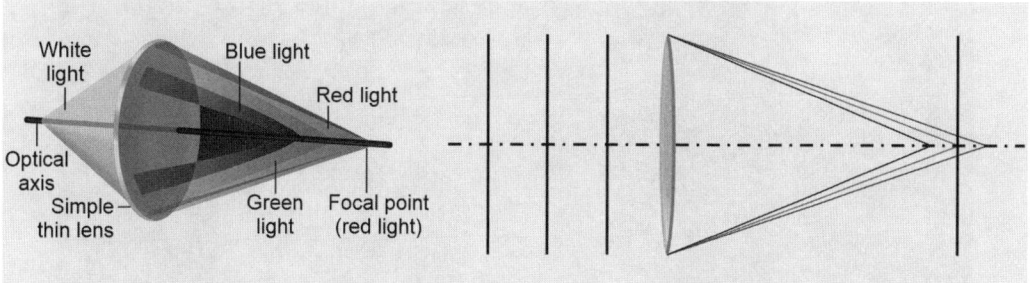

Fig. 3.9: Axial chromatic aberration.

Manufacturing Error

Lens defects due to manufacturing errors are imperfections or irregularities that occur during the production of optical lenses. These errors can have a significant impact on the optical performance and quality of the lens. The common defects are listed below:

Bubbles

Bubbles are small voids or pockets of gas trapped within the lens material during the melting stage of manufacturing process **(Fig. 3.10)**. They can scatter light and create visible imperfections in the lens, impacting optical clarity. The presence of bubbles is typically considered a manufacturing defect and can lead to a lens being rejected during quality control checks.

Stones

Stones are unmelted solid inclusions which may come from frit or from the wearing of the refractory material used in the construction of melting tank. Similar to bubbles, stones can also lead to localized distortions in the lens and may cause optical aberrations or reduced transparency. High-quality lens manufacturing processes involve meticulous cleanliness and control to minimize the presence of inclusions.

Striae

Striae are thin, thread-like structures or lines that can form within a lens due to uneven stress distribution during the lens manufacturing process **(Fig. 3.11)**. These stress-induced irregularities can affect the lens's optical properties by causing birefringence, where light passing through the lens is split into different polarization states, leading to optical distortion. Striae are often visible under polarized light and can reduce image quality.

Stress

Stress in lenses can refer to the presence of mechanical stress or strain within the lens material **(Fig. 3.12)**. This stress can result from various factors, including the lens manufacturing process, changes in temperature, and external forces. One of the most common reasons for stress in lenses is molten lens is cooled too rapidly that results in outer surface being cooled faster than inner portion. Stress within a lens material can cause birefringence, which is the property of

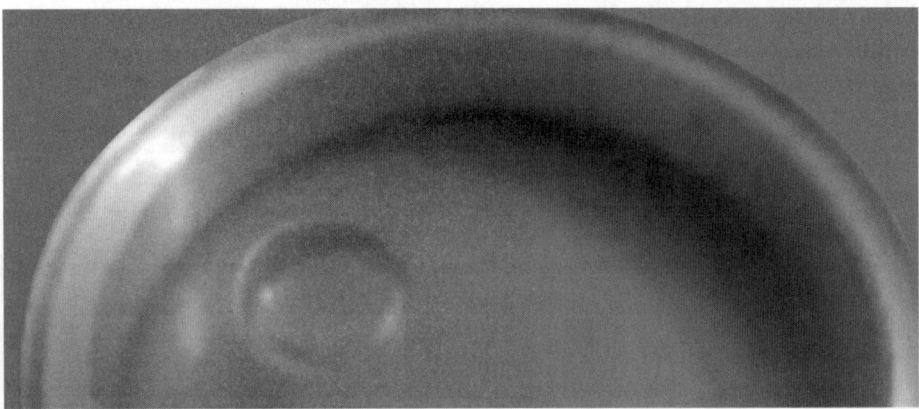

Fig. 3.10: Bubbles.

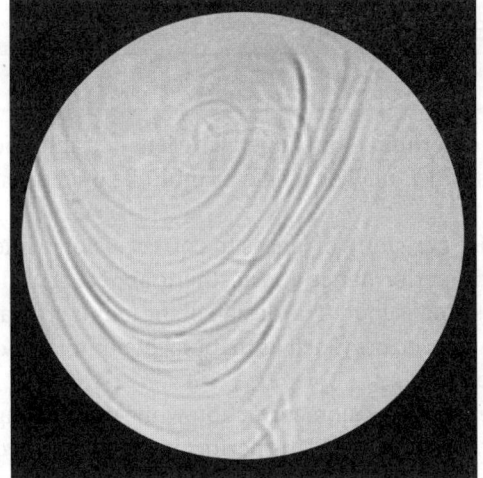

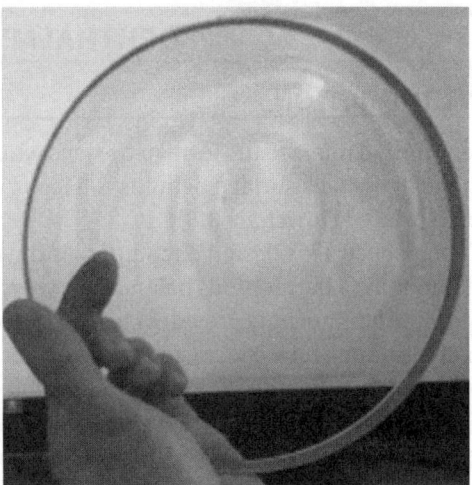

Fig. 3.11: Striae in lens. **Fig. 3.12:** Stress in lens.

having different refractive indices for light polarized in different directions. Birefringence can lead to double refraction and affect the polarization of light passing through the lens.

Cloudiness

Cloudiness is usually caused by precipitated material during cooling **(Fig. 3.13)**.

Lens Design Flaws

Lens design flaws occur when the lens design deviates from the principle of "Best form lens" which refers to an idealized lens that has a specific curvature to provide perfect balance between vision and comfort. These lenses are theoretical constructs and serve as benchmarks for comparing and evaluating the performance of real-world lenses. The deviations from best form lens may lead to error in lens design and eventually create discomfort and disturbed vision.

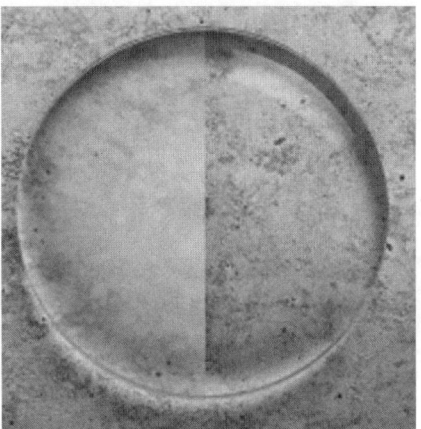

Fig. 3.13: Cloudiness.

Physical Damage

Physical damage to lenses can significantly impact their optical performance and structural integrity. Some common types of physical damage that can occur to lenses:

Scratches and Surface Damage

Physical damage to the lens surface, such as scratches or abrasions, can degrade image quality and clarity. These defects scatter light and can cause visual disturbances.

Warping

Lenses may warp due to temperature changes or physical stress, causing distortions in the image they produce.

OPHTHALMIC LENS DESIGNS

INTRODUCTION

Lens design refers to the form of the lens which is determined by shape of the lens surface. The shape of the lens surface denotes the lens curves which may be single or multiple on a given lens surface **(Flowchart 3.8)**.

In essence, lens design encompasses the precise curvature of lenses to correct vision while maintaining a harmonious balance between optical performance and aesthetic appeal. A well-designed lens not only provides clear vision but also looksgood. The design of the lens is crucial in determining how effectively it can correct refractive errors (such as myopia, hyperopia, and astigmatism) and provide clear, comfortable vision.

The primary goal is to create lenses that deliver precise vision correction while minimizing optical aberrations and ensuring wearer comfort. Absolute best lens performance is achieved and the lens behaves as given by the "Focal Power of the Lens". As we move away from the optical center, the lens performance deteriorates **(Fig. 3.14)**.

Currently, there are five most common designs of ophthalmic lenses:
1. Spherical lens
2. Aspheric lens
3. Atoric lens
4. Bifocal lens
5. Multifocal lens

Spherical Lens

In mathematics, a sphere is a three-dimensional geometric object that is perfectly round in shape. It is often defined as the set of all points in three-dimensional space that are equidistant from a fixed center point. This fixed point is known as the center of the sphere, and the constant distance from the center to any point on the sphere's surface is called the radius.

Flowchart 3.8: Lens design.

Lens forms → Shape of the 2 lens surfaces → Their curves → Single or multiple curve

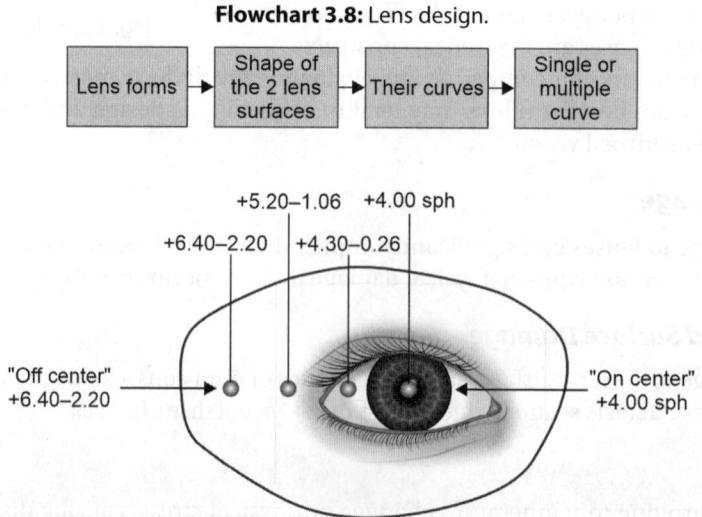

Fig. 3.14: Optical performance of lenses from different portions of the lens.

In geometry, a sphere is a three-dimensional geometric object that analogue to a two dimensional circle. In our daily life, we can see baseballs, tennis balls, and many more examples that are spheres.

A spherical lens in ophthalmic optics refers to a lens surface design in which the surface has the same power in all meridians **(Figs. 3.15A and B)**. It also has the same curvature from the center to the edge. The spherical surface may be on the front, the back or on both surfaces.

The basis of spherical lens designing is the 'best form lens' which is based on the "base curve selection". There are several laws available for the selection of base curve among which Vogel's rule says that keep the basic lens prescriptions on 6.00 D base curve and adjust higher powers in plus to steeper front curves and higher minus powers to flatter front curves.
There are two main limitations of spherical lens design:
1. Thicker and bulging out lens profile.
2. Clarity from the peripheral portion of the lens is not the same as from the center of the lens.

Aspheric Lens

An aspheric lens surface design is one in which the curvature of the lens gradually flattens or steepens as you move from the optical center to the edge of the lens. An aspheric design offers an advanced lens profile that looks flatter and provides wider field of clear vision **(Fig. 3.16)**. Contextually, the term "Aspheric" denotes rotationally symmetric surfaces. The wearer enjoys following advantages over spheric lenses:
* Sharper vision in any angle of view
* Optimization of oblique vision
* Better stereo-vision
* Wider field of clear vision

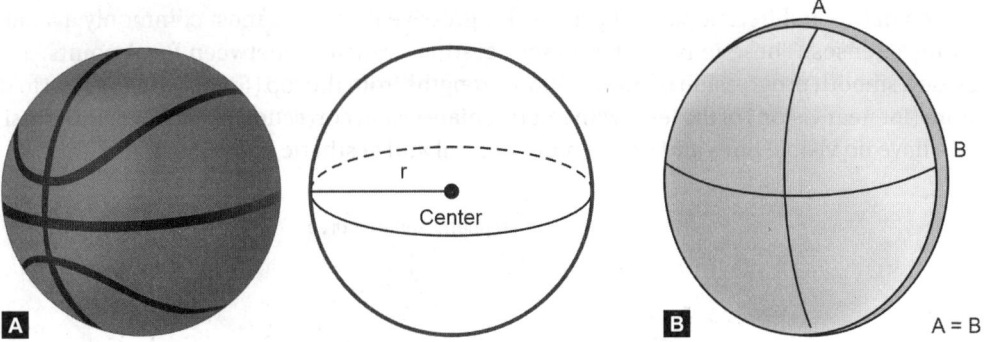

Figs. 3.15A and B: (A) Sphere; (B) Spherical lens surface.

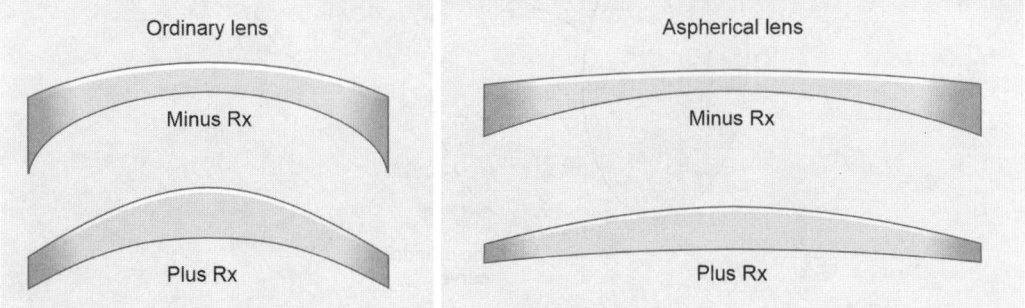

Fig. 3.16: Aspherical lens profile.

Atoric Lens

Like aspheric is an advancement over spherical lenses, atoric is an extension over the aspherical lens surface. Atoric lens design optimises both the sphere and cylinder power of the lens. While the aspherical lens is a rotationally symmetrical aspherical lens, atoric lenses are customized to be non-rotationally symmetrical **(Fig. 3.17)**. Literally, atoricity refers to varying the amount of asphericity from one meridian of the lens to another. This ensures that nearly all wearers enjoy the same wide field of vision, especially those with astigmatism. The wearer enjoys unrestricted field of clear vision, regardless of the power meridian of the lens, since the optical aberrations associated with each power meridian are corrected individually.

Bifocal Lens

Bifocal lenses are indeed referred to as "double focal" or "dual focus" lenses because they incorporate two different optical powers within a single lens. This dual focus allows individuals with presbyopia to see clearly at both near and far distances. The top portion of the lens is typically set for distance vision, while the lower portion is designed for near vision, such as reading or close-up work. This dual-focusing capability makes bifocal lenses a valuable solution for people who require correction for both far and near vision in a single pair of eyeglasses.

Multifocal Lens

Multifocal lenses are designed to provide multiple focal points within a single lens. These lenses are particularly useful for individuals with presbyopia, a common age-related vision condition that affects the ability to focus on objects at different distances. Multifocal lenses allow wearers to see clearly at various distances, including far, intermediate, and near vision, without the need to switch between different pairs of glasses. Progressive lenses are most commonly available multifocal lenses. These lenses offer a more gradual transition between focal points. They provide a smooth progression of prescription strengths from the top (for distance vision) to the bottom (for near vision) of the lens, with intermediate vision correction in between. Progressive lenses have no visible lines and offer a more natural and aesthetic appearance.

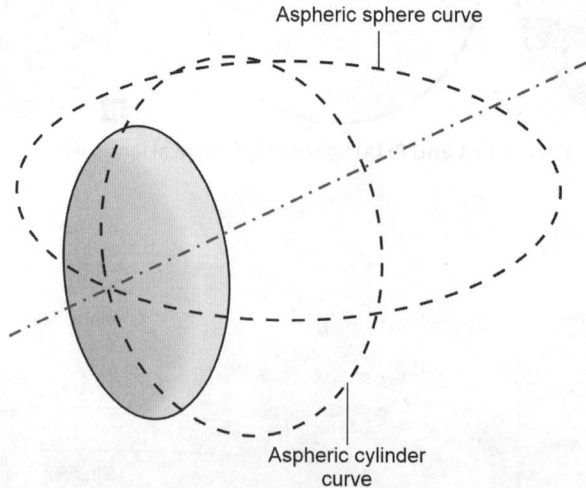

Fig. 3.17: An atoric surface with a differing amount of asphericity applied to the sphere and cylinder meridians.

TYPES OF OPHTHALMIC LENSES

ASPHERIC LENS

In the context of spectacle lenses, aspheric lenses are specially designed lenses with one or both surfaces featuring non-spherical curves. These non-spherical curves are carefully calculated and applied to the lens surface to improve optical performance and reduce various aberrations, such as spherical aberration and oblique astigmatism, and thereby improve the peripheral visual performance of the lenses. In terms of "lens designing", the term "aspherical" usually refers to a surface that is rotationally symmetrical, but at the same time not spherical. A change in curvature is noticed over the lens surface, rather than constant curvature like a spherical surface. The change is the same in all direction or meridians of the lens.

In case of plus lenses, the periphery of the front surface is flattened and in case of minus lenses, the periphery of the front surface is steepened. Using the "asphericity", the lens designers are able to produce thinner and flatter lens that also provide peripheral vision comparable to the best form lens. The off-axis performance of the lens improves considerably. The lens looks flatter which makes the eyes look more natural due to reduced magnification or minification. Also flatter lens fits better ensuring the attractive look of the spectacles, thereby, offering the subjects a wider variety of frames to choose from. If the aspheric lens design is coupled with high index material, it will definitely provide thinner, lighter and flatter lens that looks cosmetically the best **(Fig. 3.18)**.

Aspheric lenses represent the ultimate in optics. Using the aspheric curves in a lens produces two benefits—better vision and improved cosmetics. The dispensing of aspheric lenses requires more precise positioning by the dispenser. A poorly fitted aspheric lens can adversely affect its all benefits. Precise monocular PD measurements together with fitting height are essential to place the pole of the lens in front of pupil. **Table 3.7** shows the features, advantages and benefits of the aspheric lenses.

HIGH INDEX

The refractive index is an optical property of a lens material. The refractive index of a material is a measure of how much light slows down as it passes through the material compared to its speed in a vacuum. In the context of lenses, the refractive index is important because it

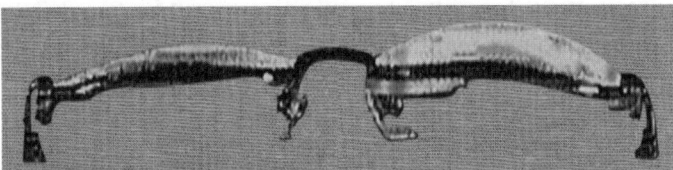

Fig. 3.18: Comparison between aspheric and spheric surface.

Table 3.7: Aspheric lenses.		
Features	*Advantages*	*Benefits*
Reduced spherical aberration	Rays of light passing through the lens periphery are brought to near correct focus	The wearer enjoys wider field of clear vision
Enhanced aesthetic appeal	Thinner and flatter lens profile	The lens fits well into the frame and reduces magnification of eyes

determines how much the light is bent (or refracted) when it passes through the lens. Different lens materials have different refractive indices, and this property plays a crucial role in optics, including the design and performance of lenses. For example, in eyeglasses, the choice of lens material can affect how light is focused and how images are formed. Lens designers take into account the refractive index of the materials used to create the lens to achieve the desired optical properties, such as focal length, magnification, and aberration correction. BS 7394-2-2007 has classified the lens material from normal to very high index as shown in **Table 3.2**.

High index lenses are basically selected to reduce the edge thickness in minus lenses and reduce the center thickness in plus lenses. This is because high-index lens materials have a higher refractive index compared to standard lens materials, which allows them to bend light more efficiently. By using high-index materials, lens designers can achieve the same optical power with less lens material, resulting in thinner and lighter lenses. However, high-index lens material is usually associated with lower Abbe value which means that the effect of chromatic aberration as shown in **Figure 3.19** increases with the increase in refractive index of lens material. If the chromatic aberration is significant enough, the lens wearer will likely see some reduction in vision quality, and possibly colored ghost images around objects.

MULTIFOCAL LENSES

Multifocal spectacle lenses are a type of lens designed to provide clear vision at multiple distances. They are often used by individuals who have presbyopia, a common age-related vision condition that makes it difficult to focus on close-up objects. Multifocal lenses eliminate the need for constantly switching between different pairs of glasses for various activities, such as reading, using a computer, or seeing objects in the distance. Progressive addition lenses are very common multifocal lenses available in the industry. Progressive lenses, also known as no-line bifocals or varifocals, provide a seamless transition from one prescription to another without any visible lines. These lenses offer a gradual change in prescription as you move your eyes up or down the lens. They have become increasingly popular due to their aesthetic advantages and the absence of visible lines.

BIFOCAL AND TRIFOCAL LENSES

Bifocal spectacle lenses are specialized lenses designed to provide clear vision for individuals who require correction for both distance and near vision. These lenses have two distinct optical powers within a single lens, allowing wearers to see objects at two different distances without the need to switch between different glasses. The upper portion is typically designed for distance vision, while the lower portion is intended for near vision.

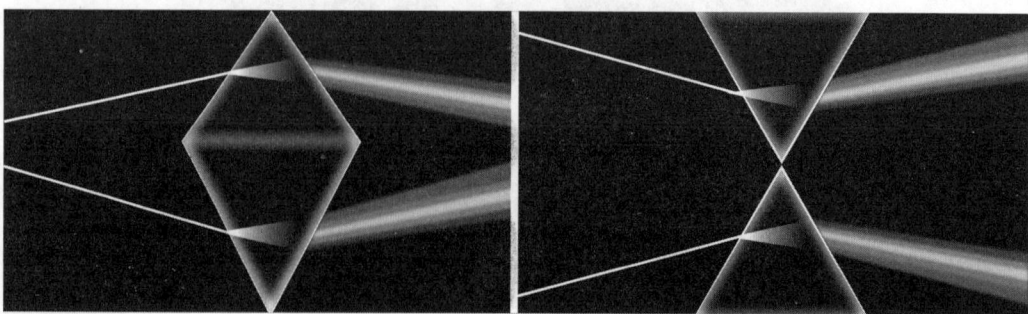

Fig. 3.19: Chromatic aberration through Cx and CC lens.

Bifocal lenses can be obtained in four basic constructional types—fused bifocals, solid bifocal, cemented bifocal and split bifocal. Most of them, except the fused bifocals are almost extinct from the real world. Hence, we will restrict our discussion concentrated to fused bifocal lenses only. The first fused bifocal was the fused kryptok invented by Borsch in the year 1908. In countries where glass lens still represent a sizeable section of the market, the fused bifocal remains the most common form of bifocal design. The round segment is still in production for some markets but no doubt, the most commonly used segments are D-shaped flat top or the C-shaped curved top as shown in **Figures 3.20A to C**.

The segment is permanently bonded onto the convex surface of the lens by heat fusion process and the required addition depends upon:
- The refractive indices of the two glass materials.
- The depression curve.
- The curve worked on the segment side of the lens.

Trifocal spectacle lenses are specialized eyeglass lenses designed to provide clear vision for individuals who require correction for three different focal points: distance, intermediate, and near vision. They are divided into three segments as shown in **Figure 3.21**.

1. **Upper segment:** The upper segment is typically designed for distance vision correction. It helps wearers see clearly when looking at objects in the distance, such as road signs or TV screens.
2. **Intermediate segment:** The middle portion of the lens is for intermediate vision, which is ideal for tasks like using a computer, reading a sheet of music, or working on crafts. It provides a clear focus at arm's length.
3. **Lower segment:** The bottom segment is intended for near vision, making it suitable for reading books, newspapers, or fine print.

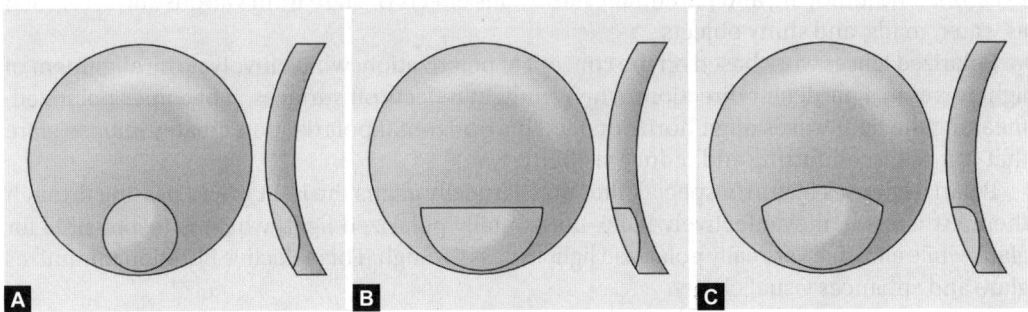

Figs. 3.20A to C: Fused bifocal design: (A) Round segment; (B) D segment flat top; (C) C Segment curved top.

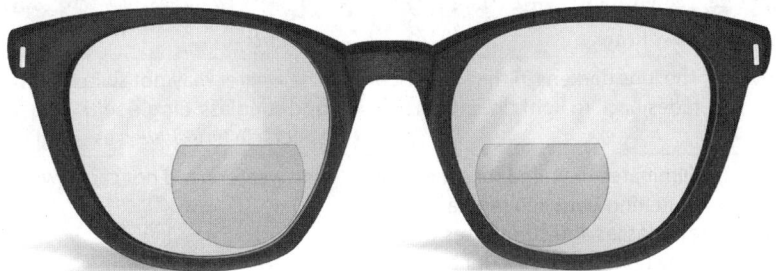

Fig. 3.21: Trifocal lens.

PHOTOCHROMATIC LENSES

Photochromatic lenses are light sensitive lenses. They were developed by Corning Glass Works in 1964. Photochromatic materials are those which act reversibly to light. The photochromatic behavior of these lenses is due to silver halide microcrystals which are formed by precipitation and subsequent heat treatment at a temperature between the annealing strain point and the softening point of glass.

These silver halide photochromatic glasses are believed to be truly reversible and immune to fatigue which means without degradation in their performance. They can go through numerous darkening and clearing cycles without a substantial decrease in their performance. However, the rate of fading in the dark and the darkening rate can be influenced by temperature. Warmer temperatures tend to promote a faster fading process in the dark. This means that in higher-temperature environments, the lenses may clear more quickly when you move from a bright to a dark area.

Fused multifocal lenses are not practical in photochromatic glasses as the high temperature during fusing completely destroy the photochromic mechanism. If fused bifocal lenses are needed than it is possible to use clear glass button component with an overlay of 2 mm thick photochromic glass. The high temperatures involved in the fusing process can potentially damage or disrupt the photochromic molecules within the lenses, rendering them less effective or completely non-functional.

Table 3.8 shows the key features and benefits of photochromatic lenses.

POLARIZED LENSES

Polarized lenses are a remarkable innovation in eyewear designed to significantly improve visual comfort and clarity, especially in high-glare environments. These lenses are engineered to combat the annoying and potentially hazardous effects of glare from various surfaces, such as water, roads, and shiny objects.

Polarized lenses work based on the concept of polarization, which involves the alignment of light waves in a particular direction. When sunlight reflects off surfaces, it becomes polarized, meaning the light waves align horizontally. This horizontal polarization creates intense glare that can be discomforting and reduce visibility.

Polarized lenses feature a special filter that vertically aligns the light waves passing through them. As a result, they effectively block horizontally polarized light, which is responsible for glare, while allowing vertically polarized light to pass through. This selective filtration minimizes glare and enhances visual clarity.

There are several types of polarized lenses designed for different applications and specific needs. These lenses vary in terms of polarization orientation, materials, and coatings.

Table 3.8: Photochromatic lenses—key features and benefits.

Features	Advantages	Benefits
Light sensitive lenses	The lens darkens in the sunlight and fades back to light tint indoors	The wearer may not switch between spectacle and sunglass. Single solution serves both spectacle lens as well as sunglass lens
Convenience and comfortable	Eliminates the need for constantly switching between regular eyeglasses and sunglasses when moving between indoor and outdoor settings	The wearer need not carry two products

Chapter 3: Mechanical Optics, Lenses and Lens Prescription

- **Linear polarized lenses:** These lenses have a linear polarization orientation, meaning they allow light oscillating in a specific direction (e.g., horizontally or vertically) to pass through while blocking light with perpendicular polarization. Linear polarized lenses are commonly used in sunglasses to reduce glare from horizontal surfaces like water, roads, or car hoods.
- **Circular polarized lenses:** Circular polarized lenses are designed for 3D movie viewing and certain photography applications. They use circular polarization to separate images for the left and right eyes, creating a 3D effect when viewed through circular polarized eyewear.
- **Tilted polarized lenses:** Some polarized lenses are tilted or oriented at an angle other than vertical or horizontal polarization. These lenses may be used in specialized applications where precise control of light orientation is needed.
- **Photochromic polarized lenses:** These lenses combine the properties of photochromic lenses (which change tint based on UV exposure) with polarization. Photochromic polarized lenses darken in response to UV light, providing glare reduction in varying light conditions. They are commonly used in outdoor sports and activities.
- **Gradient polarized lenses:** Gradient polarized lenses have varying levels of polarization across the lens surface. They may be darker at the top and gradually become less polarized or clear at the bottom. These lenses are useful for activities where overhead sunlight is intense (e.g., driving) while still allowing clear vision at the bottom of the lens.
- **Mirrored polarized lenses:** Mirrored polarized lenses have a reflective coating on the outside surface of the lens. The mirror coating reduces glare and provides additional protection from intense sunlight by reflecting some of the incoming light.

Principle of Polarized Lenses

Light is a transverse electro-magnetic wave motion in which the vibration takes place in all direction. These displacements can be polarized by passing light through certain filters.

The coating materials used are designed to interact with light waves at the molecular level, allowing them to selectively transmit and reflect specific polarization orientations.

The principle of polarized lenses is based on the selective filtering of light waves to reduce glare and improve visibility in specific conditions. Polarized lenses work by allowing light waves of a certain polarization orientation to pass through while blocking or attenuating light waves with different orientations.

The principle of polarized lenses is to selectively filter light waves based on their polarization orientation to reduce glare and enhance visibility. By effectively blocking horizontally polarized light (glare) while allowing vertically polarized light to pass through, these lenses improve visual comfort and clarity in bright and reflective conditions.

Advantages of Polarized Lenses

By selectively filtering out horizontally polarized light (glare) while allowing vertically polarized light (natural light) to pass through, polarized lenses improve:
- Visual clarity
- Contrast
- Color perception
- Comfort in bright and reflective environments.

How is Polarizing Filters Made?

Polarized lenses are manufactured using various methods and materials to achieve their optical properties:

Film Lamination Method

The thin film consists of uniform thin sheets of optically cast polyvinyl alcohol which are stretched to arrange the complex molecules in long parallel chains. This stretching aligns the PVA molecules in a specific direction, which is crucial for polarization. The film is then impregnated with iodine. Iodine molecules interact with the aligned PVA molecules to enhance the polarization effect. Film so prepared is called H-Polaroid. The polarizing film is cut and shaped to match the size and shape of the lens needed for the eyewear frame. The cut film is sandwiched between two layers of transparent material, often made of glass or plastic. Adhesive is used to bond the layers together.

Dichroic Coating Method

Dichroic polarizing filters are typically made using specialized coatings composed of multiple thin layers of materials. Various techniques, such as vacuum deposition and sputtering, are used to deposit these materials as thin layers onto a substrate (e.g., glass or plastic). These coatings are designed to interact with light waves at the molecular level, allowing them to selectively transmit specific polarization orientations and colors. Common materials used in the construction of dichroic polarizing filters include calcite, quartz, and tourmaline, can be used to create dichroic effects. These crystals naturally split light into different polarization states and can be incorporated into optical components.

TINTED LENSES

Tinted spectacle lenses are eyeglass lenses that have been treated or coated with a specific tint or color. These tinted lenses serve various purposes and can be customized to meet different needs.

A spectacle lens is said to be tinted if the transmission of light is deliberately decreased by any means, either over the whole of the visible spectrum and its neighboring regions, or merely a part of it. They offer selective absorption for each wavelengths of the spectrum, and this determines their tints. Such absorption may be fixed or variable. Fixed absorption is the case with all traditional fixed tinted glasses, whereas, photo chromic glasses offer variable absorption where transparency varies according to light conditions.

Spectacle lenses may be tinted in three different ways—integral tinting, surface treatment and dye tinting.

Integral tinting is usually used for glass lens material. Various oxides were added to the batch materials to give the lens a specific color. For example, cerium is added to the batch mix would give rise to pinkish tint while cobalt oxide would give rise to blue tint lens. By adding the various metallic oxides or other compounds to the glass constituents, the absorption can be deliberately increased in almost any desired way, both within and beyond the visible spectrum. If the absorption is uniform within the visible spectrum, the tint imparted to the material will be grey or neutral. Selective absorption gives rise to a definitive hue. Thus, a relatively higher absorption in the red region of the spectrum would produce a greenish tint.

An absorptive coating can be applied to a clear glass lens using a metallic oxide in a vacuum process. This approach offers several advantages:
- ❖ These coatings maintain a consistent density, regardless of the lens prescription they are applied to. This ensures that the coating's effectiveness remains constant, no matter the corrective power of the lens.
- ❖ Lenses with metallic oxide coatings exhibit predictable transmission properties, providing a consistent and reliable level of light transmission.

- These coatings are applied to the lens surface using a vacuum process. They often resemble mirror reflectors.
- Metallic oxide coatings can be applied uniformly across the entire lens surface or as a gradient. A gradient coating offers a distinctive look, similar to a reflector mirror, which can be visually appealing and functional.
- These coatings are particularly effective for sunglasses, as they reduce glare, enhance visual comfort, and provide UV protection. The mirror-like appearance also adds a stylish element to the eyewear.

Resin lenses can be tinted by immersing in a container of dye. The container is put in a unit that allows heat to be transferred to the dye. The longer the lenses remain in the dye, the more dye will be absorbed, thus making them darker. The dye penetrates the lens material and becomes the part of it. It cannot be rubbed off. Red, yellow and blue are the three primary dyes form with which almost all other colors can be made. For example blue and yellow can be mixed together to make green.

PROTECTIVE LENSES

Eyes are delicate and vulnerable organs that require protection from various potential hazards. Protecting your eyes is crucial for maintaining good eye health and preventing injuries. The potential hazards that can pose a risk to eyes are listed below:

Ultraviolet (UV) Radiation Protection

Prolonged exposure to UV radiation from the sun can lead to various eye problems, including cataracts, macular degeneration, and photokeratitis, which is painful corneal sunburn. UV protection is essential when spending time outdoors. Lenses with UV protection are designed to block or filter out harmful ultraviolet (UV) radiation from the sun. Most tinted lenses protect eyes from UV rays. Tinted lenses may be made to vary in the density of their color in different parts (gradient lenses). However, the choice of the color of tinted lenses, grey, brown, blue, green or pink is however, not often made upon scientific grounds alone and the aesthetic factor often predominates. Many polarized lenses also offer UV protection and photochromatic lenses automatically darken in response to UV exposure, providing UV protection when needed. Lens materials with inherent UV protection are a convenient option for individuals who want to ensure their eyes are shielded from harmful UV radiation. Polycarbonate and Trivex lenses are examples of lens materials that often come with built-in UV protection. These materials are known for their natural ability to block a significant amount of UV rays, making them popular choices for prescription and non-prescription sunglasses. New MR 8 lenses have also been advertised to have inbuilt properties to protect eyes from UV rays. There are short and long terms adverse effect of UV rays. The short-term adverse effects of UV Rays include sunburn, photokeratitis and eye irritation, while the long terms effects are observed as early development of cataracts, age-related macular degeneration (AMD), pterygium and cancerous affect around the eye adnexa. Basal cell carcinoma and squamous cell carcinoma are the two most common types of skin cancer that can develop around the eye adnexa due to chronic UV exposure. These cancers typically start on the skin's surface but can potentially invade nearby tissues if left untreated. They are usually slow-growing and can be treated successfully when detected early.

Infra-red Radiation Protection

Workers in industries like welding and healthcare may be exposed to infrared radiation that can harm the eyes. Specialized eye protection, such as welding helmets with protective shields, should be used to mitigate these risks. Infra-red rays are harmful to the eyes, and when absorbed in quantity may produce cataract and retinal lesions of the nature of burns. Sunlight contains a large quantity of these heat rays, but rarely enough to do harm unless the sun is looked at directly, when the lesions of eclipse blindness are produced. In some industries, there is considerable exposure to infra-red, as for example, in the smelting of metals and the making of glass. Crooke's sage-green glass, as we have seen, which eliminates 95% of the infra-red as well as the ultra-violet and a proportion of the luminous spectrum, forms an ideal protection in this respect. Another method of dealing with the problem is the use of reflecting glass made by depositing layers of metals such as gold, silver or platinum. Reflecting lens prevent heat absorption by lens and thus can be employed as a protection against infra-red rays.

Glare Protection

Glare is a visual sensation characterized by excessive and uncontrolled intensity of light that can cause discomfort, visual impairment, or even pain. It occurs when there is a significant contrast between the brightness of a light source and the surrounding environment. Glare can also be caused because of light reflected of the surface. Glare cause both discomfort as well as disability. Reducing glare is important not only for visual comfort but also for safety, as glare can decrease visibility and impair one's ability to react to changing conditions. Dark tinted lenses can be effective in minimizing the effects of glare, especially when it comes to reducing discomfort glare caused by bright sunlight. Some tinted lenses, especially LT 85% may also include anti-reflective coatings to further reduce glare caused by reflections from artificial lighting or oncoming headlights when driving at night. Polaroid lenses are very effective in protection of eyes from light reflected of the smooth surfaces such as concrete road or an expanse of water. Reflected light is partially polarized in a plane parallel to the reflecting surface so that the glare from extensive smooth surfaces such as a concrete road or an expanse of water is lessened. Because of this, polaroid spectacles may be of value to motorists, yachtsmen and fishermen and since they are colored they tone down the ordinary light in addition.

Blue Light Exposure

Light is necessary for vision but light can damage the sight of organ itself. This is very much applicable to shorter wavelength blue light. Light is necessary for vision, as the visual process in our eyes depends on the detection of light by specialized cells called photoreceptors. However, it is also true that prolonged or excessive exposure to certain types of light, particularly blue light, can potentially have harmful effects on the eyes.

Blue light is a short-wavelength, high-energy component of the visible light spectrum. It plays a role in our ability to perceive colors and contrasts, and it is also involved in regulating our circadian rhythms, helping to control our sleep-wake cycle.

With the increasing use of digital devices such as smartphones, tablets, and computers, many people are exposed to high levels of blue light emitted by screens. Prolonged screen time, especially in the evening, can potentially disrupt sleep patterns and lead to eye strain, known as digital eye strain or computer vision syndrome.

There is ongoing research to determine the potential short and long-term effects of blue light exposure on eye health. Some studies suggest that excessive exposure to blue light, especially from artificial sources like digital screens, may contribute to eye problems such as digital eye strain in short-term and possibly play a role in the development or progression of conditions like age-related macular degeneration (AMD) in long run.

To mitigate potential risks associated with blue light exposure, especially from screens, many people use blue light blocking lenses. There are two ways of incorporating the blue light blocking properties into the lenses. One common method is to apply a special blue light blocking coating to the surface of the lens. This coating is often referred to as an anti-blue light coating. It is a thin layer of material that is added to the lens during the manufacturing process. This coating is designed to selectively filter out a portion of the high-energy visible (HEV) blue light that is emitted by digital screens and other artificial light sources. The effectiveness of the coating depends on the specific materials used and the manufacturing process. Another method is to incorporate blue light blocking properties directly into the lens material during manufacturing. This means that the lens material itself has blue light blocking capabilities. These lenses are sometimes referred to as blue light blocking or blue light filtering lenses. Both coating and lens material options can effectively reduce the amount of high-energy blue light that reaches your eyes from digital screens and other sources.

Physical Trauma Protection

Accidental physical injuries to the eye can occur during sports, recreational activities, or even day-to-day life. Activities like sports, construction work or mechanical injury can result in eye injuries, so wearing appropriate protective gear such as helmets or safety goggles is crucial. Lenses designed to provide protection against physical trauma or mechanical injuries, such as impacts or dust, debris, and flying particles are commonly referred to as safety lenses or protective lenses. These lenses are specifically engineered to withstand potential hazards in environments where there is a risk of projectiles, debris, or other physical impact that could harm the eyes. Safety lenses are made from materials that are more durable and impact-resistant than regular eyeglass lenses. Polycarbonate and Trivex are two popular materials used for safety lenses due to their high impact resistance. These lenses are designed to minimize the risk of shattering upon impact, reducing the likelihood of eye injury from flying debris or objects. In addition to the impact-resistant material, safety lenses might also have coatings or treatments to enhance their performance, such as scratch-resistant coatings and anti-fog treatments. They are commonly used in various industries, including construction, manufacturing, sports, and laboratory work, where there is a higher risk of eye injuries.

It is important to note that while safety lenses provide a higher level of protection compared to standard eyeglass lenses, they may not offer complete protection in all situations. Workers and individuals exposed to potential eye hazards should also consider using additional protective gear, such as goggles or face shields, depending on the nature of the hazards they encounter.

Light Sensitivity

Some individuals with specific eye conditions or sensitivities may find certain tints more comfortable or beneficial. For example, people who are sensitive to bright lights (photophobia) may prefer tints that reduce glare and brightness, regardless of their refractive error.

SPECTACLES FRAMES: HISTORY, NOMENCLATURE, TERMINOLOGY AND CLASSIFICATION

HISTORY OF SPECTACLE FRAMES

Spectacle frames have a long history and have evolved from crude and heavy contrivances to the comfortable devices of modern times. The earliest evidence that has been recorded dates to the 13th century, when evidence of the use of a lens set in a rim attached to a handle **(Fig. 3.22)**, known as 'Manokel', was observed in a statue in the cathedral of Konstanz. It probably predates the spectacle frame proper.

Riveted frames, developed in 14th century are the oldest known frame type **(Fig. 3.23)**. These riveted frames had two monocles riveted together with an iron rivet. These riveted frame-type structures were made of metal or wood. They were very simple, and they were often held by pinching the bridge of the nose or holding them by hand. These riveted frames, dated around the period of 1350, were found in the choir of the monastery of Wienhausen. Wienhausen is a municipality in the district of Celle in Lower Saxony, *Germany*.

Riveted frames were soon competing with newer and far easier to use Bow frames. The two eye-wires were connected together by a fixed arching central bridge and not iron rivet. They were so called because of their curved bridge, some of which were carefully crafted to behave like spring, improving the comfort as they rested directly on the nose **(Fig. 3.24)**. They were made of iron, bronze, horn or bone.

Experiments continued with different options for positioning the frames on the nose. In the 15th century, threads were added to the eye-wire to hold the frame in front of the eyes. Bonnet frames **(Fig. 3.25)** were suspended from a bonnet or cap. Others were tied up with ribbon or threads to the ears. The eye-wire has two holes pierced in both temporal sides. A thread passed from the holes around the ears, which kept the frame in place **(Fig. 3.26)**.

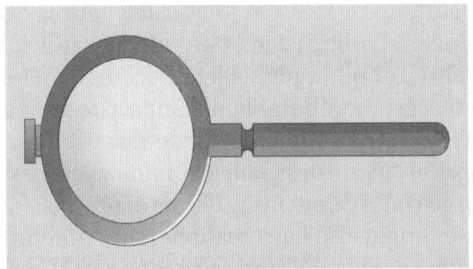

Fig. 3.22: Manokel.

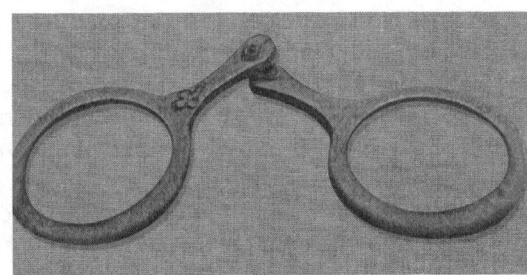

Fig. 3.23: Rivet frame.

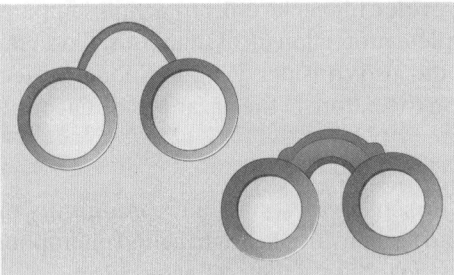

Fig. 3.24: Bow frame.

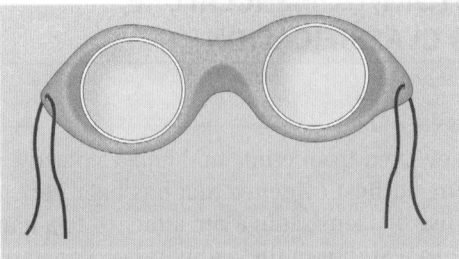

Fig. 3.26: Thread frame.

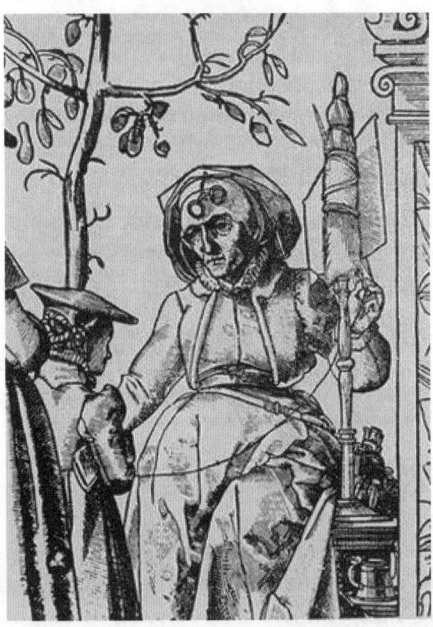

Fig. 3.25: Bonnet frame.

Further development of eyewear continued and efforts were directed towards developing the ways to place frames on the nose and eye-wire in front of the eyes. It was around 16th century some bow frames were developed to have a spring on the nasal side of the bridge. The purpose of the spring was to create a pressure on the nose so that the frame is held in place **(Fig. 3.27)**. Headband frames **(Fig. 3.28)** consisted of a metal band which surrounded the head were introduced. Each lens could be moved separately along the band and suspended before an eye. Belt frames were the first that were attached to the head **(Fig. 3.29)**. The lenses, held in horn rims, were fitted into a wide leather belt, which was worn around the head above the ears.

The 17th and 18th centuries saw significant development in the development of frames with the introduction of "temple spectacle frames," where arms curled around the ears, providing a more secure fit. Several types of temples were developed, and the spectacle frames became more elaborate in design **(Fig. 3.30)**. Temple frames featured two sides attached on either side that curled around the ears, providing a more secure and comfortable fit for the wearer. Temples with round end sides, temples with loop-end sides, double hinged sides, sliding sides, and many more types were experimented with. The temples were connected to the eye wire through screws and hinges, allowing them to pivot and fold inward. This hinge mechanism enabled the wearer to open the temples for use and fold them back when not needed, making the glasses easier to store and carry. Many of these frames were elaborately decorated with engravings, inlays, or other embellishments, showcasing the craftsmanship of the era. The hinges also offered some adjustability, allowing wearers to customize the fit by altering the angle and position of the temples. This was an important feature for comfort and proper fit. It was

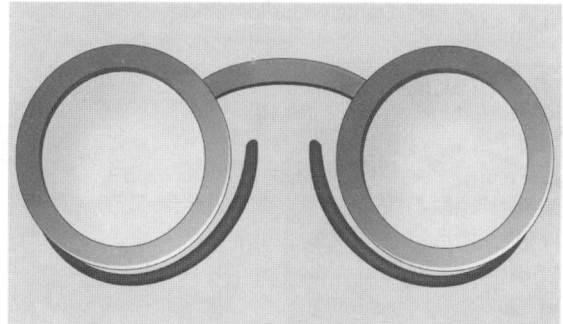

Fig. 3.27: Bow frame with spring which grip the nose.

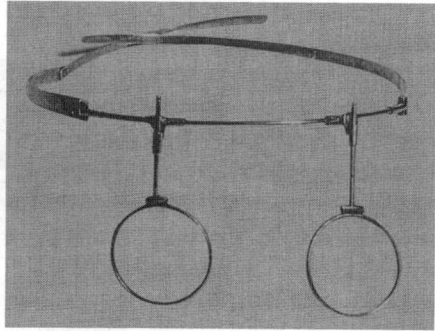

Fig. 3.28: Headband frame.

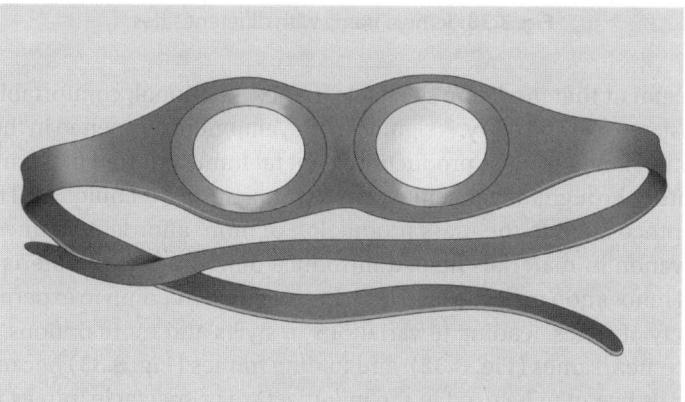

Fig. 3.29: Belt frame.

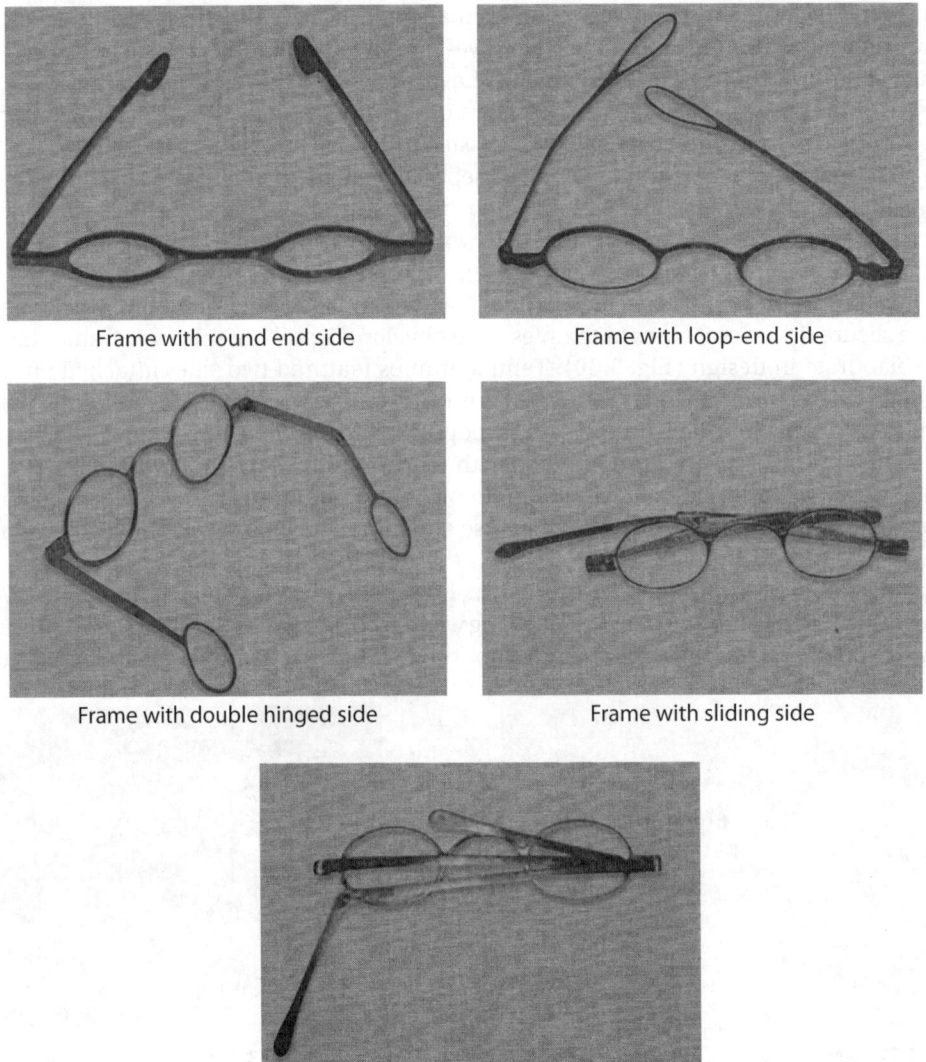

Frame with round end side

Frame with loop-end side

Frame with double hinged side

Frame with sliding side

Frame with double hinged side

Fig. 3.30: Temple frame with different sides.

a crucial advancement that made the spectacle frames functional, comfortable, and versatile, making them easier to use and carry. A significant development happened in the materials used for manufacturing frames as mass production of metal frames started in Germany.

The 19th century brought advancements in manufacturing techniques. The standardized manufacturing process led to the mass production of more affordable frames for a variety of purposes. Innovation in materials helped introduce new alloys and materials like steel and aluminium, and innovation in design and artisans provided freedom to experiment with frame design in a variety of styles, leading to variations in styles and more options. Rimless frames **(Fig. 3.31)**, pince-nez frames **(Fig. 3.32)**, and folding frames **(Fig. 3.33)** became popular.

Plastic materials began to be used in the manufacture of spectacle frames in the early 20th century, around the 1930s. Celluloid acetate material was introduced, which allowed for a

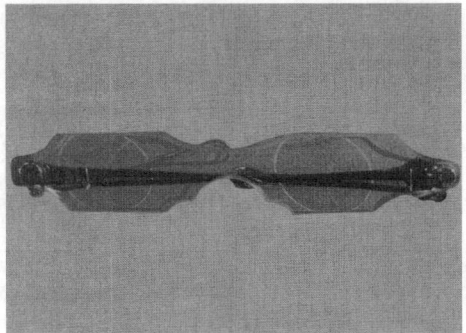

Fig. 3.31: Rimless frame.

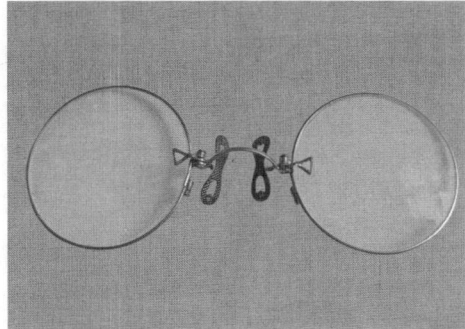

Fig. 3.32: Pince-nez frame.

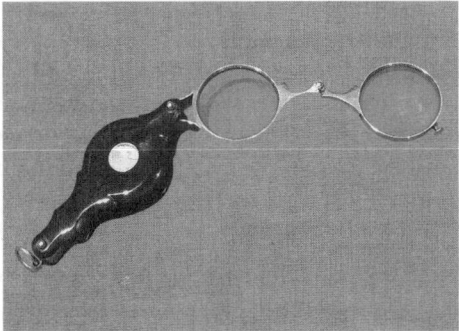

Fig. 3.33: Folding frame.

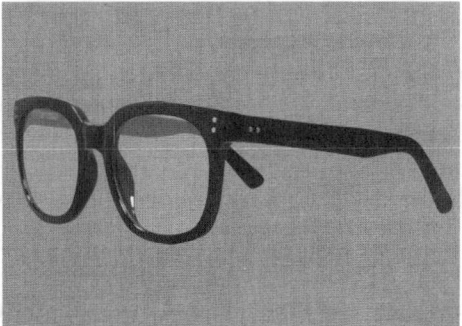

Fig. 3.34: Library frame.

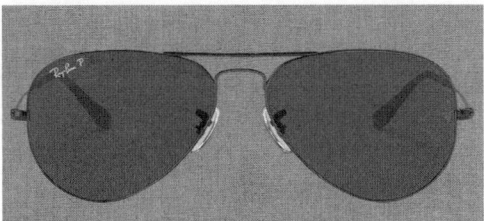

Fig. 3.35: Ray-ban shape.

wider range of shapes and colors. Rimless frames with hockey end sides, round shapes, oval shapes, PRO (Pantoscopic round ovals), and octagonal shapes were introduced. Library frames **(Fig. 3.34)** consisted of a heavy front, and the broad sides were made of plastic and tortoiseshell. In 1935, Bausch and Lomb introduced the Aviator shape in the USA **(Fig. 3.35)**. In 1945, the first semi-rimless frames were made of stainless steel, in which the lens is held in position by clamps that fit into slots made in the lens edge **(Fig. 3.36)**. An upswept shape was introduced in the plastic frame **(Fig. 3.37)**. In 1954, nylon and polyamide frames were produced. In 1965, Optyl introduced a new frame material. Optyl was a type of thermosetting plastic that offered several advantages over traditional frame materials like acetate or metal. Optyl is hypoallergenic, making it suitable for individuals with sensitive skin or allergies to certain materials commonly used in eyewear. One of the unique properties of Optyl was its memory effect. It could retain its shape even after deformation, such as bending or twisting. This made it more resilient and less likely to break or warp. Titanium frames emerged as a lightweight and hypoallergenic alternative

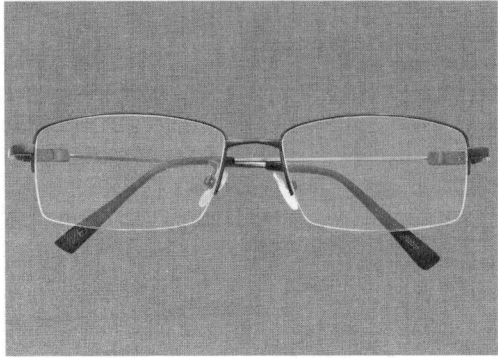

Fig. 3.36: Semi-rimless frame.

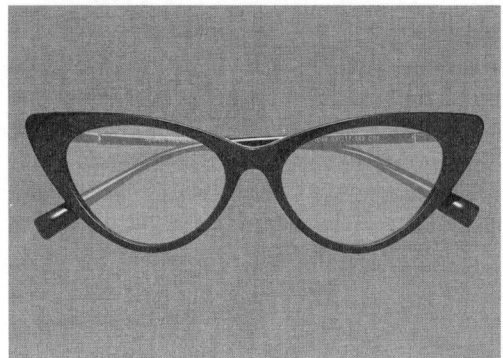

Fig. 3.37: Upswept shape frame.

The 21st century has seen eyeglasses become a significant fashion accessory. Frames are available in a wide array of materials, including stainless steel, acetate, titanium, and even wood. Designer eyewear brands gained prominence, offering frames with unique designs and features. Bespoke and couture frames have been developed, allowing individuals to choose from a variety of frame shapes, colors, and sizes. With the introduction of 3D printing technology in frame production, eyewear technology is continuously heating up.

NOMENCLATURE AND TERMINOLOGY

Spectacle frames comprise of two main parts, containing multiple sub-parts within their construction. The two main parts are:
1. Frame front
2. Frame temples

The frame comes in many different styles, shapes and materials which have their own specific names and utility. Detail knowledge of the parts as shown in **Flowchart 3.9** is very important to understand their functional importance for spectacle dispensing.

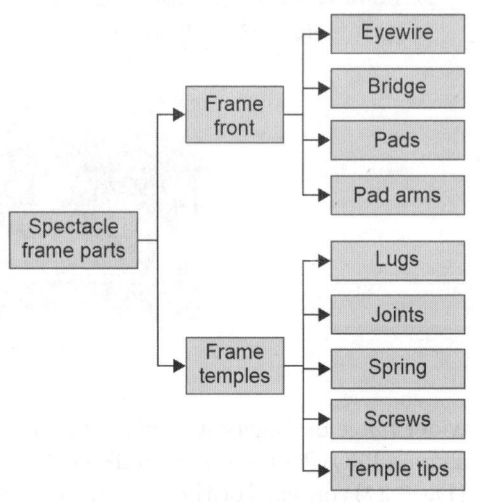

Flowchart 3.9: Parts of spectacle frames.

Frame Front

The part of the frame that houses the lens and allows the wearer to see through them is called frame front **(Fig. 3.38)**.

Eyewire

The eyewire or rims are the part of the frame front that surrounds the lens. The eyewire thickness depends upon material and design of the frame. The thicker eyewire or rim of plastic frames hides the lens thickness within itself and are designed without any joints, whereas eyewire or rim forming in metal frames is designed with joints where the upper and the lower rims meet at the closing blocks and are joined together with screws.

There is a continuous recess within the rim of the frame front is what holds the edge of a lens in place. The angle of the cut is usually at 120° at a depth of about 1.5 mm which makes the optimum angle and depth to receive the beveled edge of an optical lens **(Fig. 3.39)**. The groove

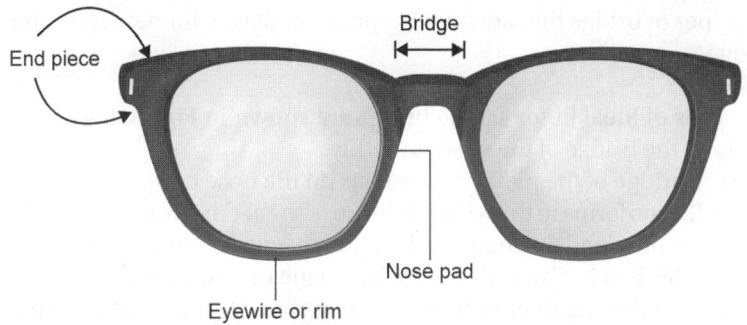

Fig. 3.38: Frame front.

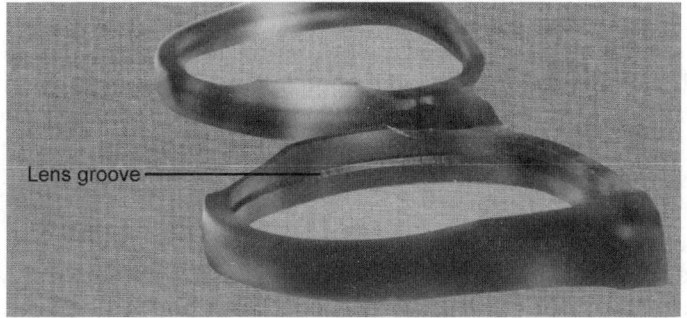

Fig. 3.39: Groove for fitting lens.

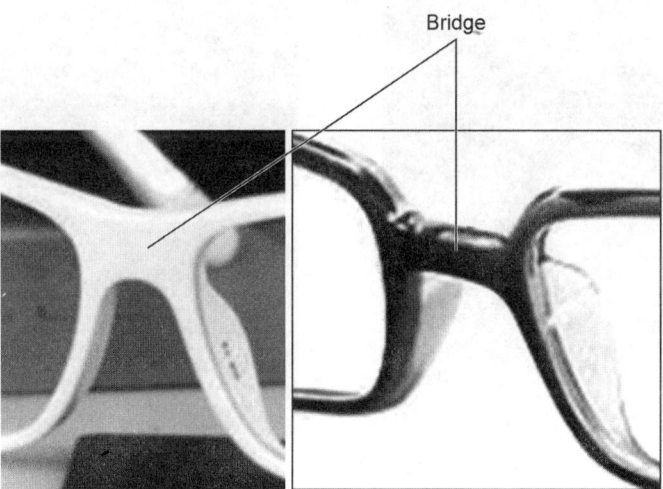

Fig. 3.40: Bridge of the frame.

seamlessly connects with the lens edge, ensuring a dependable union without the necessity for screws or adhesives.

Bridge

The bridge of the frame connects the right eyewire of the front to the left eyewire of the front. In plastic frames, it is shaped to act as the bearing surface on the wearer's nose **(Fig. 3.40)**. The width of the bridge determines the frontal angle in case of plastic frame.

There are two types of bridge that are quite common in plastic frames. They are:
1. Saddle bridge
2. Keyhole bridge

The key features of ideal fit for saddle bridge are shown in **Figure 3.41**. It is shaped like a saddle and follows the bridge of the nose smoothly.
* The base of the bridge of the plastic frame rests on the nose crest.
* The bridge width conforms to the width of the nose so that the frontal angle of pads is parallel to the sides of the nose and the total weight of the spectacle frame is distributed on the wider bearing surface both in horizontal and vertical plane of nasal flank.
* Keyhole bridge makes contact only at two points on the sides of the nose as shown in **Figure 3.42**.

Pads

Pads or nose pads are attached to the pad arms to rest on the nose and provide cushion to bear the entire weight of the metal frame such that the metal rims of the front does not come in contact with skin. They are made of either rigid plastics or silicone material but have a metallic insert for the attachment to pad arms. There are different types of pads as shown in **Figure 3.43**.
* Rocking pads
* Adjustable strap pads
* Fixed form pads

Fixed form pads do not allow any sort of adjustments possibility, whereas rocking pads allow making necessary adjustments for splay angle, frontal angle and vertical angle.

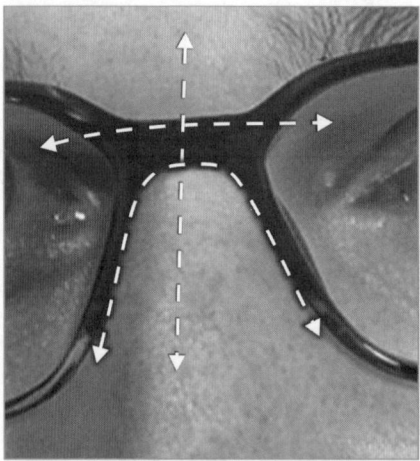

Fig. 3.41: Ideal fitting of saddle bridge.

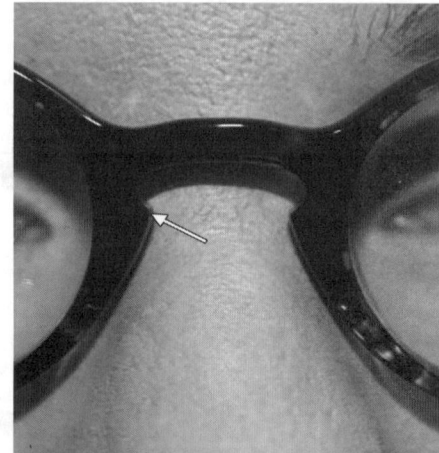

Fig. 3.42: Keyhole bridge.

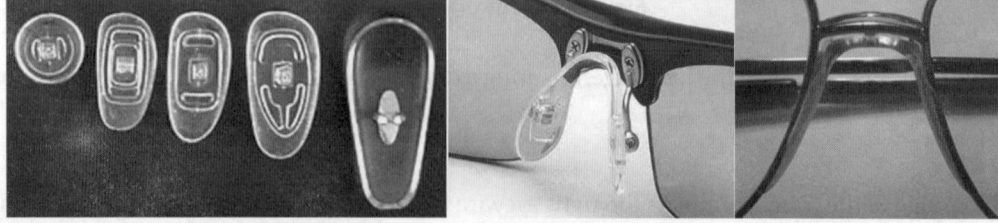

Rocking pads Adjustable strap pads Fixed form pads

Fig. 3.43: Different types of pads.

Pad Arms

The two small pads are attached to the eyewire with pad arms. These pad arms are located just under the bridge on the nasal side of the eyewire and are attached with point soldering **(Fig. 3.44)**. Pad arms allow modification for vertical angle of nose pads.

Temples

Temples, also known as earpieces, arms or sides are the second most important part of the frames that extend over and/or behind the ears to hold the frame in place, preventing the frame slipping **(Fig. 3.45)**. The temples are joined with the end piece of the front by joints A. The portion of the temple from A to B in **Figure 3.45** is the thickest, portion of the temple that is the nearest attachment to the front is known as butt. The portion on the temple from C to point D where it first bends down to go over the ear at point C is called the bend. The portion BC that lies between the butt and the bend is called the shaft and the portion near the joint is referred to as end piece. While dispensing two different fitting adjustments can be done using temples—temple curve and temple bend.

Lugs

Lugs are also known as end piece. They are extension at each end of the frame front to which the joints or sides or temples are attached **(Fig. 3.46)**. This is the portion from where pantoscopic angle of the frame is modified.

Joints

Joints are the means of attachment for the sides with the front on which they can pivot **(Fig. 3.47)**. All the joints are made of two pieces—one is attached to the end pieces of the front and another is attached to temples.

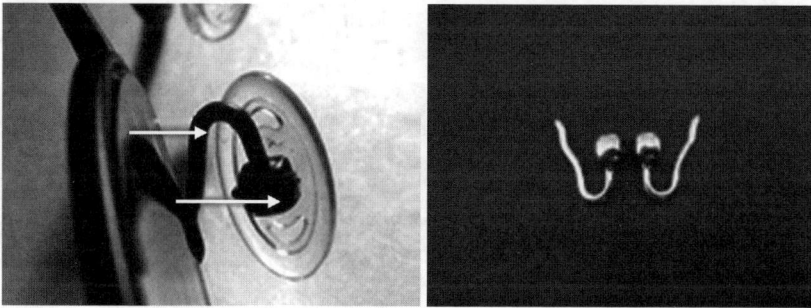

Fig. 3.44: Pad arms.

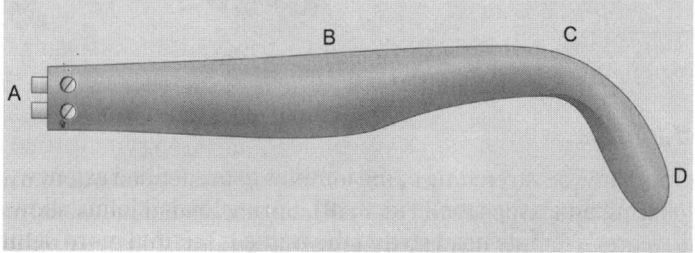

Fig. 3.45: Temple of spectacle frame.

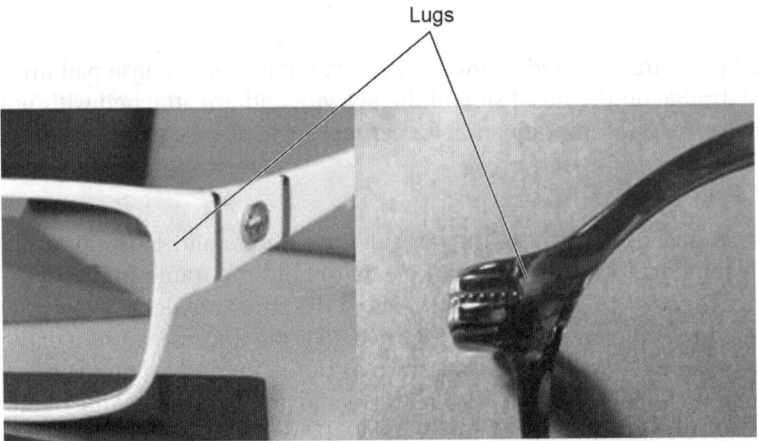

Fig. 3.46: Lugs.

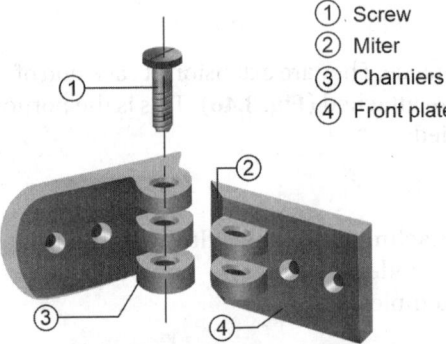

① Screw
② Miter
③ Charniers
④ Front plate

Fig. 3.47: Joints.

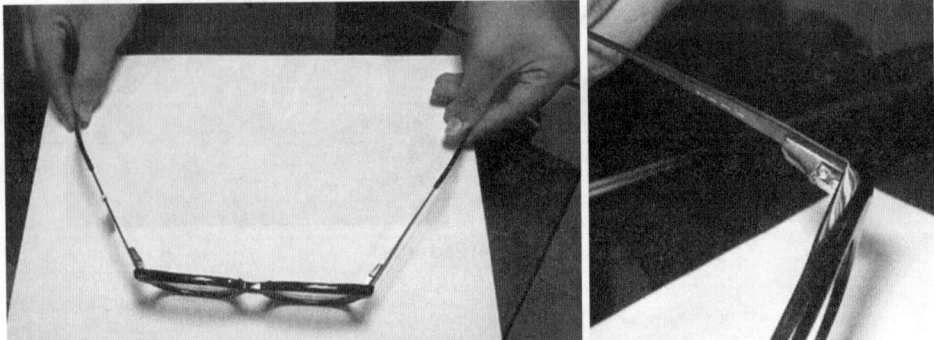

Fig. 3.48: Spring loaded joints.

Spring Loaded Joints

Spring loaded joints allow outstretching of the temples to predefined extent without damaging the joints and ensuring an elastic stop **(Fig. 3.48)**. Spring loaded joints allows the temples to press against the wearer's temple head so that the frame is secured more tightly and to enable the wearer to use the spectacle frame more comfortably without slipping tendency.

Screws

Screws are the smallest part of the frames **(Fig. 3.49)**. Some manufacturer places silicone on the screw thread and when the screw is tightened, the silicone expands between the thread of the closing block and the screws, thus ensuring good friction.

Temple Tips

Temple tips are usually removable plastic sleeves that slip over the ends of metal temples **(Fig. 3.50)** to provide comfort for the wearer. In case of plastic frames, the temple tip is the part of the temple that goes behind the ears.

CLASSIFICATION

Spectacle frames are made in different shapes and styles with varieties of materials. They may be classified in various ways based on different criteria such as material, style, shape, and function as shown in **Flowchart 3.10**.

Material

Broadly, two types of materials are used to manufacture spectacle frames—metals and plastics. Frames can also be made by combining both the material together. Besides, precious materials like gold, platinum, horn wood, etc., can also be used to manufacture frames.

Metal Frames

These frames are made from materials like stainless steel, titanium, aluminum, or other metal alloys. They are known for their durability and lightweight design.

Plastic Frames

Plastic frames are made of materials like nitrate, acetate or cellulose propionate, plastic frames are popular due to their versatility in design and color options.

Combination Frames

These frames combine both metal and plastic elements, offering a mix of durability and style.

Style

In the context of spectacle frames, "style" refers to the design, aesthetics, and visual characteristics of the frames. It encompasses various elements that determine the overall

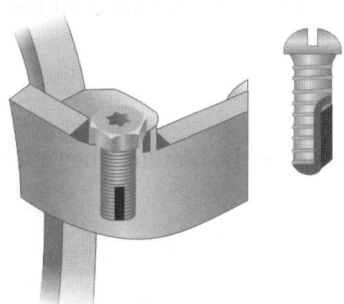

Fig. 3.49: Screws.

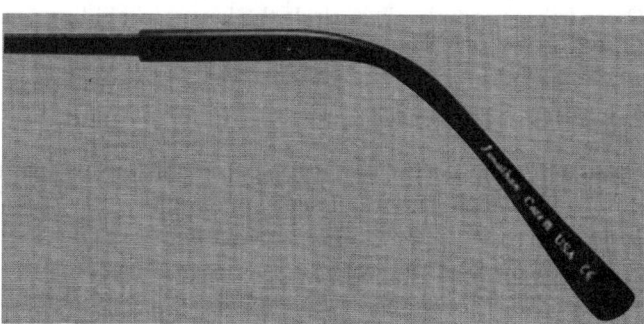

Fig. 3.50: Tips.

Chapter 3: Mechanical Optics, Lenses and Lens Prescription

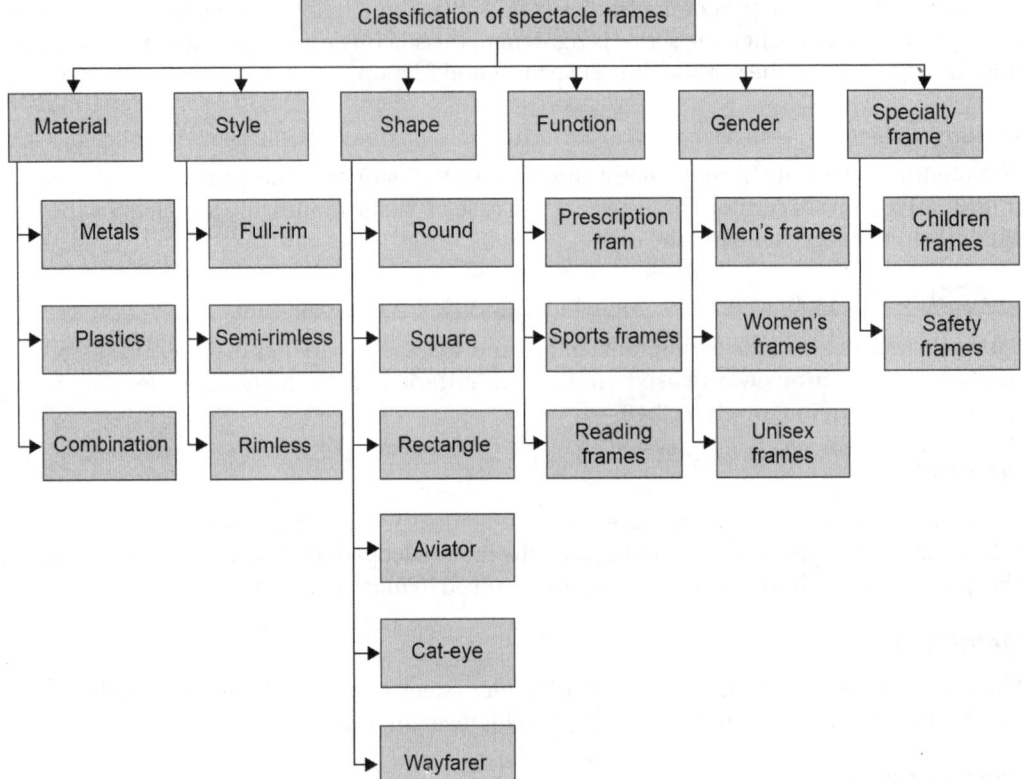

Flowchart 3.10: Classification of spectacle frames.

appearance and appeal of the eyeglasses. The style of spectacle frames is a highly subjective choice, and individuals select frames that resonate with their personal preferences, fashion sense, and lifestyle. The style of eyeglasses can make a significant impact on a person's overall appearance and can makes spectacle frame a key accessory in expressing one's individuality and fashion identity. Spectacles frames can be of different styles. Currently, the popular frame styles are:

Full-rim Frames

These frames completely encircle the lenses, providing a classic and bold look. They are often sturdier and can accommodate a wide range of prescription types.

Semi-rimless Frames

These frames have a rim on the top part of the lenses but are rimless on the bottom. They offer a more lightweight and minimalist appearance.

Rimless Frames

Rimless frames have no rim around the lenses, offering a nearly invisible look. They are very lightweight and often chosen for their subtle appearance.

Shape

Frame shape is a crucial aspect of personal style. The choice of shape of frame is important for several reasons. Frame shape can affect the field of vision, especially for individuals with strong prescriptions. Certain frame shapes may be better suited for specific activities or purposes. Frame shapes are also important for face shape compatibility. Frame shapes can be influenced by fashion trends, and choosing a current or timeless shape can help individuals stay in line with their fashion preferences. Based upon shapes spectacle frames can be classified as follows:

Round Frames
Circular or oval-shaped frames are a timeless classic that can give a retro or intellectual look.

Square Frames
Square or rectangular frames are known for their sharp and angular appearance, providing a modern and professional look.

Aviator Frames
Originally designed for pilots, aviator frames have a distinctive teardrop shape and are often associated with a sporty or adventurous style.

Cat-Eye Frames
Cat-eye frames have an upswept outer edge, creating a feline-inspired look. They are often associated with a retro and glamorous style.

Wayfarer Frames
Wayfarer frames are characterized by their bold and angular design. They have a distinctive look that is both classic and trendy.

Functional Classification

Prescription Frames
Prescription frames, also known as dress wear frames are designed to hold prescription lenses, helping individuals correct vision issues such as nearsightedness, farsightedness, and astigmatism.

Sports Frames
Sports frames are eyeglass frames designed specifically for athletes and individuals engaged in sports and physical activities. These frames are engineered to provide a secure and comfortable fit while offering protection and durability in high-impact situations. The key features of sports frames are as follows:
- They are highly curved frame, wrapping around the face to shield the eyes from wind, dust, and debris. This design also provides better peripheral vision and reduces glare.
- Sports frames are designed to withstand impact, protecting the eyes from potential injuries that can occur during sports like baseball, basketball, or cycling.
- Some sports frames incorporate ventilation features to prevent fogging of lenses during strenuous activities.
- Sports frames are often made of rubberized nose pads and temple tips that prevent slipping during physical activities.

❖ Certain sports frames come with interchangeable lenses to adapt to various lighting conditions.

Reading Frames

Reading glasses are a specific type of prescription frame designed for close-up reading or other near-vision tasks.

Gender-wise Classification

Men's Frames

These frames are typically designed with larger sizes and more conservative styles and colors like brown, black, grey, dark tortoise colors. However, there are men's frames in crystal and light transparent colors also. The common shapes that are mostly seen in men's category are square, rectangle, and aviator.

Women's Frames

Women's frames often feature smaller sizes and a wider range of colors and styles. Cat-eye shape is one of the most popular women's styles. However, they are made in varieties of shapes and colors.

Unisex Frames

Unisex frames are designed to be worn by people of any gender and often have neutral or versatile designs. Wayfarer shape is commonly used by both genders with equal preference.

Specialty Frames

Specialty spectacle frames refer to eyeglass frames that are designed for specific purposes, conditions, or activities. These frames are often engineered with unique features, materials, or design elements to address the specialized needs of the wearer. Some of the popular specialized frames are as follows:

Children Frames

Frames designed for children are typically smaller in size and more durable to withstand the rigors of active play.

Safety Frames

Safety frames are designed to protect the eyes in hazardous work environments and may meet specific safety standards. These frame may be made of polycarbonate material in full wrap style similar to sports frames.

TYPES OF FRAME MATERIAL

When the spectacle frames were developed, they were mostly made of precious materials like tortoise shell, gold or buffalo horn. It is only after the advances in manufacturing technology of mass-production, wide varieties of materials were tried with an objective to improve the machinability of the material, reduce the cost of production, and improve craftsmanship. Mostly plastic and metal family of materials as shown in **Flowchart 3.11** is used to manufacture the spectacle frames.

Chapter 3: Mechanical Optics, Lenses and Lens Prescription

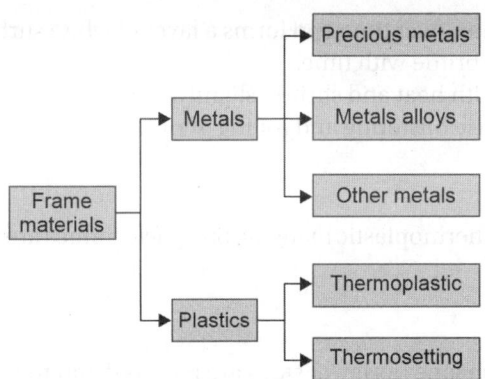

Flowchart 3.11: Types of materials used for spectacle frames.

PLASTIC FRAMES

Plastic material is the most commonly used material for mass production of spectacle frames. Plastics are synthetic polymers and may be grouped into two broad categories: Theromoplastic and thermosetting.

Thermoplastic materials are linear polymers, they flow on heating. Thermosetting materials are crosslinked polymers, they do not flow on heating. Once molded and set in a shape, they cannot be reshaped or remolded. Most materials used for plastic frames manufacturing are of thermoplastic variety. Among all the plastic materials used for spectacle frame manufacturing, the following are most common:

Celluloid Nitrate

Celluloid nitrate is a thermoplastic material. Spectacle frames are made from flat sheets of celluloid material.

Advantages

- ❖ The material polishes well.
- ❖ The strong machinability of the material makes it easy to work with.

Disadvantages

- ❖ The color of the material fades quickly.
- ❖ Material dries up soon and becomes brittle.
- ❖ The material is highly inflammable.
- ❖ It softens faster with heat and excessive heating causes blistering and rolling of rims.

Celluloid Acetate

Celluloid acetate is a thermoplastic material. Spectacle frames are made from flat sheets of celluloid material.

Advantages

- ❖ The material polishes well.
- ❖ The material is easy to work with.

Colors can be produced in multiple layers. Enormous range of colors is possible. Carving reveals different colors.

Disadvantages
- The material deteriorates over time and forms a layer of white surface.
- It cracks and becomes brittle with time.
- The material softens with heat and shrinks slightly.
- Excess heating will cause blistering and rolling of rim.

Celluloid Propionate

Celluloid propionate is a thermoplastic material. Spectacle frames are made by forced injection molding process.

Advantages
- Cost of production is cheaper as fewer steps are required and the waste is less.
- Wide colors are possible with dip coating process.
- The material is very durable for longer period of use.
- The material is very heat sensitive.
- The material is not well-suited for stretching or shrinking.

Disadvantages
Material uses more plasticizers which make it more sensitive to heat.

Nylon

Nylon is a thermoplastic material. Spectacle frames are made by forced injection molding process.

Advantages
- The material is easy to mold to frame shapes.
- Nylon is very ideal for eyewear. It provides minimal weight with high strength.
- It provides stability of shapes even in hot environment.
- Nylon material can be used to make thinner eye wire frames.
- They also provide better anatomical fit at the nose.
- It is possible to make transparent and glossy surface finish.
- Frame coloring is possible by dip coating procedure. Final touch of coloring may be given by printing, which can also make sophisticated patterns.

Disadvantages
Nylon material dries out due to low humidity. It is, therefore, recommended that the wearer soak the frame in water overnight on a periodic basis. This will prolong frame life and deter breakage.

Carbon Fiber

Carbon fiber frames are another type of material used to manufacture frames by injection-molded technology. The material has a better balance between light weight, strength and durability. The most common application of this material is in making combination frame with a carbon front and a metal temple or metal front and carbon temples. These frames deliver the look of an ultra thin plastic frame while exhibiting many of the characteristics of a metal frame.

Advantages

* Carbon fiber frames exhibit good shape retention, light weight and strength.
* Since carbon is black, coloring of these frames is achieved through enameling process.

Disadvantages

Changes in the carbon portion are not readily achieved. Hence pantoscopic and retroscopic adjustments should be provided from the metal portion of the end piece rather than the carbon material itself.

Optyl

Optyl is an epoxy resin. The material was specially developed to manufacture spectacle frames. Frames are made from this material by a process of casting and then curing. After the finishing operations, frames are dyed in liquid colors. Polishing is done by immersing in a bath of polyurethane.

Advantages

* The material is very light in weight.
* The material allows to maintain rigidity and stability in its "set or adjusted" state.

Disadvantage

The material is very brittle.

METAL FRAMES

Metal frames are usually made of metal alloys specially developed to suit the skin. In fact, most base metals oxidize and corrode easily and react variably. In order to avoid this problem, alloy of two or more metals is made in which the major component is one type of metal. The aim of making alloy is generally to make the material less brittle, hard and resistant to corrosion or have a more desirable color and luster. Metal by its nature are malleable that allows working with its shape through the pressure and torque applied gently using plier. A metal spectacle frame uses various combinations of metal materials to create the most functional design. One metal may be chosen for an end piece because of its rigidity, while on the same frame a different flexible metal is chosen for the temple, and yet another metal may be chosen as a final finish because of its hardness or luster. In general, following metal materials are commonly used for spectacle frames:

* **Precious metals gold:**
  * Silver
  * White gold
* **Metal alloys:**
  * Rolled gold
  * Nickel alloys
  * Monel alloys
* **Other metals:**
  * Titanium
  * Aluminum
  * Stainless steel

Precious Metals

Gold and silver are most common precious metals used for exclusive metal eyewear. Apart from its value and noble appearance gold has lot of other merits. Gold is highly resistance to tarnishing and corrosion and can be shaped to any style and thickness with ease. The only disadvantage is that the gold in its purest form is very soft and has to be alloyed with other metals to add needed strength and hardness. Gold alloyed with other metals is known as carat gold and is designated as so many carats according to the proportion of gold in the alloy. 24 ct is termed as pure gold, and the purity goes down to 18 ct, 12 ct and 9 ct. The higher qualities are more resistant to corrosion and are more valuable. The proportion of other metal in the alloy determines the effective color appearance of the gold frames. A pink effect is obtained by increasing the proportion of copper. White gold is obtained by replacing silver with nickel and copper with zinc. A white finish can also be obtained by electroplating gold material with another precious metal rhodium. Other precious metals used are palladium and rhodium which are silvery finish, hard and very expensive.

Metal Alloys

- **Rolled gold:** Rolled gold is designed to provide most of the advantage of gold at cheaper cost. A thin plate or plates of gold is welded to a block of base metal. The adjoining surface is carefully milled to ensure even contact. After the materials have been bonded together the block is subjected to cold-rolling process in order to reduce the gold layer to desired thinness The material is then drawn or formed into wire, strip or tubing having an even covering of carat gold. Bronze and nickel silver are mostly preferred alloys. The gold content depends upon two things— the purity of gold cladding and the proportion of gold covering to base metal. The usual way of expressing the gold quality is "1/10th 10 ct" which implies that the skin is made of 10 ct gold and accounts for 1/10th of the total weight of the whole material. The end product is eventually gold plated to improve the appearance of final product.
- **Nickel silver:** The nickel silver contains as little as 12–25% nickel and mostly copper. The proportion of silver may be very negligible or sometimes no silver. Mechanically, this is an excellent metal alloy for spectacle frames and is fairly resistant to corrosion. If not plated or coated it rapidly turns green in contact with bodily fluids. It can be easily worked to any shape and soldered. It is, therefore, the most common material for the spectacle frames. Nickel silver alloy is also used very commonly for making joints and side's reinforcement of plastic frames.
- **Monel alloy:** This is similar to nickel silver, but contains 68% of nickel. The higher nickel content reduces the rate of corrosion.

Other Metals

Titanium is probably closest to the most ideal metal material for the spectacle frames because of its following properties:
- Mechanically very strong.
- Corrosion resistant and is not affected by perspiration.
- Light weight and hypoallergenic in its purest form.

Currently, they are very expensive for spectacle frames which do not seem to be associated with the manufacturing costs. It is relatively difficult to plate with more attractive metals such as gold. Sometimes they are colored by a process called "ion plating" which is very much similar to vacuum coating of lenses.

It should be noted titanium frames are seldom made completely with pure titanium material. Screws, nose pads and side tips are frequently excluded. There are other descriptors, such as

Chapter 3: Mechanical Optics, Lenses and Lens Prescription

β-titanium in which only about 75–80% is titanium, the rest being either aluminum, chromium, iron, molybdenum, niobium, zirconium, etc.

Aluminum is very light and soft and in its pure form it is hypoallergenic and is highly resistant to corrosion. Aluminum parts are always quite thick for a metal frame, due to the softness of the material. Being a good conductor of heat, aluminum is noticeably cold to the touch. It can be beautifully decorated by a process known as anodizing.

Stainless steel is relatively difficult to work with and is highly resistant to corrosion. It is relatively uncommon material for spectacle frame, although their use is increasing.

TYPES OF HUMAN FACES AND CHOICE OF FRAMES

There is nothing more important than how your eyewear looks on your face. A good-looking frame makes the wearer feel good, sophisticated, polished, snazzy, attractive, stylish, and confident. Theoretically, there are several factors that influence frame selection, but in the real world, facial shapes dominate the most while selecting the appropriate frame shape. The first act that a patient does is put the frame on his eyes and sees how it looks on his face. The fundamental laws that govern the choice of the frames are shown in **Flowchart 3.12**.

The shape of the frame should contrast with facial shape, so that it can balance the proportion. It should maximize the positive aspects of facial features and/or minimize the negative aspects of the face. The overall size of frame should be in scale with face width. The goal should be to find a frame shape that emphasizes the complimenting lines of face.

One of the most ideal ways to select an appropriate frame shape for a given face is to analyze the face shape by comparing the length of the face to its width **(Fig. 3.51)**. Then observe the bone structure and cheeks below the eyes and match the frame shape that emphasizes the complimenting lines of face.

The following guidelines may help for different facial shapes.

TYPES OF HUMAN FACES

Oval Face

Oval face is considered to be perfect ideal facial shape for most spectacle frame shapes. The perfect oval shape of the face has a length that is one and half times the width, with no obvious

Flowchart 3.12: Laws of spectacle frame selection.

Law 1	The frame matches to the lens prescription of the wearer to provide the desired optical function.
Law 2	The frame looks good on the wearer's face.
Law 3	The frame provides the maximum wearing comfort.
Law 4	The frame style matches to the lifestyle of the wearer.

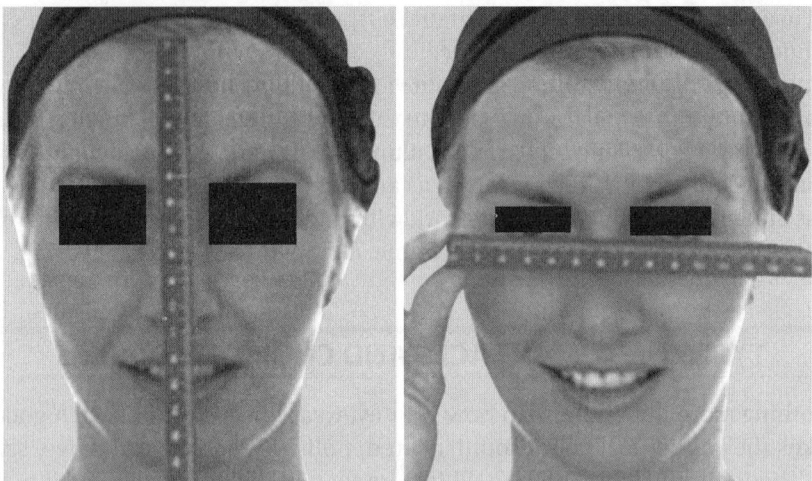

Fig. 3.51: Measuring facial width and length.

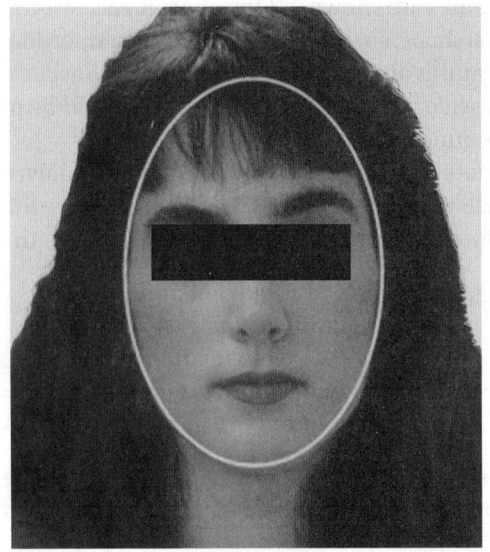

Fig. 3.52: Oval face.

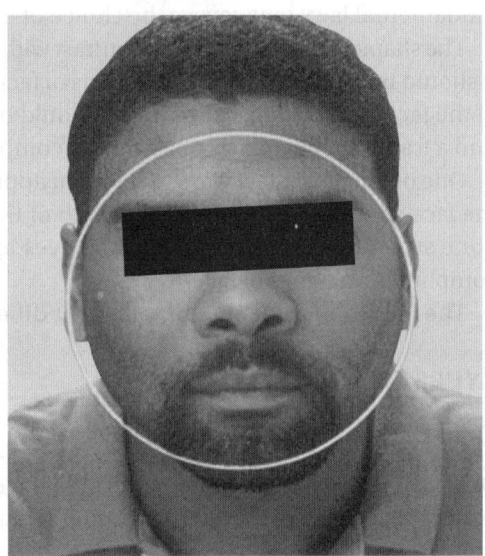

Fig. 3.53: Round face.

angles **(Fig. 3.52)**. Almost all types of frame shapes compliment with the oval shape face. The thumb rule while selecting the frame is "maintain oval's natural balance".

Round Face

Round face is characterized by almost similar proportion of length and width **(Fig. 3.53)**. In such case the shape of the frame should make the face look longer and thinner. Frame shape with wider "A" measurement than "B" measurement will create an effect that creates angles or horizontal lines and makes the facial shape appear longer and thinner. Rectangular shapes will be the most ideal that will cover the full facial width. Wider bridge will also add to size and clear bridge widens the look of eyes. Dark colored temples add width. Metal frame with rocking pads will keep away the lower rim from fuller cheeks.

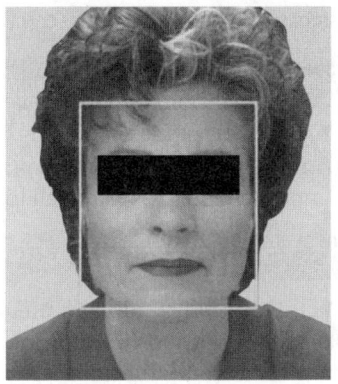 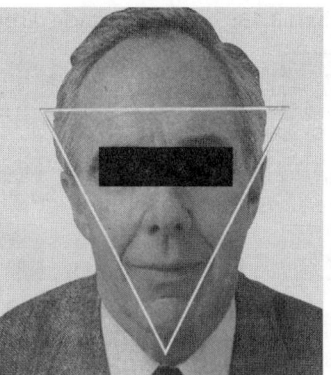 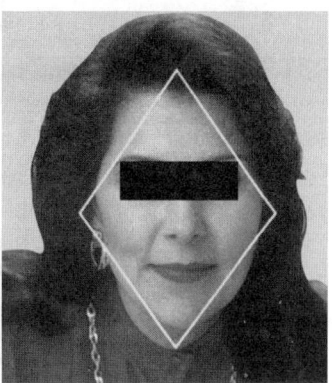

Fig. 3.54: Square face.   **Fig. 3.55:** Triangular face.   **Fig. 3.56:** Diamond face.

Square Face

The width of the face is wider in relation to its length in case of square face **(Fig. 3.54)**. Square shaped faces are also characterized by strong jaw line, broad forehead and broad cheek bones and wide chin. The frame shape should make the face look longer. Select frame with weight on the top of the frame. This will give a look of lengthening the face. Oval shape frames with top or center joint will suit better. Decorations and dramatic designs at the upper temporal corner will lengthen the face. Narrow shape with larger "A" measurement will be better option.

Triangular Face

The face has wider forehead and higher cheek bones and narrow chin and jaw lines **(Fig. 3.55)**. The ideal selection of frame shape will draw the attention away from the forehead and will balance the narrow jaw with the frame shape. Taper shape from top, cat's eye shape or aviator shape frames may suit. Light and delicate styles are better. This is the difficult facial shape to select the frame for. Top heavy frame, i.e., thicker top rim or metal front with top plastic mount should be good.

Diamond Face

The diamond shaped face is the rarest face shape. The shape of face is narrow at the eye line and the jaw line with a small forehead and chin **(Fig. 3.56)**. Cheekbones are high and raised. The frame shape should widen the forehead and jaw and minimize the appearance of cheekbones. Choose frames that are heavy on top but avoid low temples joints frames. Rimless, square frames or straight top frames may work. Select square or straight top with bottom curved frames.

COSMETIC AND FUNCTIONAL DISPENSING OF SPECTACLES

The dispensing of spectacles or prescription glasses refers to the process of providing patients with the appropriate eyeglasses based on their prescription and individual visual needs. The entire process of spectacle is a 12 step procedure as shown in **Flowchart 3.13**.

DISPENSING OF SPECTACLES

Prescription Verification

The dispensing process begins with verifying the prescription provided by an optometrist or ophthalmologist. The prescription specifies the type and strength of lenses needed for each eye.

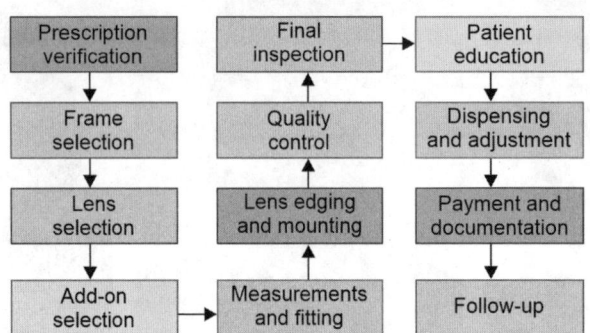

Flowchart 3.13: Steps of spectacle dispensing.

Frame Selection

Patient or customer selects a frame from the available options. The frame should not only fit comfortably on the face but also be compatible with the prescription and look good cosmetically.

Lens Selection

Based on the prescription and any specific visual requirements or preferences of the patient, the optician helps select the appropriate type of lenses. This may include single vision lenses for distance or reading, bifocals, trifocals, or progressive lenses for multifocal correction. While the lenses serve the fundamental objective of the dispensing, the choice of lens is also critical for cosmetic values.

Add On's Selection

The optician discusses lens material options in terms of lens material and lens design and then recommends add on's like fixed tints, changing tints, anti reflection coating, blue light filter etc. These add-ons are useful to enhance the lens performance and minimize the possibilities of any disadvantages that may be associated otherwise.

Measurements and Fitting

Precise measurements are taken to ensure that the lenses will be properly centerd in the selected frame. These measurements include the pupillary distance (PD) and segment height (if applicable). The frame may also be adjusted for a comfortable fit on the face.

Lens Edging and Mounting

Once the frame and lens selections are finalized, the lenses are cut and shaped to fit the frame. They are then mounted securely in the frame.

Quality Control

Before dispensing, the glasses undergo a quality control check to ensure that the lenses are correctly aligned, the prescription is accurate, and there are no defects.

Final Inspection

The optician or technician inspects the finished eyeglasses to ensure that they meet the patient's expectations in terms of appearance and functionality.

Patient Education

The patient is educated about the proper care and maintenance of their new glasses, including how to clean the lenses, adjust the frame if needed, and recognize signs of lens damage or wear.

Dispensing and Adjustment

The patient is provided with their new glasses, and the optician makes any necessary final adjustments to ensure a proper fit and alignment. This includes checking the comfort of the nose pads, temple arms, and overall balance of the glasses.

Payment and Documentation

The patient pays for the eyeglasses, and the optician provides a receipt or documentation of the purchase, which may be used for insurance reimbursement or warranty purposes.

Follow-up

The optician may schedule a follow-up appointment to address any concerns or issues the patient may have after wearing the glasses for a period of time.

Vision is by far the most important sense and, unfortunately, the most neglected aspect of overall well-being. We have allowed it to happen by underestimating the importance of vision in terms of occupation, lifestyle, and general health and by not having evidence that visual and occupational performances are interrelated, and they also have direct effects on lifestyle and behavioral performance. However, this would seem evident when we look at the preventive and protection sides of dispensing, which also fall into the realm of dispensing. It is, therefore, prudent to look at the process of dispensing as an integral part of holistic eye and vision care. In this holistic approach, both the functional and cosmetic aspects of dispensing should be taken into consideration. This approach not only ensures that patients receive effective vision correction but also helps them feel confident, comfortable, and satisfied with their eyewear, ultimately contributing to their overall well-being and quality of life.

FUNCTIONAL ASPECT SPECTACLE DISPENSING

Functional aspect of spectacle dispensing focuses on selecting lenses based on understanding of prescription and lifestyle needs that include occupation, recreation and general life activities. The above information can be gathered at twelve stages of dispensing as mentioned above in different ways and at different times during the patient's visit to the practice. It is best to discuss and understand the prescription at the beginning of the patient's visit and discover lifestyle needs by asking questions related to occupation, hobbies, recreation and unique needs of the patient which may be related to either his occupation or for his leisure time. Most practitioners focus more on occupational needs and in the process they tend to forget discussing about recreation and other leisure time activities. While prioritizing the occupational needs of their patients when prescribing eyeglasses or other vision correction solutions is important, it is equally important to consider and discuss recreational and leisure-time activities. This comprehensive approach to vision care ensures that individuals can enjoy a balanced and fulfilling life both at work and during their free time, enhancing their overall well-being. Having the complete information helps you and the patient through the appropriate frame and lens selection. You may gather lifestyle information by asking open-ended questions starting with "What," "Why" or "How." For example, "How much time do you spend at a computer each day?" Their answers serve as a treasure chest of information for you to use.

Once you obtain the necessary lifestyle information, the process of selecting lenses and frames begins. It is recommended to first select the lenses, then the frames. The lenses are the most important part of eyewear as they fulfil the objective of providing better vision. With today's premium lens products and lens enhancements, you have the ability to address all three elements of dispensing—enhancement, prevention and protection.

Enhancement

Vision is enhanced by the use of lenses and vision is maintained by the use of lenses. You patient need to see clearly and react quickly. This is important for visual satisfaction. The visual satisfaction transpires when an individual develops a positive feeling with his eyewear, he is able to cope with his occupational and recreational needs unconsciously and he continues with it comfortably for a prolonged period of time. **Flowchart 3.14** shows the different stages of visual satisfaction. Anti reflection lenses further helps enhancing the light transmission that not provide improved visual performance but also aids during night driving.

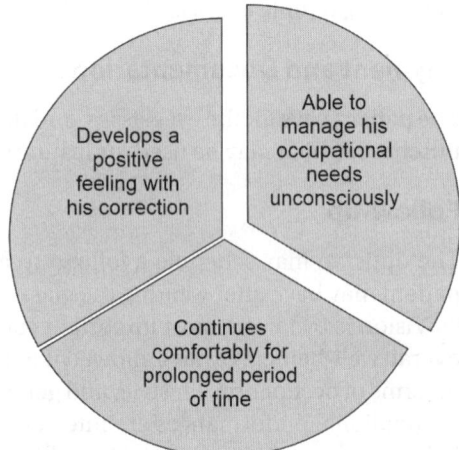

Flowchart 3.14: Visual satisfaction triad.

Prevention

The preventive side of dispensing is still at nascent stage. Although the idea has gained more attention and awareness in recent years, it seems there are still significant challenges and opportunities for further development in this field. The ultimate goal is to shift the focus from treating illnesses after they occur to preventing them in the first place, which can lead to better health outcomes and reduced healthcare costs in the long run. There is a lot of evidences now that, non-ionizing radiations contributes to early eye aging especially cataract and macular degeneration. The soft adnexa is also susceptible to the effects of sunlight and are a common site for basal and squamous cell carcinoma. The external eye also often shows signs of over exposure to sunlight which includes pinguecula and pterygium. The prevention of UV rays and high energy shorter wavelength of blue light are very critical for long term ocular health. Myopia control lenses are useful lenses for kids.

Protection

Accidental physical injuries to the eye can occur during sports, recreational activities, or even day-to-day life. Activities like sports, construction work, or mechanical injuries can result in eye injuries, so dispensing polycarbonate lenses is crucial. Polycarbonate lenses are also essential for kids. Polycarbonate and Trivex are two popular materials used for safety lenses due to their high impact resistance. These lenses are designed to minimise the risk of shattering upon impact, reducing the likelihood of eye injury from flying debris or objects. Immediate protection from glare caused by excessive and uncontrolled intensity of light that can cause discomfort, visual impairment, or even pain Glare can also be caused by light reflected off the surface. Glare causes both discomfort and disability. Reducing glare is important not only for visual comfort but also for safety, as glare can decrease visibility and impair one's ability to react to changing conditions. Tinted lenses can be effective in minimising the effects of glare, especially when it comes to reducing discomfort caused by glare caused by bright sunlight.

Some tinted lenses, especially LT 85%, may also include anti-reflective coatings to further reduce glare caused by reflections from artificial lighting or oncoming headlights when driving at night. Polaroid lenses are very effective in protecting the eyes from light reflected off smooth surfaces such as concrete roads or an expanse of water.

Occupation Dispensing

The visual satisfaction is maximum when an individual acquires the task specific automatic processes that enable efficient and sustained acquisition and processing of spatial information. This is possible when the eye is able to fixate, converge and focus quickly. In comparing one task with another, several factors must be considered:
- Visual acuity which depends upon viewing distance, object size and illumination
- The contrast of the object with its background
- Required perception of motion
- Influence of reflection of light from the object
- Repetitiveness and time spend on the task

There occupation specific lenses like anti fatigue lenses, and regressive lenses that work effectively. More solutions can be customized to suit individual's specific needs and budget.

Once you finish the selection of lenses and frames, dispensing measurements are taken precisely. The accuracy and sufficiency of measurements are critical for successful dispensing. It is also important that you make sure that you have the relevant information needed to order the lenses to the laboratory for procurement before the patient leaves your practice. There are three broad categories of lenses used for spectacle manufacturing: finished stock lenses, prescription lenses, and customised lenses. Dispensing measurements vary accordingly. Fitting rituals, which include interpupillary measurements and fitting height, are sufficient for most finished stock categories, while for prescription and customised lenses, more measurements may be needed.

The uncut lens is checked for surface and material blemishes, such as scratches, veins, bubbles, strie, greyness or waves and its power verified using focimeter. If the lens is found perfect, optical center and axis are marked with glass pencil. The lens is then placed upon a protector with its axis along the require direction and a horizontal line is drawn through the optical center.

The actual fitting of lenses into frame is known as glazing and this includes two processes – cutting and edging. In the classic procedure of cutting, a lens cutting machine engraves a deep line with a diamond upon the glass of the required shape and size. The glass is then broken off at this line by nippers and subjected to edging by which the edge is smoothed and if necessary bevelled by rotating carborundum wheel.

Hand edging is now, rare in practice. The whole procedure of reducing the lens to the required shape and size is automated to ensure end to end work and cutting as a distinct process is eliminated. Lastly, in the process of glazing the lenses are inserted and fitted into the frames.

A final checking completes the process. The optical center in relation to papillary distance measurement and the axis of cylinder are checked. Faults or scratches are eliminated and any strain in the lens detected by special means. During the process of glazing, strains may be put on the lenses which may induce the phenomenon of double refraction. Such strain can be detected by a strain tester whereby the lens is examined by a polarizing apparatus.

The spectacle is ready for delivery. The patient is reminded to collect the spectacle. On his visit the spectacle is finally checked on his face. At first the fitting is checked. The fitting assessment is a sequential process which starts with assessment of front positioning followed by horizontal angle, vertical angle and then nose pad fitting and standard alignment.

The patient is educated about the proper care and maintenance of their new glasses, including how to clean the lenses, adjust the frame if needed, and recognize signs of lens damage or wear and is also briefed about follow ups.

The spectacles are the commonest way of correcting refractive errors, it is vitally important for them to be dispensed accurately with zero error. There is a certain area of tolerance that is earmarked for different power ranges. Several countries of the west have regulations set up by the government that define the level of tolerance. Therefore, it is imperative that opticians be careful to deliver in accordance with the guidelines set by the regulatory bodies.

COSMETIC ASPECT SPECTACLE DISPENSING

Good looks are the snare that everyone likes to be caught in. The statement suggests that an attractive appearance can be alluring and captivating, attracting the interest and admiration of others. Cosmesis, which reflects the real desire of everyone, becomes very important for several reasons, as the use of eyewear is a functional need as well as an expression of their personality and a way of social recognition. The ugly will detract from the pleasure of using, thus jeopardising the benefits. Moreover, good-looking objects are often seen as good-task-performing. It is no coincidence that the introduction of multiple frame styles, shapes, and colors has part of its appeal in the beauty of its design.

When an individual who has been prescribed refractive correction by his health care provider takes the prescription to the optician, the first remark that he makes is, "Show me the frames.' And when the optician asks for the lens prescription, often the reply is, 'First, let me see the frame'. Such behavior is quite common when individuals are getting prescription eyeglasses. Most people prioritise the style and aesthetics of their eyeglass frames. They want frames that not only correct their vision but also suit their personal style and face shape. Therefore, their initial focus is on finding frames that they like. Once they find frames they like, they are more willing to provide their prescription details. This is because the prescription needs to be tailored to the selected frames to ensure the lenses fit properly. The opticians are now tuned to this order of preference and are trained to assist customers in finding frames that meet their style preferences and accommodate their prescription needs. It's important for the final glasses to not only correct vision but also be something the individual feels comfortable wearing and confident in.Eyeglasses have become a fashion accessory in addition to their functional role. Some individuals want to make a fashion statement with their frames, which can be an important aspect of their overall style.The cosmetic aspect of dispensing predominates. The frame should look good and complement the facial shape, complexion and style of the wearer besides meeting the functional needs.

The cosmetic approach entails:
- Study of facial shape
- Study of facial complexion
- Study of hair color
- Study of frame ergonomics
- Study of frame shapes
- Study of frame styles
- Study of frame material and color

Facial Shape

There is nothing more important than how your eyewear looks on your face. A good looking frame makes the wearer feel good, sophisticated, polished, snazzy, attractive, stylish and confident. Theoretically, there are several factors that influence the frame selection, but in practice facial shapes has a dominant weightage while selecting the appropriate frame shape. The shape of the frame should contrast with facial shape, so that it can balance the proportion. It should maximize the positive aspects of facial features and/or minimize the negative aspects of the face. The overall size of frame should be in scale with face size. The goal should be to find a frame shape that emphasizes the complimenting lines of face. One of the most ideal ways to select an appropriate frame shape for a given face is to analyze the face shape by comparing the length of the face to its width. Then observe the bone structure and cheeks below the eyes and match the frame shape that emphasizes the complimenting lines of face. **Table 3.9** gives an interesting perception as to frame shape and style selection.

Facial Complexion and Hair Color

The choice of frame color depends upon the user's skin and hair color. Men usually look good in dark colors. Brown, black, gray and dark blue are popular color for men whereas red, pink and aqua are more popular in females. Females usually prefer lighter tones. Black is equally common for both especially young male and female.

Face color may be cool or warm. Cool color has blue or pink undertones whereas warm color has peaches or cream undertone or yellow cast. Everyone looks good in their own color tone. Frame color should complement facial color complexion. Colors may be solid or vertically gradient or horizontally gradient. Solid color has a shortening effect, i.e., the apparent length of the face seems shortened when you put on solid color frame. Gradient colors, specially vertically oriented gradient colors have a face lengthening effect, making them more compatible for wider face.

Hair colors are also taken into consideration while selecting the frame color. Black, white and brown for hair color is taken as cool colors and golden and dirty gray is taken as warm color. Warmer color frames look good with golden hair. Pink tone best suits brown hair.

Frame Ergonomics

There are certain important elements of frame design that create the intended relationship between the structures of the frames and the wearers. They are engineered to maintain a

Table 3.9: Perception regarding frame shape and style selection.

Facial shape	Face description	Preferred frame shape	Perceived notion
Oval	Most balanced facial shape	Almost all frame shape compliments	Maintain the oval's natural balance
Round	Similar proportion of length and width	Rectangle shapes, wide bridge, dark temples	Makes the face appear longer and thinner
Square	Wide face with strong jaw line, broad forehead, cheek and chin	Oval frame shape, decoration at upper temporal corner, larger "A" measurement	Lengthen the apparent look of the face
Triangular	Wide forehead, high cheek bones, narrow chin and jaw lines	Cat's eye shape and Aviator shape, Top heavy Design	Will draw the attention away from forehead and will provide a balanced look
Diamond	Narrow at the eye line and jaw line, small forehead and chin	Rimless, square frames or straight top frames	Widen the forehead and minimize the appearance of cheekbones

balanced and secure fit, crafted to ensure comfortable contact at the bridge of the nose and behind the ears, and to provide an innovating new look to the overall design of the frame. The temples are attached to the extension of the front of the spectacle frame termed as lug. Temples are side bars that run from the joints across the sides of the head, thus holding the spectacle to the face. Temples interject an artificial dividing line that divides the frame front into two halves. The lower the line shorter the face appears and higher the line longer the face appears when viewed from the sides. If the temples are attached high on the frame front **(Fig. 3.57)**, there is more facial area below the line and face appears lengthened. If the temples are attached lower on the frame, there is less distance from this line to the bottom of the chin and therefore, face appears shorter **(Fig. 3.58)**. Temple thickness also affects the look of the facial length with broad temples reducing the apparent facial length and thinner temples increasing the apparent facial length. The position of the joints in the vertical plane along the front also affects the fit of the frame. Low joint frames cause greater fitting problem than high joint frames because their center of gravity may result in somewhat precarious balance. Moreover low joints affect the inferior temporal field of view while high joints normally do not. A center joint temple may affect the

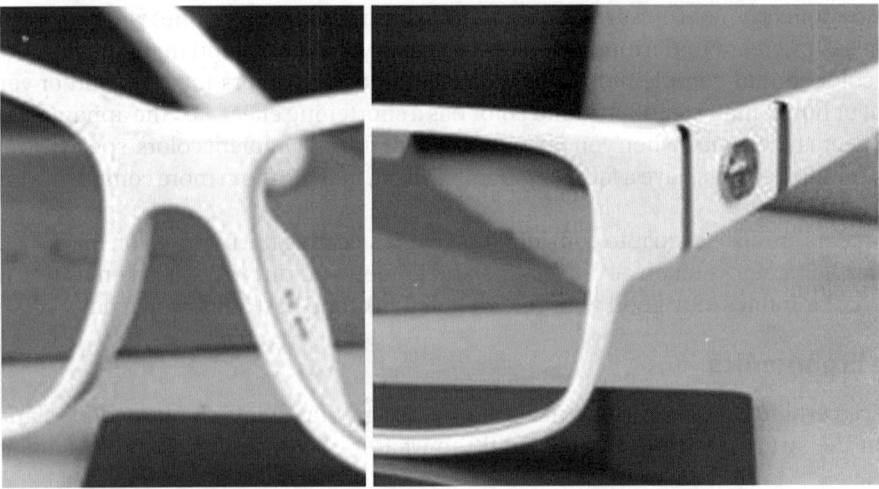

Fig. 3.57: Top joint frames.

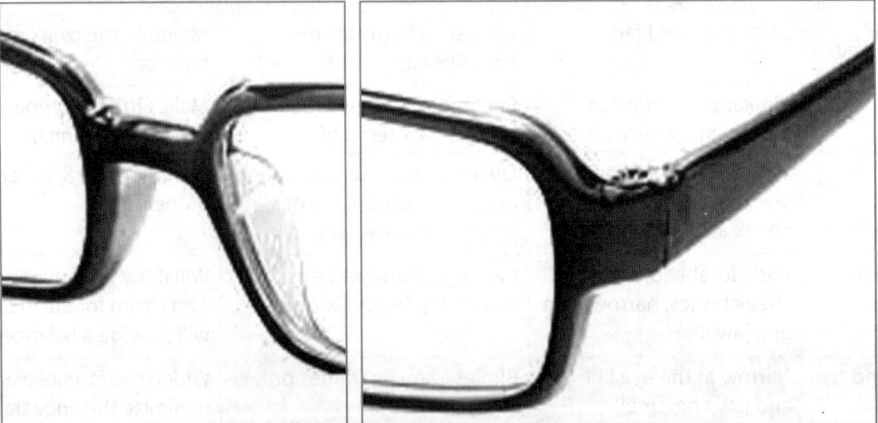

Fig. 3.58: Temple joints little above datum line.

temporal field of view. The angle of sides of low joint frames differs noticeably from other two types in that it usually has to have a negative value. Thus, it has a lot of impact on choice of the appropriate frame selection. Bridge style can also be selected to hide the negative aspects of the nose. In order to lengthen the look of the nose, choose a frame that exposes as much of nose as possible. The keyhole bridge exposes most of the nose because it rests on the sides and not on the crest. To shorten the look of nose, choose a frame with a low or solid colored bridge and avoid a keyhole bridge, or a high bridge, or a clear bridge. To narrow and lengthen a wide nose use a clear or metal bridge that sits close to the nose and use nose pads on metal frames.

Frame Styles and Shapes (Flowchart 3.15)

Rimless frames are subtle and work well for most face shapes, especially if you want a minimalistic look. These are lightweight and unobtrusive, making them suitable for everyday wear and professional settings.

Full rim frames provide structure and can be suitable for round or oval faces. They offer more durability and are better for activities where your glasses may undergo stress, like sports or outdoor activities.

Supra frames typically have a more retro or vintage look and can suit square or heart-shaped face. These frames can add a touch of style and are often chosen for fashion-forward or artistic looks.

Aviator shape frames typically have a teardrop shape and work well with a variety of face shapes, especially oval, round, or heart-shaped faces. The soft curves of aviator frames can balance out angular features.

Square frames are excellent for round and oval faces as they add structure and angles to the face. Avoid square frames if you have a square face shape as they may emphasize your existing strong angles.

Oval frames are quite versatile and complement most face shapes, but they particularly suit square and heart-shaped faces due to their soft, rounded edges.

Pillow frames, with their gentle curves and slight angularity, can work well on oval and heart-shaped faces.

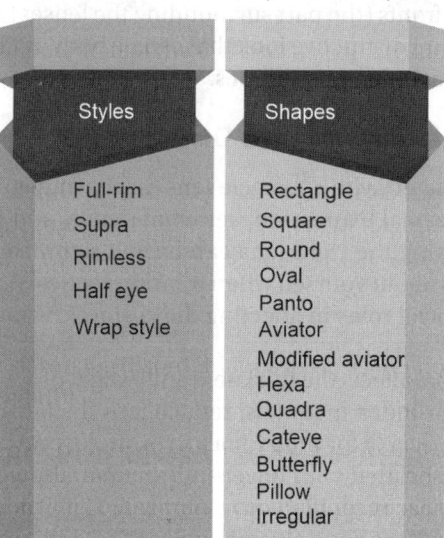

Flowchart 3.15: Frame styles and shapes.

Cat's eye frames are known for their upswept outer edges, making them a great choice for balancing the features of round and square faces. They are particularly flattering for heart and oval face shapes.

Frame Material and Color

Plastic frames with their wide range of colors and patterns provide wide range of options and convey depending upon design, patter, thickness, and color. Thick, bold plastic frames with a classic shape, such as square or rectangular, can create an intellectual or academic appearance. They are often associated with a serious and studious image. Bright and vibrant colors, unique patterns, or modern frame shapes can give you a stylish and trendy appearance. Certain plastic frame styles, like cat's eye or round frames, can evoke a retro or vintage vibe, adding a touch of nostalgia to your look. Thin plastic frames can provide a minimalist and understated appearance. They are a great choice if you prefer a clean and simple aesthetic. Plastic frames with unusual or asymmetrical designs can add a playful and artistic element to your style. Bright and bold plastic frames can make you appear more youthful and energetic. They can add a pop of color to your outfit and personality. If you want your glasses to be a bold fashion statement, opt for oversized plastic frames or frames with embellishments like studs or unique textures.

Metal frames offer a distinct look and feel compared to plastic frames. They have their own unique characteristics and can convey various styles and impressions.

Metal frames are often associated with a sleek and minimalistic appearance. Thin, lightweight metal frames can give you a sophisticated and understated look. Metal frames, especially in classic shapes like rectangular or round, can project a professional and timeless image. They are commonly chosen by individuals in formal or corporate settings. Metal frames with intricate designs, or engraved details, can add an element of elegance and sophistication to your appearance. Contemporary metal frames often incorporate modern design elements and materials, creating a fashionable and up-to-date style. If you prefer a subtle and unobtrusive look, metal frames can blend seamlessly with your facial features, drawing less attention to your eyewear.

Combine the durability of metal with the design versatility of plastic. Offer a unique and stylish look. Combination frames, which feature both plastic and metal elements, offer a unique and stylish choice that combines the best of both materials. These frames often feature metal temples (arms) and plastic fronts (the part surrounding the lenses) or vice versa. Combination frames provide a versatile and distinctive look that can be both modern and stylish. The mix of materials allows for creative design possibilities.

Cosmetic Values Associated with Lens Dispensing

The cosmetic values associated with spectacle lens dispensing go beyond vision correction. They encompass style, personal expression, self-confidence, and the enhancement of one's overall appearance. Choosing the right lens can have a significant impact on how you are perceived and how you feel about yourself when wearing glasses. Both the material and design of spectacle lenses play crucial roles in affecting the cosmetic values associated with wearing spectacles.

The choice of lens material affects the thickness and weight of the lenses. Thinner and lighter lens materials, such as high-index materials, reduce lens thickness, making the lenses more cosmetically appealing, especially for individuals with strong prescriptions.

Thicker lenses, often associated with lower-index materials, can result in a "Coke-bottle" effect, making the eyes appear magnified or minimized. High-index materials can minimize this effect, contributing to a more natural appearance.

Chapter 3: Mechanical Optics, Lenses and Lens Prescription

The shape of the lenses can impact the wearer's cosmetic appearance. Progressive lenses, which provide seamless vision correction for near, intermediate, and distance vision, have a no-line design, avoiding the cosmetic drawback of visible bifocal or trifocal lines.

Applying anti-reflective (AR) coatings to the lenses can improve cosmetic values by reducing glare and reflections on the lens surfaces. This not only enhances the wearer's vision but also makes the lenses less distracting to others.

Lens design includes options for tinting which can affect the cosmetic appearance of eyeglasses. Tints can be used for cosmetic purposes, like adding a fashionable color to the lenses.

Some advanced lens designs, such as digitally surfaced lenses, can be customized to the frame shape and wearer's facial features, optimizing cosmetics by reducing lens thickness.

The edge thickness of lenses, particularly in rimless or semi-rimless frames, is critical for aesthetics. Proper edge thinning or bevelling can create a sleek, polished look.

the flatter lens profile of aspheric lenses has made them increasingly popular among eyeglass wearers. They not only provide a wider field of clear vision but also offer cosmetic and comfort benefits, making them an attractive choice for those seeking both visual clarity and aesthetics in their eyeglasses.

Aspheric lenses are preferred for their ability to provide a more cosmetically appealing appearance.

The flatter profile of aspheric lenses helps minimize the "fishbowl effect," where the eyes appear magnified or diminished when viewed from the side.

Last but not the least, a well-fitted spectacle frame is essential for both aesthetics and functional performance.

Properly fitted frames ensure that the lenses are correctly positioned in front of your eyes, optimizing your field of vision and allowing you to see clearly without distortion or blurriness.

Frames that fit well distribute the weight of the glasses evenly across your nose and behind your ears. This minimizes pressure points and discomfort, making it more comfortable to wear your glasses throughout the day.

Frames that fit well not only feel comfortable but also look better on your face. Ill-fitting frames can appear crooked or uneven, detracting from your overall appearance.

In today's modern world the value of cosmetic look plays a significant role in many aspects of life. The emphasis on appearance and personal style has increased due to various factors including social media, celebrity culture and widespread availability of fashion and beauty content. Personal branding has become crucial particularly for entrepreneurs, influencers and public figures. The overall impact is that a good balance between functionality and cosmetics while spectacle dispensing cannot be avoided.

MEASUREMENT FOR ORDERING SPECTACLES: IPD AND VD

When ordering prescription eyeglasses, two important measurements are IPD, i.e., interpupillary distance and VD, i.e., vertex distance. These measurements ensure that the spectacle lenses are well centerd and the prescription power of lens is determined based on required vertex distance.

INTERPUPILLARY DISTANCE

Pupillary distance is the measure of distance between the center of the pupil of one eye to the center of the pupil of the other eye measured in millimetres as shown in **Figure 3.59**. It can also be measured from outer limbus edge of one eye to the inner limbus edge of other eye as shown in **Figure 3.60**.

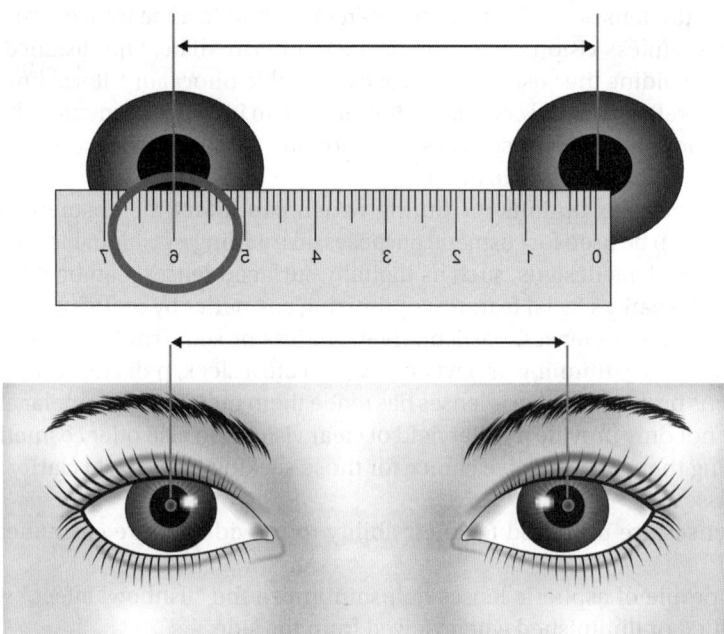

Fig. 3.59: Anatomical IPD.

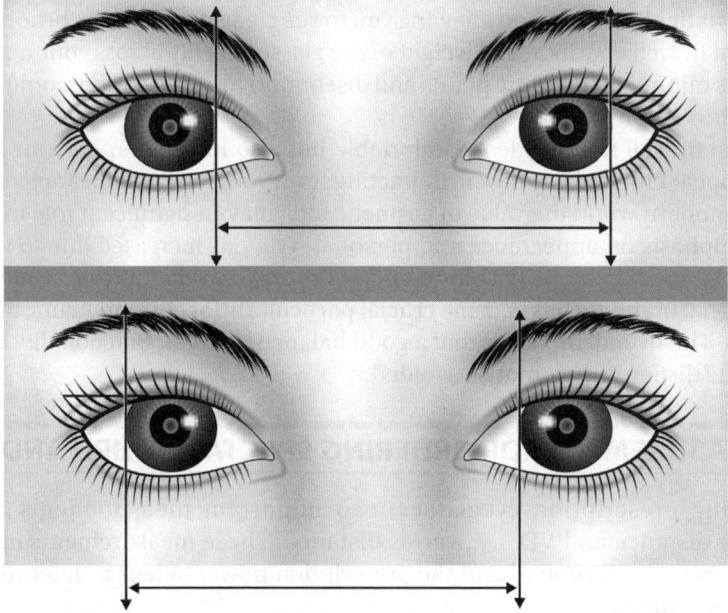

Fig. 3.60: Measuring IPD from limbus to limbus.

Since pupil is displaced 0.3 mm nasally, limbal measure will be approximately 0.5 mm greater than the measure found using pupil center. The measurement of pupillary distance varies with the gaze angle of the patient. When a person looks at closer distance, his eyes turn in towards each other. As he lifts his eyes to look at longer distance the two eyes move away from each other. Pupillary distance for distance vision is measured when the patient looks in the straight ahead gaze direction when the eyes look at infinity and pupillary distance for near viewing gaze is measured when the patient looks at a distance of 40 cm. For this reason IPD for distance viewing angle is larger than IPD for near viewing angle. The amount of difference may vary between 4 and 5 mm. Digital pupillometer is used to take papillary distance measurement. Most pupillometer measures the IPD taking the geometrical center of the pupil as reference point. Essilor pupillometer uses the corneal reflex as reference. The vertical hairline is aligned to the center of the corneal reflex. An internal light source produces an image by reflection on each cornea, and the vertical line within the device is moved until coincided with the corneal reflex. The measurement so taken is assumed to correspond to the subject's line of sight. The line of sight is defined as a line passing through the center of the pupil to the object of regard. This is the line that desirably passes through the optical center of the lenses and is the basis upon which the measurement of IPD rests. The advantage of using pupillometer is the measurements taken are not subject to parallax errors. The sequential procedure of using pupillometer is as under:

- Dispenser and the patient should be at the same level.
- Take distance IPD monocularly and near IPD binocularly. Set the viewing distance 40–50 cm for near PD measurement and infinity for distance PD measurement using viewing distance adjustment lever.
- Hold the pupillometer from the dispenser side and put the forehead rest against the forehead of the patient with rubber removable pads on nose. You may ask the patient to hold the instrument for support.
- Ask the patient to keep both eyes open.
- For monocular distance PD use the eye occluding lever to occlude LE first to measure RE pupillary distance and then RE to measure the LE pupillary distance.
- Ask the client to focus on the target light and move the left or right eye monocular PD adjustment lever, to align the centric line with the corneal reflex.
- When measurement is over, all measurement would appear on the digital display. The result of monocular distance PD and total distance will automatically be recorded on the instrument.

VERTEX DISTANCE MEASUREMENT

Vertex distance is the distance between the front surface of the cornea and the back surface of the eyeglass lens. It is also measured in millimeters (mm). VD is crucial because the prescription power of the lens depends on this distance. When the VD changes, it can affect the effective power of the lens. Typically, eyeglass prescriptions are written for a standard vertex distance of 12 millimeters, which is an average distance between the front of the eye and the back surface of the lens. However, in some cases, the actual VD may differ, and adjustments may be needed to ensure the correct prescription power.

Digital device like visio-office takes this measurement automatically. In the absence of visio-office simple millimetre ruler as shown in the **Figure 3.61** can be used.

The process is very simple. Put the frame on the patient's eyes and ask the patient to turn his face sideways. Place the scale next to the frame and measure the distance from the front of the cornea to the back surface of the lens as shown in the **Figure 3.62**.

The vertex distance, which is measured in millimeters, serves as the reference for positioning the front of the frame on the face.

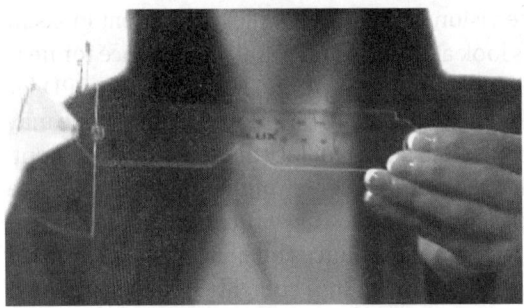

Fig. 3.61: Millimetre ruler.   Fig. 3.62: Measuring vertex distance.

Flowchart 3.16: Special dispensing measurements.

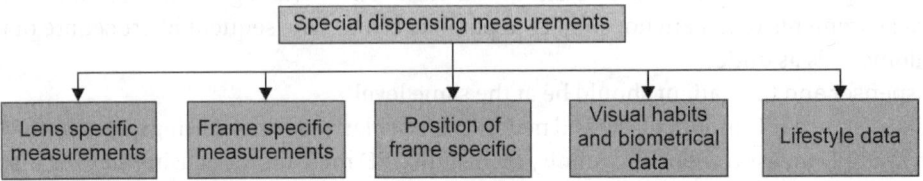

SPECIAL MEASUREMENT FOR FITTING SPECIAL TYPES OF LENSES

Fitting special types of spectacle lenses often requires additional measurements and considerations beyond the standard measurements taken for regular eyeglasses. These specialized measurements help ensure that the lenses are tailored to the individual's unique visual needs and specific requirements. The list of measurements for fitting specialty spectacle lenses is not static and can evolve as new lens technologies and designs are developed. Advances in optics, materials, and digital technology continue to drive innovation in eyewear. As a result, new types of specialty lenses with unique features may indeed introduce new measurements or considerations for dispensing. Eye care professionals, such as optometrists and opticians, are continually incorporating new measurements into their practice to incorporate the latest advancements in eyewear. They receive training and stay updated on new lens options to ensure they can provide the best possible solutions for their patients' changing needs.

The current list of special measurements includes several new measurements that can be grouped under four broad categories as shown in **Flowchart 3.16**.

SPECIAL DISPENSING MEASUREMENTS

Lens Specific Measurements

These measurements pertain directly to the characteristics of the lenses and their optical properties. In addition to the interpupillary distance and fitting height it includes four other measurements as shown in **Flowchart 3.17**.

Base Curve

Base curve is the curve from where the other curves of the lens are determined. It is an important measurement for lens designing as it determines a balance between optics and cosmetics of the lenses. It is measured on the front surface of the lens while taking other dispensing measurements using Geneva lens measure watch.

Flowchart 3.17: Lens specific measurements.

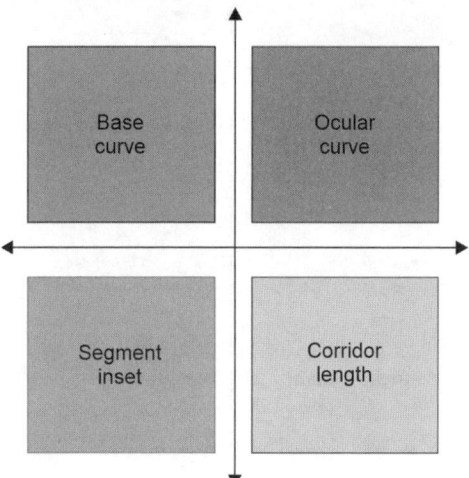

Ocular Curve

Ocular curve is the curve of the back surface of the lens. It is important measurement in high lens prescription as it affects vertex distance and effective lens power. It is also measured using Geneva lens measure watch. An incorrect ocular curve measurement can lead to visual discomfort, including issues like poor vision and/or difficulties in adapting to the new eyeglasses.

Segment Inset

Segment inset is particular important for round shape bifocal lenses as the position of the near segment is important for near vision for the line of sight to pass through the center of the near segment. When the near segment of a bifocal lens is correctly inset, it ensures that the wearer has an equal and balanced field of clear vision in either side of gaze in the horizontal direction.

Corridor Length

The corridor length in a progressive lens refers to the vertical distance or area within the lens which determines the position of near viewing zone within the frame to the allow the wearer clear and comfortable near vision. It is the portion of the lens that progressively changes from the distance prescription to the near addition power. A properly selected corridor length ensures that the wearer can read and perform close-up tasks with ease and accuracy.

Frame Specific Measurements

These measurements focus on the eyeglass frame itself and its compatibility with the lenses. These measurements are shown in **Flowchart 3.18**.

A Measurement

The "A" measurement in frame sizing typically refers to the horizontal lens width. It is an important measurement that helps determine the size of the lenses. Specifically, the "A" measurement represents the width of each individual lens from one edge to the other, excluding the frame's thickness. 'A' measurement is essential for ensuring that the eyeglasses not only

Flowchart 3.18: Frame specific measurements.

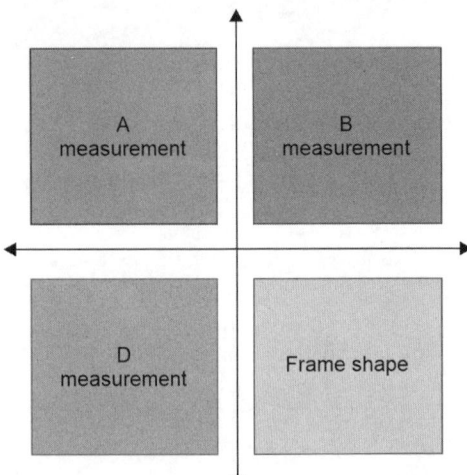

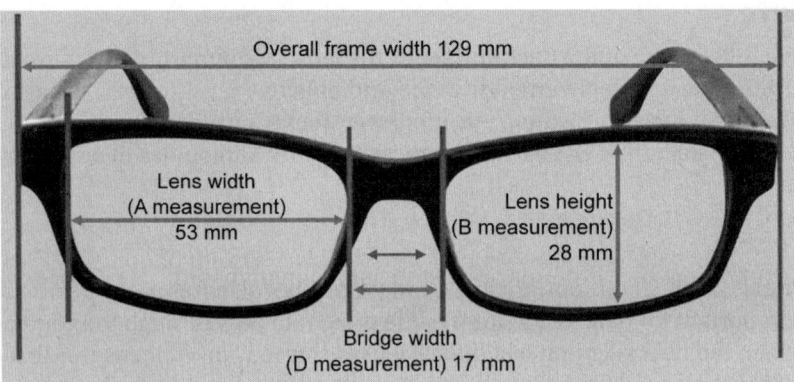

Fig. 3.63: A Measurement, B Measurement and D Measurement of the frame.

provide wider field of clear vision but also fit comfortably, look aesthetically pleasing, and meet the wearer's specific needs, including their prescription requirements and lifestyle **(Fig. 3.63)**.

B Measurement

The "B" measurement in frame sizing typically refers to the vertical lens height. It represents the distance from the top to the bottom of each lens in a pair of eyeglasses or sunglasses. Like the "A" measurement, the "B" measurement is expressed in millimeters (mm) and is an essential factor in determining the size and fit of the lenses in a frame.

D Measurement

The "D" measurement in eyeglass frame sizing, often referred to as the "DBL" (Distance Between Lenses), is critical because it directly affects the fit, comfort, and visual performance of the eyeglasses. This measurement represents the distance between the centers of the lenses. "D" measurement helps align the lenses with the wearer's pupils. This alignment is essential for maintaining optical clarity and ensuring that the wearer's gaze passes through the center of the lenses, minimizing distortions and visual discomfort.

Frame Shape

The frame shape plays a crucial role in determining how the lenses are positioned in front of the wearer's eyes. Accurate lens positioning is essential for optimal visual performance. It ensures that the optical centers of the lenses align correctly with the wearer's pupils, reducing distortions and maximizing clarity.

Position of Frame Specific Measurements

These measurements determine the precise positioning of the frame and lenses on the wearer's face. They are crucial for optical performance and comfort. They are shown in **Flowchart 3.19**.

Pantoscopic Tilt

Pantoscopic tilt is an important consideration in eyeglass lens design because it affects both the visual performance and wearer's comfort. Pantoscopic tilt refers to the angle at which the front of the frame tilts downward or upward in relation to the wearer's face **(Fig. 3.64)**. It plays a significant role in lens design and fitting of frame. Pantoscopic tilt influences the positioning of the lenses in front of the wearer's eyes. The angle at which the lenses are oriented can affect the optical center alignment, helps optimize the visual experience, and can affect the effective lens power perceived by the wearer, especially in progressive lenses.

Face Form Wrap

Face form wrap, also known as wrap angle or face form angle, refers to the curvature or angle of the frame as it wraps around the wearer's face **(Fig. 3.65)**. It affects lens design and eyeglass fitting on wearer's face. The following points of consideration are important to understand the effect of face form wrap:

* Frames with a significant face form wrap can provide better coverage and protection for the eyes, particularly against glare, wind, and dust. This wrap-around design can enhance peripheral vision by reducing side glare and light intrusion.

Flowchart 3.19: Position of frame specific measurements.

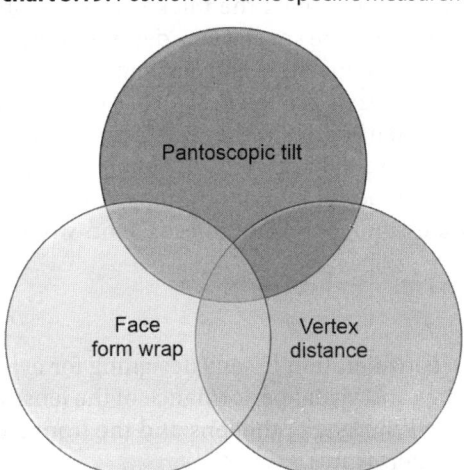

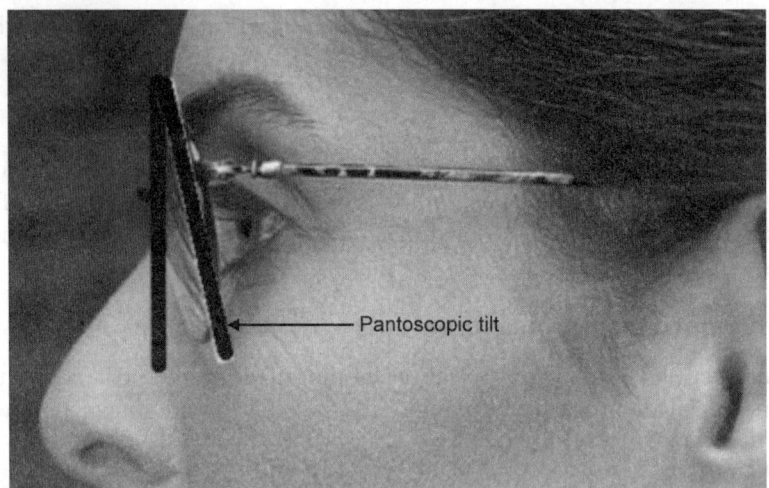

Fig. 3.64: Pantoscopic tilt.

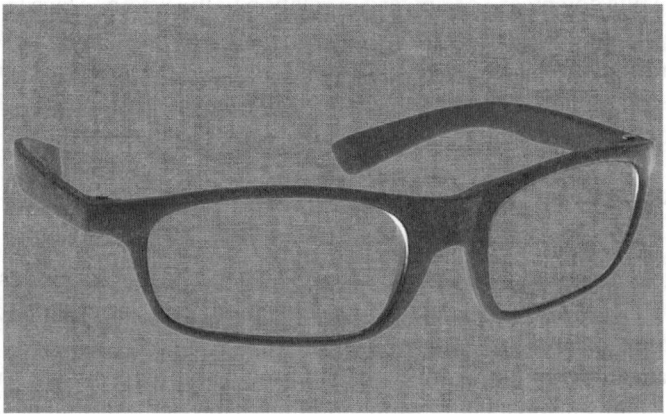

Fig. 3.65: Face form wrap.

- The angle of the frame wrap can impact the thickness of the prescription lenses. Frames with a strong wrap angle may require special lens designs or materials to accommodate the curvature, which can affect lens thickness and aesthetics.
- The face form wrap angle is closely related to the base curve of the lenses. The base curve refers to the curvature of the lens itself. Frames with a pronounced wrap angle often require lenses with a specific base curve to fit properly and maintain optical clarity.
- The wrap angle can increase peripheral aberrations, including spherical aberration and astigmatism. Eyecare professionals consider these factors when designing lenses for wrap-around frames.

Vertex Distance

Vertex distance is a crucial consideration in lens designing for eyeglasses because it directly impacts the optical properties and visual performance of the lenses. Vertex distance refers to the distance between the back surface of the lens and the front surface of the wearer's eye, typically measured in millimeters (mm).

The vertex distance affects the effective power of the lens as experienced by the wearer. Lenses are designed and prescribed to provide their specified power at a specific vertex distance. Deviations from this distance can result in a change in the perceived lens power. Errors in vertex distance measurement can lead to suboptimal vision correction, potentially causing eyestrain, headaches, or reduced visual clarity. Vertex distance considerations are essential for individuals with presbyopia, an age-related condition that affects near vision. Proper vertex distance ensures that progressive or multifocal lenses provide the intended near vision correction.

Visual Habits and Biometrical Data

These measurements take into account the wearer's visual habits and individual ocular characteristics **(Flowchart 3.20):**

Dominant Eye

In a binocular vision system, the dominant eye is an important role in vision particularly in situations that require binocular vision and depth perception.

The dominant eye is typically responsible for central vision tasks, such as fixating, focusing and reading. It is crucial for identifying details in the center of the visual field. It provides the clearest and most detailed view of objects that are directly in front of the viewer. When it is paired with the other eye which may be called non-dominant eye it helps to provide depth perception or stereopsis. This helps individuals judge distances and perceive the three-dimensional nature of objects in their surroundings. When both eyes send slightly different images to the brain, there can be some visual confusion or overlap of images. The dominant eye's image takes precedence in the brain's processing, reducing the potential for visual conflicts.

When reading or performing near tasks, such as using a computer or crafting, the dominant eye is more actively engaged in providing clear, close-up vision. This is because saccades are important for reading and every saccade starts with fixation which is the primary function of dominant eye. A well-coordinated interplay between the dominant and non-dominant eye is essential for comfortable and efficient reading. When the dominant eye accurately establishes the point of fixation, it allows for clear and stable vision, reducing visual fatigue and improving

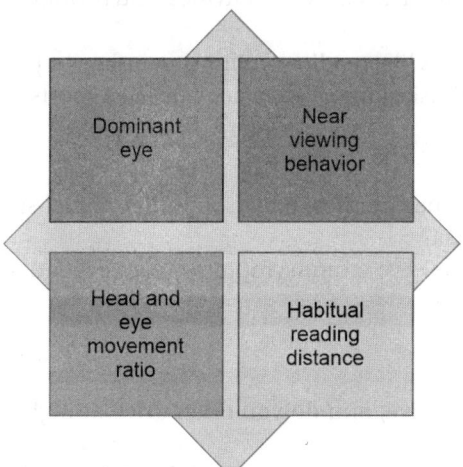

Flowchart 3.20: Visual habits and biometric data.

reading comprehension. Binocular vision ensures that the eyes move in harmony and that the images from both eyes are seamlessly combined in the brain to create a single, coherent visual perception.

Opticians and eyecare professionals use this information to optimize eyeglass prescriptions, lens designs, or visual training techniques to enhance the reading experience for individuals.

Near Viewing Behavior

"Near viewing behavior" typically refers to the visual and physical behaviors people exhibit when looking at objects or text up close, such as when reading a book or using a computer. This behavior can include a variety of actions and responses by the eyes and the body to focus on and process information at a close distance. Understanding and optimizing near viewing behavior is important for maintaining visual comfort and preventing eye strain, especially in a digital age where many people spend a significant amount of time engaged in activities that require close-up vision. Some of the examples of near viewing behavior are head and eye movement ratio; reading distance, gaze angle, lateral offset, etc.

Lifestyle Data

Lifestyle data consider the wearer's lifestyle and specific needs and involves assessing the relative visual demands between distance, near and intermediate viewing zones. Predefined set of questions pertaining to occupation and leisure time activities together with hobbies and habits are asked. The process aims to match the optics of the lens design to wearer's lifestyle. The immediate advantage is noticed as reduced number of dissatisfaction as primary occupational needs is not immediately affected that minimizes the levels of frustration. The following questions may be considered:

Occupation and Work Habits

- What is your occupation, and what are your typical visual tasks at work?
- Do you spend a significant amount of time working on a computer or other digital devices?
- Are you frequently involved in detailed or fine-print tasks at work?

Hobbies and Leisure Activities

- What are your favorite hobbies or leisure activities, and do they involve close-up or distance vision?
- Do you engage in activities like reading, crafting, painting, or playing musical instruments?
- Are you an outdoor enthusiast involved in activities like sports, hiking, or biking?

Digital Device Usage

- How often do you use smartphones, tablets, or other digital screens for tasks like texting, browsing, or social media?
- Do you experience digital eye strain symptoms (e.g., eye fatigue, headaches) after using digital devices?

Driving Habits

- How frequently do you drive, and do you often drive at night or in challenging weather conditions?
- Are you comfortable with your current glasses while driving, or do you encounter difficulties?

Reading Habits

❖ Do you read extensively, and if so, what type of reading material (books, newspapers, and digital screens) do you prefer?
❖ What is your preferred reading posture and distance?

Indoor and Outdoor Activities

❖ Are you more active indoors or outdoors, and what types of environments do you frequent?
❖ Do you need eyewear for both indoor and outdoor use?

FITTING OF LENSES IN VARIOUS TYPES OF FRAMES

Inserting lenses into frames is an art and it needs proper tools and equipment. The optician needs to have a complete working table and a trained fitter who can consistently perform the job. The working table should be fully equipped with all tools and equipment needed for lens insertion and other necessary materials used during fitting procedures. Spectacles frame warmers, screwdrivers, nut drivers, a set of specially designed pliers, vice, polishers, files, flat top platform, ultrasonic cleaners, stress tester and pad popper are some of the basic tools and equipment needed. In addition, there are some consumables that should also be always available readily. Bonding agents, loose screw set, spare nose pads, nylon threads, nail polish and edge markers are common amongst them.

LENS INSERTION INTO ZYL FRAMES

Arrange heating unit, a bowl filled with water, a set of screwdrivers, a wiping cloth and tissue papers on a working table with adequate light on top.

Now you are ready for inserting the lens into the frame front **(Fig. 3.66)**. Before you apply heat to the frame front, hold the lens in your hand at an angle and position that allows you to insert the lens immediately on heating. This is important to ensure minimum time lag after the frame is heated because zyl frames cool very rapidly and lose their pliability instantly.

If the lens curvature is more than the eyewire curve, it is advisable to apply little heat and reshape the upper and lower sections of the eyewire so that it conforms to the meniscus of the lens edge.

Now apply uniform heat to the eyewire from all around and make sure that the thicker portions, i.e., nasal and temporal eyewires are heated little more. Care should be taken to heat both the front and back of the eyewire alternately to avoid overheating while using air blower. The salt bath contains two components—salt and talcum powder. Salt conveys heat while talcum powder prevents salt from lumping and sticking to the frame. When the salt pan is used, make sure that you stir the salt to equalize the temperature and then push some of the salt into a mound in one portion of the pan. Place the section of the frame to be heated just beneath the salt mound as parallel to the surface of the salt as possible. Remember to place only the section that is to be heated, leaving the rest out of the salt. Move the frame continuously and very slowly while under the salt to avoid salt granule sticking to dry frame. If salt sticks to a dry frame, additional talcum powder should be added to the salt. If you are using warm heater, keep moving the frame front in such a manner that the heat is applied to back, front and entire eyewire uniformly. Keep checking the pliability of the eyewire by curving the eyewire to prevent overheating.

Now push the lens into the front eyewire. Insert the temporal edge of the lens into the inner edge of the frame from the back. Keeping the thumbs on the back surface of the lens and

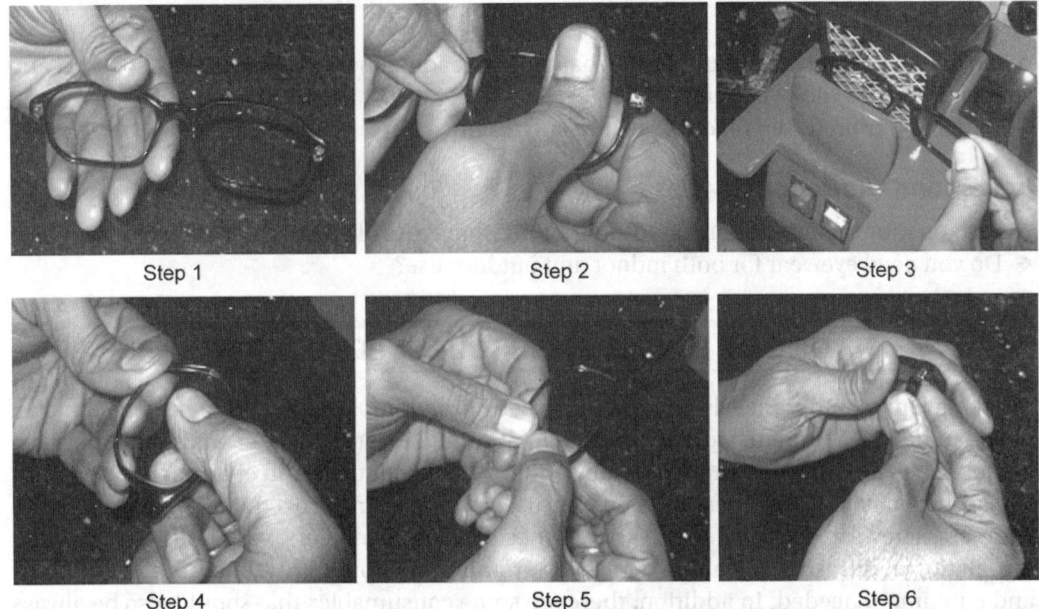

Fig. 3.66: Sequential steps for lens insertion in plastic frame.

fingers on the nasal edge of the frame eyewire, snap the lens into the frame from the nasal side by pressure of both thumbs and fingers. If the frame has pads, take care not to bend or break it. Alternately, insert the upper temporal edge of the lens into the frame groove from the front, then push the lens holding it from the nasal edge into the eyewire so that the entire edge of the lens is in the frame.

Finally, pull the lower portion of the eyewire around the lower lens edges. After inserting the lenses into the frame, plunge the frame and lenses into ice water to "set" them except when the frame material is optyl, as this can have exactly the opposite effect on lens tightness.

The following care must be taken while inserting the lens into the frame:
- Make sure that there are no marks made by the lens against the softened plastic or by undue stretching of the plastic.
- If the frame cools down before the lens is inserted fully, it is advisable to remove the lens totally before reheating the frame.
- While pulling the eyewire, care must be taken that your pulling force is straight and make sure that the eyewires are not rolled out. The rolling of the eyewire will turn the groove at an angle, and will spoil the front appearance of the frame. A rolled eyewire does not secure the lens tightly that results in constant complain of lens falling out of the frame front.
- If the lower eyewire is rolled forward, i.e., front side is slanted down and in spite of all attempts to straighten it, it still remains a problem, reinsert the lens from back side of the frame.

LENS INSERTION INTO SUPRA FRAMES

Nylon monofilament cord is used to secure lenses to semi-rimless chassis. In order to fit the lens, the cord is attached to the mounting arm.

A groove is cut into the lens edge. This groove is the channel into which the monofilament cord is fitted **(Fig. 3.67)**.

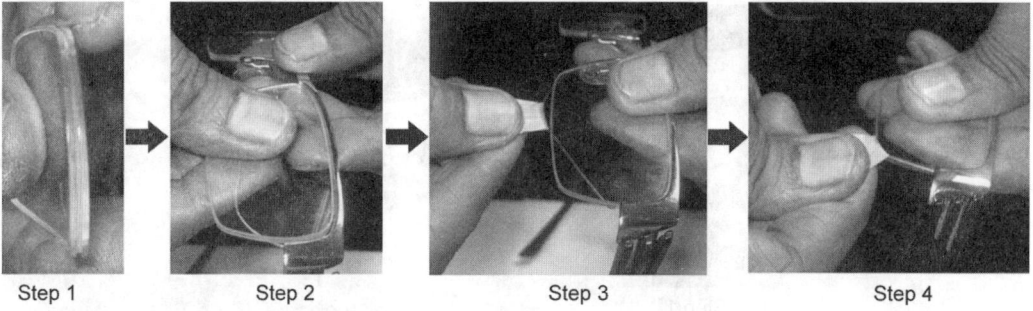

Fig. 3.67: Sequential steps for lens insertion in supra frame.

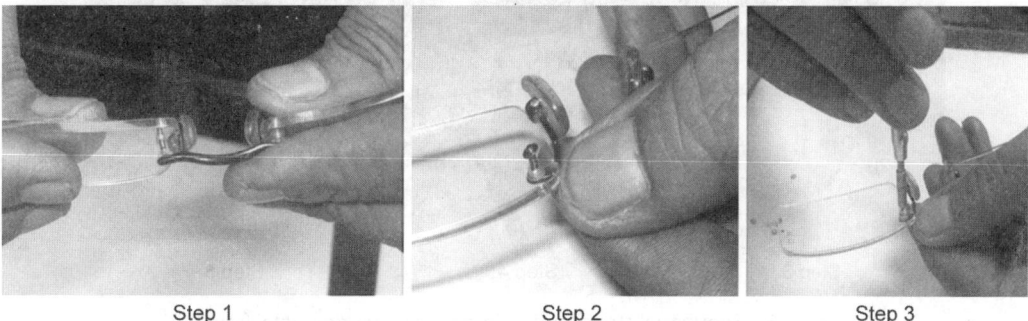

Fig. 3.68: Sequential steps for lens insertion in screw mounting rimless frame.

The lens is inserted into the loop created by the monofilament cord using a ribbon to pull the line around the lens circumference. They secure the lenses completely around like a rim but without dealing with screws, hex nuts, filing, messy glues or special riveting tools and mounting pins.

The cord is susceptible to temperature change and can shrink over time and snap, but it can be easily changed.

LENS INSERTION INTO RIMLESS FRAMES

Rimless frames are designed with no eyewire surrounding the lenses. Lenses are suspended and secured using several mounting methods including screws and hex nuts, fixing pins, bushing and cementing.

The mounting of lenses using screws and nuts begins with drilling holes through the lenses and then follows the following process **(Fig. 3.68)**.
- First lens is placed on the mounting.
- Screws are inserted through each hole.
- Nuts are used to secure the lens in place.
- This process is repeated for the second lens.
- Excess screw length is cut away with cutter pliers and filed smooth.
- A plastic washer may be used under the screw's head to cushion the pressure on the lens front and a plastic bushing may be used around the screw for the same purpose laterally.

LENS INSERTION INTO FULL-RIM METAL FRAMES

Before inserting the lenses into metal frame make sure that meniscus curve of the top and bottom of the lens matches to the upper and lower eyewire of the frame front **(Fig. 3.69)**.

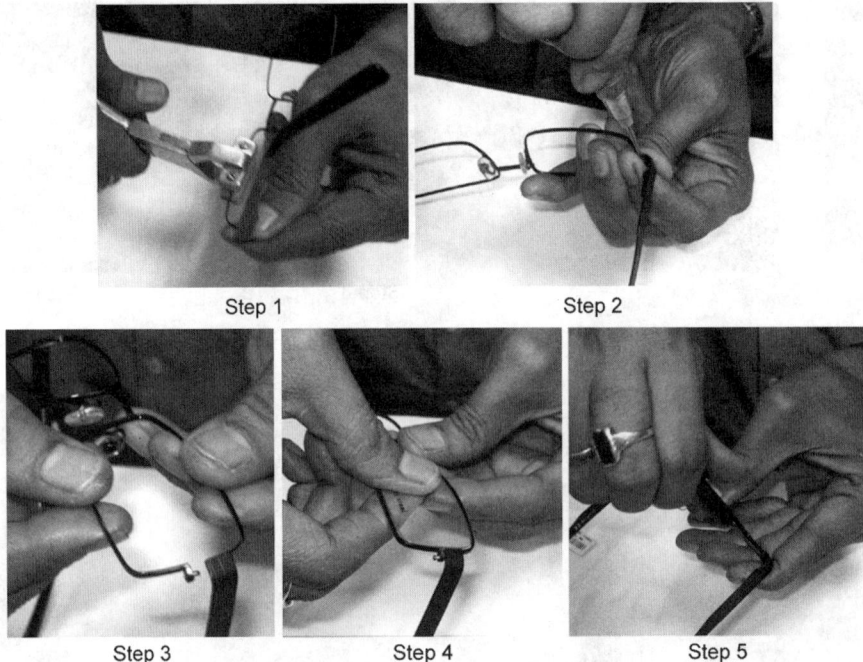

Fig. 3.69: Sequential steps for lens insertion in full-rim metal frame.

If there is any mismatch the lens will not fit squarely in the eyewire groove. It means using eyewire forming pliers to reshape the eyewire rim is important.

Now remove the eyewire screws completely, put the lens within the eyewire and replace the eyewire.

Do not simply loosen the screws and put the lenses. It may cause lens chipping.

SPECTACLES INTOLERANCE

Often in the practice, it has been seen that there are occasional unhappy patient returning to the practice and complaining of discomfort with their new spectacle. Discomfort is a condition characterized by episodic or persistent adverse sensations related to spectacle wear, either with or without visual disturbance, resulting from reduced compatibility between the spectacle and the visual system which can lead to intolerance, unusual feelings, and discontinuation of spectacle wear. Spectacle related discomfort is the subjective experience of the patient that the patient feels while using his new spectacle, makes him uncomfortable to use or incapacitates him to perform certain tasks. In essence, it creates non-tolerance to spectacle and implies that patient is a symptomatic patient. The reasons for intolerance to spectacle may be many—some may be because of the practitioners, some may be because of optician and some may be patient himself.

REASONS FOR INTOLERANCE

Intolerance Because of Patient Himself

This intolerance can be influenced by a combination of psychological and physiological factors of the wearer himself.

Psychological

The psychological reasons for discomfort with spectacle arise from the inter-relationship of the personality of the patient. Fatigue, stress and headaches are part of everyday life and elements of dissatisfaction are certainly present when desirable performance is not achieved. However, there are situations when it has been observed that symptoms do not appear in proportion to the intensity with which they have been presented. It varies from individual to individual in the most surprising manner without any reason. The explanation to many such cases lies in the fact that it is the individual who is purposive or resolute rather than his eyes.

Intensity of new experience, consciousness about new glasses and lack of initial confidence and attitude to pinpoint the smallest defect in the glasses may contribute to headache. This is a difficult situation to manage as they strongly believe that their discomfort is because of new lenses. A professional optician must also be prepared to solve such problems on daily basis that may occasionally defy logic and require enormous patience. Some of the patients are very apprehensive about the performance of their new spectacle and in the process, they try and find deficiencies and attribute the reason to their new spectacle.

It is not uncommon for some people to have a negative reaction to wearing new glasses, even after they have been accurately prescribed and made to fit. This reaction can be influenced by various factors, and as a result, individuals may try to find faults or express dissatisfaction. Negative emotions, stress, or anxiety can exacerbate negative reactions to new glasses. People may focus on any minor discomfort or inconvenience, magnifying their dissatisfaction.

Physiological

- Accommodative dysfunction may cause intermittent blur vision at distance. It may be momentary when the person looks up from his work or it may last several hours after near work, causing difficulties driving home from work.
- The patient may have undiagnosed anomalies of muscle balance. Horizontal phoria may cause ocular fatigue, double vision and pulling sensation in the eyes. This is because eyes need to make extramuscular effort to maintain the fusion. The first time wearer of low degree ametropia may feel pulling sensation in their eyes. This is usually short-lived as the eyes struggle to adjust with the new correction during the initial days of use.
- Vertical phoria may be induced which may cause light sensitivity, difficulties with glare and reflection. In some cases, a binocular vision disorder may also result in light sensitivity and glare.
- The sensitivity to glare is amplified because of light scattering within the eyes because of changes in the optical media.
- Aniseikonia is often associated with Anisometropia which is still somewhat difficult to assess. Anisometropic correction may lead to unusual spatial orientation.
- Dry eyes may also cause intermittent blurred vision at near viewing distance.
- The patient's ocular condition may be such in which it is inherently difficult to correct the vision with spectacle.
- In the higher degree of ametropia even the best form lens does not entirely eliminate their disadvantages—optical, physical or cosmetic.

Intolerance Because of Practitioner

- The prescriber may have prescribed the correction incorrectly in one or both eye.
- The prescriber may prescribe near addition without considering his habitual reading distance which may result either under correction or over correction of near addition.

- The prescriber may prescribe high lens power suddenly to a patient who has never used any correction before.
- The prescriber may introduce new cylinder correction to a non-symptomatic patient.
- The prescriber may avoid prescribing prism correction just because of his ignorance.
- The prescriber may have forgotten to check the habitual correction because of which he changed the correction significantly.
- The prescriber may not spend sufficient time to explain for adaptation needed for new correction.

Intolerance Because of Optician

The dispensing of spectacles is occasionally at fault and may be responsible for some cases of intolerance. This may related solely to the frame or other aspect of the fitting as well as for lenses.
- Change in pantoscopic angle of the frame
- Change in face form wrap especially in minus lens prescription
- Change in nose pad adjustment, causing change in vertex distance
- Significant mismatch between temple widths of the frame as compare to facial width
- Improper side bend
- Incorrect frame shape and size selection
- Change in base curve, causing change in lens form
- Incorrect measurement of pupillary distance
- Ignoring the fitting height while positioning the optical center of lens
- Incorrect fitting height in case of progressive lenses
- Incorrect selection of corridor length of progressive lenses
- Change in lens tint from tinted to clear or vice versa for no reason
- A difference in the base curve in two eyes of approximately equal refraction

SPECIAL TYPES OF SPECTACLES

There are various special types of spectacles designed to address specific visual needs and preferences. These specialized eyeglasses can enhance vision and comfort for individuals with particular requirements. These are task specific spectacles and are used for specific purpose only.

TASK SPECIFIC SPECTACLES

Clip-on Spectacles

Clip-on spectacles, also known as clip-on sunglasses or clip-on eyeglass attachments, are a convenient and versatile eyewear accessory. These clip-on attachments are designed to be added to existing prescription eyeglasses or reading glasses, providing sun protection or additional functionality without the need for a separate spectacle or sunglass **(Fig. 3.70)**.

Flip-up Spectacles

Flip-up spectacles, also known as flip-up sunglasses or flip-up reading glasses, are eyewear that combines the functionality of regular eyeglasses with the convenience of easily attachable, flip-up tinted or magnifying lenses **(Fig. 3.71)**. These glasses are designed to provide versatility, allowing wearers to switch between clear vision for indoor use and tinted or magnified vision for outdoor or specific tasks without the need for multiple pairs of glasses.

Folding Frames

Folding spectacle frames, also known as foldable or collapsible frames, are eyeglass frames designed with a unique hinge mechanism that allows the frames to be folded into a compact and portable size **(Fig. 3.72)**. These frames are especially popular for individuals who require prescription eyeglasses and want the convenience of easily stowing them away when not in use.

Hearing Aid Frames

Hearing aid frames, also known as hearing aid eyeglass frames or eyeglass-compatible hearing aids, are specialized eyewear designed to integrate hearing aids seamlessly into eyeglass frames **(Fig. 3.73)**. These frames are particularly beneficial for individuals who require both hearing assistance and vision correction, offering a convenient and discreet solution.

Half-eye Spectacles

Half-eye spectacles **(Fig. 3.74)**, also known as half-eye reading glasses are primarily intended for reading or close-up tasks. Wearers can look over the lenses to see clearly in the distance, making them convenient for activities that involve switching between reading and looking at objects in the distance. These glasses come in various frame styles, materials, and colors, allowing wearers to choose options that match their personal style preferences and fashion sense.

Hemianopia Spectacles

Hemianopia spectacles, also known as hemianopic spectacles or hemianopic prism glasses, are specialized eyeglasses designed to assist individuals with hemianopia, a visual impairment characterized by the loss of vision in half of the visual field in one or both eyes **(Fig. 3.75)**. Hemianopia spectacles incorporate prism lenses to expand the visual field and compensate for the lost vision.

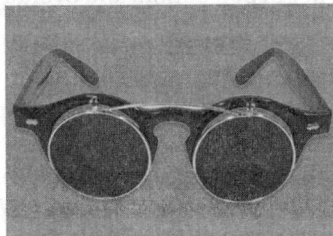
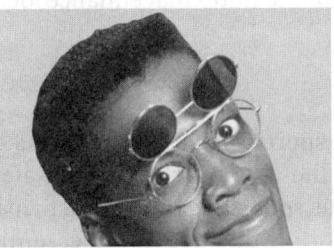
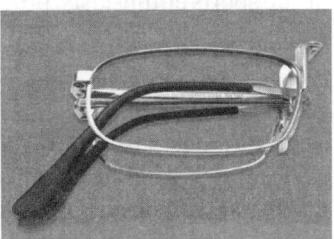

Fig. 3.70: Clip on spectacle frame.   **Fig. 3.71:** Fip-up spectacle frame.   **Fig. 3.72:** Folding frame.

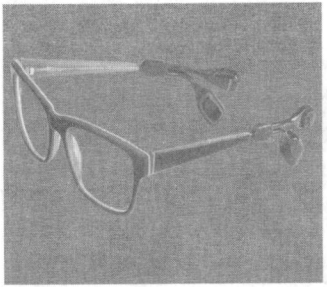
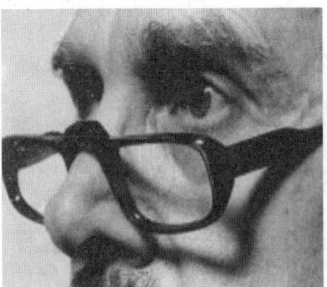
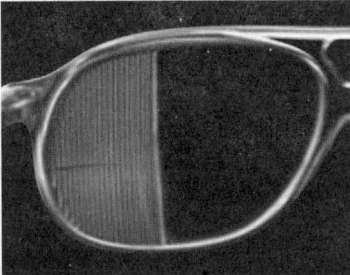

Fig. 3.73: Hearing aid frame.   **Fig. 3.74:** Half-eye frame.   **Fig. 3.75:** Hemianopia spectacles.

Pinhole Spectacles

Pinhole spectacles, also known as pinhole glasses or stenopaic glasses, are eyeglasses with multiple small, closely spaced pinhole-sized perforations or openings in the lenses **(Fig. 3.76)**. These specialized glasses are designed to improve visual clarity and reduce certain vision problems.

Ptosis Frames

Ptosis frames, also known as ptosis crutch glasses or ptosis eyelid props, are specialized eyeglasses designed to assist individuals who have ptosis, a condition characterized by drooping of the upper eyelid **(Fig. 3.77)**. Ptosis can affect one or both eyes and may be caused by various factors, including muscle weakness, nerve damage, or age-related changes. Ptosis frames provide support to lift and hold up the drooping eyelid so that the user can manage to see.

Recumbent Spectacles

Recumbent spectacles, also known as prism glasses for recumbent cycling or recumbent bike glasses are specialized eyeglasses designed for individuals who engage in recumbent cycling or other activities where the user is in a reclined or horizontal position. These glasses are unique in that they incorporate prism lenses that allow the wearer to maintain a comfortable head position while viewing the road or surroundings without straining their neck or tilting their head **(Fig. 3.78)**.

Billiard's Spectacle

Billiard's spectacles, also known as billiard glasses or snooker glasses, are specialized eyeglasses designed to optimize the vision and visual performance of individuals while playing cue sports such as billiards, snooker, or pool **(Fig. 3.79)**. These glasses are tailored to the specific needs of cue sports enthusiasts, providing features that enhance focus, depth perception, and overall game play.

Sports Frames

Sports frames, also known as sports eyeglasses or sports goggles, are specially designed eyewear designed to enhance the visual performance, safety, and comfort of athletes and active individuals during various sports and outdoor activities. These frames are engineered to withstand the rigors of sports while providing essential eye protection, clarity, and performance-enhancing features **(Fig. 3.80)**. Sports frames often feature a wraparound design that provides a snug fit around the face. This design enhances peripheral vision and minimizes

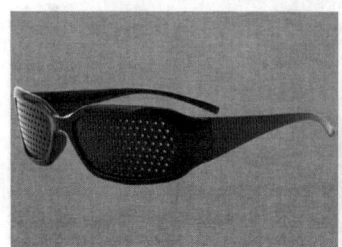
Fig. 3.76: Pinhole spectacle.

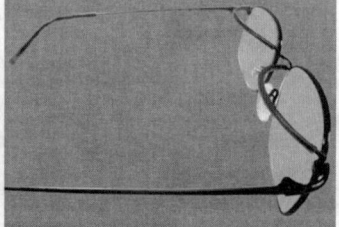
Fig. 3.77: Ptosis spectacle.

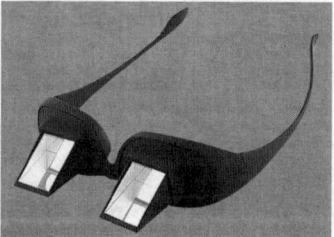
Fig. 3.78: Recumbent spectacles.

Chapter 3: Mechanical Optics, Lenses and Lens Prescription

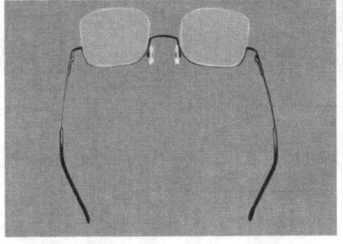
Fig. 3.79: Billiard's spectacle.

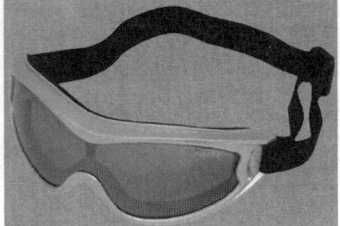
Fig. 3.80: Sports sunglass.

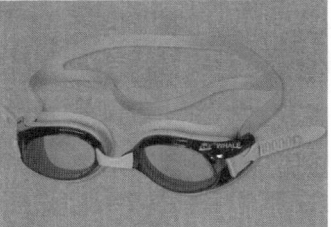
Fig. 3.81: Swimming sunglass.

wind and debris from entering the eyes, making them ideal for activities like cycling, skiing, or snowboarding. Some sports frame may also have ventilation systems that help reduce lens fogging and maintain comfort by allowing airflow around the eyes.

Swimming Sunglasses

Swimming sunglasses, also known as swim goggles with tinted lenses, are specialized eyewear designed for use in swimming and aquatic activities **(Fig. 3.81)**. These sunglasses provide eye protection from chlorine, saltwater, UV radiation, and other potential hazards in and around the water. They offer several features and benefits tailored to swimmers and water enthusiasts.

DISPENSING OF PRISMS AND PRISMATIC EFFECT OF LENS

PRISMATIC EFFECT OF LENS

The lenses are combination of multiple prisms—a convex lens is the combination of prisms placed base to base whereas a concave lens is the combination of prisms placed apex to apex as shown in **Figure 3.82**.

It implies that when the light passes through any point outside of its optical center, the effect of the prism will be noticed.

The prismatic effect of the lens typically causes light to bend towards the base of the prism, i.e., the thicker portion of the lens as shown in **Figure 3.83**. The straight forward understanding is that the accurate positioning of the optical center of the lens is obvious.

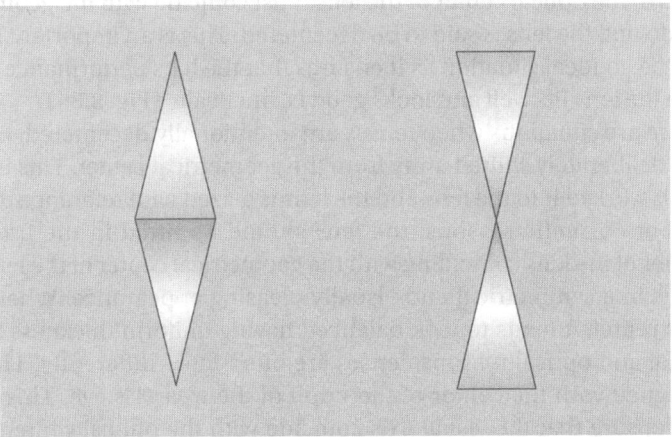
Fig. 3.82: Lenses are the combinations of various prism.

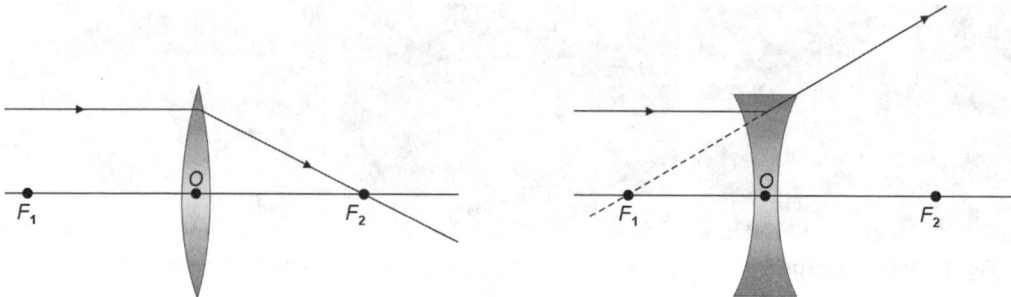

Fig. 3.83: Ray passing through any point outside of its optical center bends towards base of the prism.

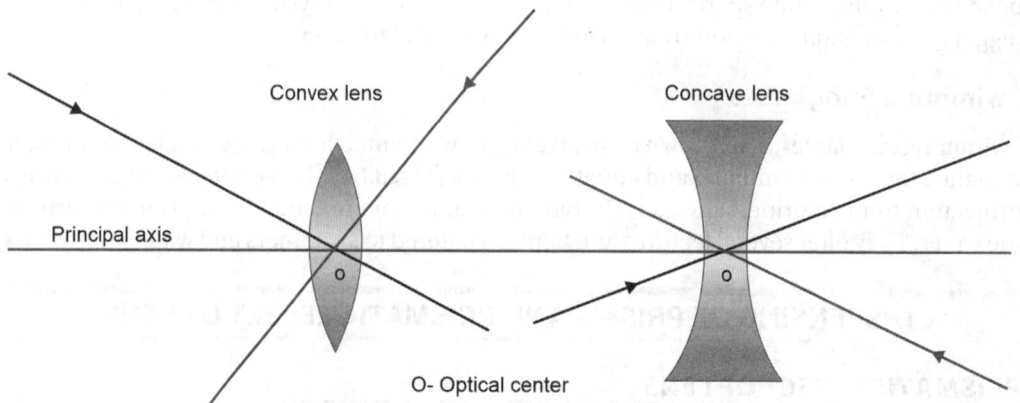

Fig. 3.84: Light passing through optical center does not deviate.

The optical center of the lens is the point in a lens where two principal meridians meet. The rays of light passing through optical center do not deviate **(Fig. 3.84)**.

It may coincide with the position of geometrical center of the lens or it may lie at any point other than geometrical center. The term 'geometrical center' of the lens typically refers to the point that is located at the exact middle of the lens and is often used as a reference point for various optical calculations for optical design and analysis.

In an uncut lens, the optical center of the lens must coincide with the geometrical center of the lens. If they do not, the lens is said to be decentered. This is an important relationship and is considered to be an ideal situation as it ensures that the lens performance is optimum and at the same time the lens fits well and looks good cosmetically **(Fig. 3.85)**.

However, there are situations when lenses are intentionally decentered, meaning that the optical center is deliberately shifted away from the geometrical center. This is often practiced when the prism is worked into the lens and the lens is glazed with reference to the decentered optical center. For cosmetic reasons, the lens should be fitted in the frame keeping the geometrical center of the lens coinciding with the geometrical center of the lens aperture. This alignment results in a symmetrical and visually pleasing appearance. When the lens aligns with the frame's center, it tends to look balanced having uniform thickness from all around. But for functional and optical reasons, lenses are often fitted differently. The optical center of the lens is aligned with the center of the pupil of the wearer's eye. This is an important arrangement to ensure that the visual axis coincide with the optical center of the lens. The visual axis is an imaginary line that connects the center of the pupil to the object being viewed

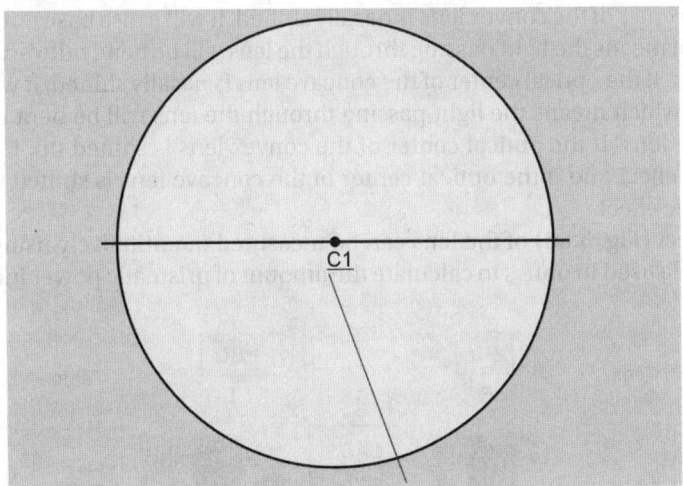

Fig. 3.85: Geometric center of lens.

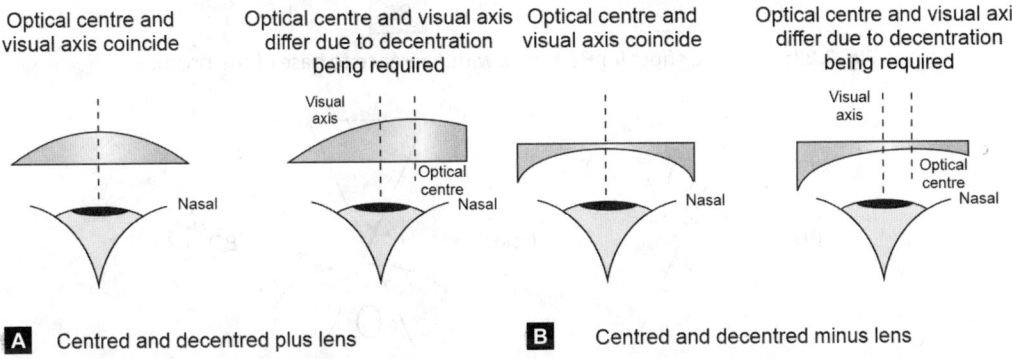

Figs. 3.86A and B: Visual axis coincides with the optical center of the lens.

(Figs. 3.86A and B). When the optical center of the lens coincides with the center of the pupil, the visual axis is also aligned with the lens's optical center. This alignment helps to ensure better and comfortable visual performance of the lens on wearer's eyes.

In practice, eyecare professionals follow lens fitting rituals and take measurements:
- Interpupillary distance of the wearer
- Fitting height

While the interpupillary distance measurement determines the horizontal position of the optical center of the lens into the frame, fitting height determines the vertical position. Using these two values they determine the position of the placement of optical center into the frame. This is done to ensure that the optical center of the lens lies just in front of the center of the pupil of the wearer so that rays of light passing through the optical axis of the lens can pass undeviated and the wearer can use the spectacle comfortably for a sustained period of time with optimum visual performance.

If there is any incongruency in the placement of optical center of the lens, it can affect how light will bend as it passes through the lens, resulting indifferent types of prismatic effect. Typically, prismatic effect is expressed as base in or base out or base up or base down effect and the direction of the base is indicated to the right eye or left eye.

If the optical center of the convex lens is nasally shifted, it will cause base out prismatic effect (**Fig. 3.87**) which means the light passing through the lens will be bend outward, away from the center of the lens. If the optical center of the concave lens is nasally shifted, it will cause base in prismatic effect which means the light passing through the lens will be bent inward, towards the center of the lens. If the optical center of the convex lens is shifted up, it will cause base down prismatic effect and if the optical center of the concave lens is shifted up, it will cause base up prismatic effect.

Prismatic effect (**Fig. 3.88**) of the lens can be measured quantitatively using Prentice Rule, which is a formula used in optics to calculate the amount of prismatic power induced by a lens.

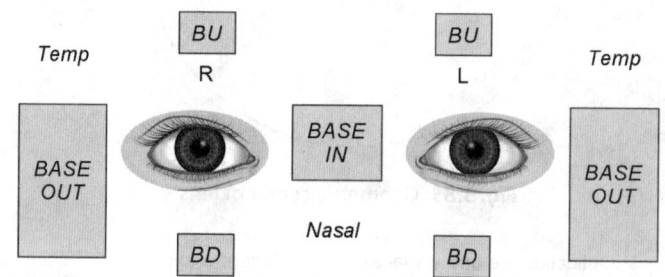

Fig. 3.87: Prismatic effect for RE and LE with reference to base of the prism.

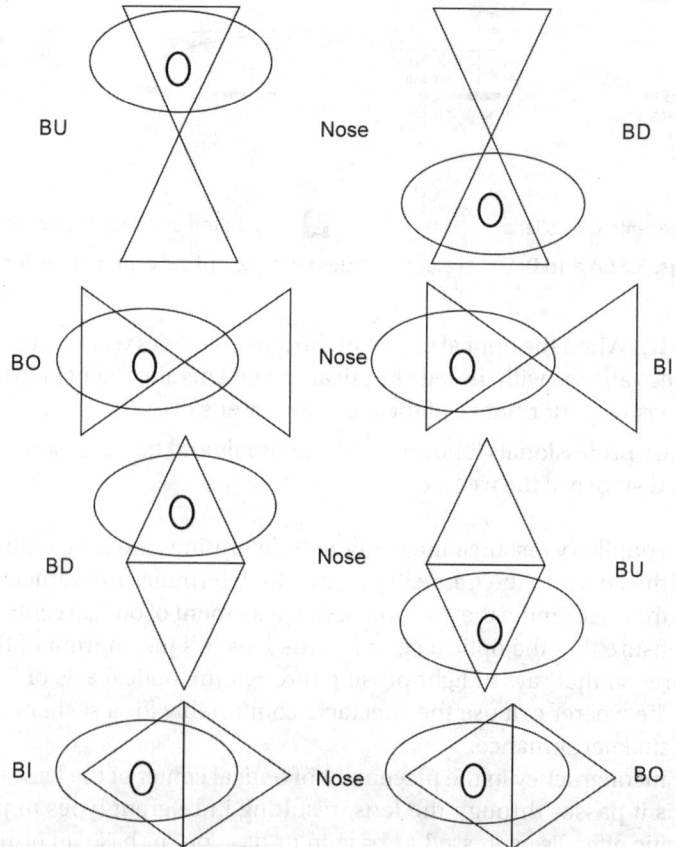

Fig. 3.88: Prismatic effect of convex and concave lenses.

The Prentice Rule states:
P = cF

Where,
P = Prism power in diopter
c = Decentration in centimeter
F = Lens power in diopter

Example: If a –1.00 Dsph lens is decenterd by 10 mm, how much prism is created by the lens?

Using, Prentice rule as under:
P = cF
P = 1 × 1
P = 1Δ

The lens creates 1 Δ prismatic effect.

The Prentice Rule tells us that the prismatic effect is directly proportional to the power of the lens and the decentration. If the optical center of the lens is displaced from the line of sight, it will induce prismatic effect proportional to both the power of the lens and the distance of decentration.

Impact of Induced Prismatic Effect

While prisms can have significant benefits in improving vision and visual comfort, their use should be tailored to the individual's unique requirements to ensure optimal result as induced prism may bring in unintended changes in the direction of light rays as they pass through the lenses. It may lead to various visual disturbances and discomfort, which may include:

- **Double vision:** One of the most common symptoms of induced prismatic effect is double vision. This occurs when the prisms cause the incoming light to diverge or converge too much, leading to the perception of two images instead of one. The brain receives conflicting signals from the eyes, resulting in double vision.
- **Muscle pulling sensation:** The induced prism can change the way the eye muscles work to maintain proper alignment. The eye muscles may have to work harder or in an unnatural way to maintain single vision. This can lead to a sensation of eye muscle strain or pulling.
- **Asthenopic symptoms:** Asthenopia refers to a group of symptoms related to eye strain and discomfort. Induced prismatic effect can contribute to asthenopic symptoms, which may include eye fatigue, headaches and general discomfort when reading or focusing on objects.
- **Reduced depth perception:** Prisms can alter the perception of depth and distance. In some cases, this alteration can result in difficulties judging distances accurately.
- **Headaches:** Induced prisms can cause headaches, especially if they force the eye muscles to work excessively or in an unnatural way to maintain alignment.
- **Increased sensitivity to glare:** Some individuals are more sensitive to glare, and vertical prism may exacerbate this sensitivity. Glare can be especially problematic when driving at night, as it can make it challenging to see clearly and can be distracting and uncomfortable.

DISPENSING OF PRISMS

If a prism correction is deemed necessary, the eye care professional will prescribe prism. Prism prescriptions are written in prism diopters (Δ) and include following information:
- The amount of prism which is given in diopter
- Prism orientation, which is about the base direction (base-in, base-out, base-up, or base-down)

The optician uses the prism prescription to design and fit the lenses. This involves determining the precise location and orientation of the prismatic effect within the lenses to ensure that the correction aligns with the patient's eye alignment issues.

The first step in prism dispensing is a crucial discussion with the patient about the prescribed prism correction. It is essential for the patient to understand the need for prism correction and the underlying reasons for its prescription. This understanding can help the patient appreciate the purpose of the prisms and their potential benefits in improving their vision. Discussing prism correction helps set realistic expectations. Patients should know what the prisms can and cannot do, as well as the expected outcomes. This can help prevent unrealistic hopes or disappointment with the results. Prism correction can be challenging to adapt initially. Patients may experience visual discomfort, distortion, or even dizziness as they adjust to the prisms. It is crucial to inform the patient about these potential adaptation issues so they are prepared and patient during the adaptation process.

The next important patient selects a frame for their glasses. The choice of frame is important as it determines how the lenses will be mounted, and the size and shape of the frame can affect the effectiveness of the prism correction. The shape of the frame is particularly important the alignment of the lenses relative to each other. Frame shape, especially when it lacks sharp features or has a round design, can introduce challenges related to lens rotation, which can affect the intended prism correction. The size of the eyeglass frame can affect the placement of the lenses in front of the eyes. If the frame is too small or too large for the person's face, it may cause the lenses to be misaligned with the eyes' visual axes. This misalignment can compromise the effectiveness of prism correction. The third important factor for frame selection is the frame style. Full-rim frames have several advantages over rimless or supra frames in the context of stability and cosmesis. However, the selection of the frame should be a collaborative decision between the eyecare professional and the patient, taking into account both functional and cosmetic considerations.

Finally, the prism needs to be incorporated which can be done in one of the two ways:
1. Prism by decentration
2. Worked prism

Prism by Decentration

The fundamental principle of spectacle dispensing is that the optical center of the lens aligns with the interpupillary distance of the patient. The non-alignment of the optical center of the lens with the patient's interpupillary distance results in decentration of the lens that gives rise to the prismatic effect. The lenses are cut eccentrically using a larger lens size and fitted into the frame to create prism by decentration. The quantitative effect of decentration will vary with the dioptric strength of the lens. General theory is that if the lens power is 1.00D and we decenter the lens by 10 mm, it produces 1D prism. Or if the lens power is 10.00D and we decenter 1 mm, it also produces 1D prism. This is a constant. This can be shown mathematically by the following equation:

$$d = 10 \times P/D$$

$$P = D \times d/10$$

where,
d = Decentration in mm
D = Diopter or lens power
P = Prism degree

Chapter 3: Mechanical Optics, Lenses and Lens Prescription

If the lens power is spherical, the above reasoning applied for decentration in any direction. However, if the lens power is cylindrical, the amount of decentration depends on the relation of the direction of decentration with that of the axis of the cylinder. As far as cylinder is concerned, any decentration in the direction of its axis has no optical effect and any decentration in the direction perpendicular to its axis has the same effect as in the case of spherical. Thus, in a lens power +2.00Dsph/+3.00Dcyl@90, if the decentration is upwards, it acts as +2.00Dsph and if the decentration is inwards or outwards, it acts as +5.00Dsph.

There may be situation when an individual may require prism in both vertical and horizontal direction. In such case, the extent of the prismatic effect is calculated such that the two components are resolved into one oblique deviation and the effect being equally divided between the two eyes.

Worked Prisms

While decentration of lenses can induce a prismatic effect, there are practical limits to how much prism can be achieved. The limitations may be imposed by the following factors:

❖ Lens power, particularly low lens power may pose difficulties. The prismatic effect induced by decentration is directly proportional to the lens power. In other words, lenses with higher power will create a more significant prismatic effect when decentrated compared to lenses with lower power. This is because low-power lenses inherently have less impact on light bending than high-power lenses.

❖ Lens size, the larger lens may provide more room for decentration and the smaller lens may have less room for decentration.

The worked prism is made by grinding the necessary curved surface on the face of prism. The prismatic effect is determined by measuring with callipers the difference in thickness at the two opposite ends of the lens. The required edge difference is calculated in millimeters using the following equation:

$$\text{Prism} \times \text{Size of lens} \times 0.019 = \text{Edge difference}$$

CONTACT LENSES

INTRODUCTION

The idea of contact lenses was conceived by Leonardo da Vinci about 1508 who suggested immersing the eyes in a hollow glass bowl containing water. Although Vinci's idea was not universally accepted as a representation of contact lenses, it may be considered as an embryonic conception of a contact lens as a refractive correction device. A somewhat similar suggestion was put forward by Descartes in 1637. Descartes said that better vision could be achieved by enlarging the size of the retinal image which can be achieved by directly applying a tube full of water directly against the eye. Descartes theory contributed significantly to the development of the telescope. The first careful observation was made by Thomas Young in 1801. His experiments proved that the cornea played no part in the accommodative process. The next suggestion came from Sir John Herschel in 1845. He proposed the mechanism by which vision could be corrected with a contact device. He postulated the fitting of a spherical glass or jelly over the corneal surface, made from an impression of the cornea. Herschel was probably the first person to describe the concept of cosmetic lenses. Herschel can be considered the 'father of contact lenses'. William White Cooper in 1859 recommended insertion of a 'glass mask' filling the fornices, in order to prevent formation of symblepharon following lime burns of the eye. In the following year, three ophthalmologists independently and simultaneously produced contact lenses in different ways for different purposes. A. E. Fick of Zurich in 1888 who introduced the term contact lens and used a blown glass from a plaster mould taken from the eye for the optical treatment of conical cornea. E. Kalt (1888) devised the first contact lens for keratoconus. He wanted to remodel the corneal curvature by using glass contact shells as splints. A.C. Muller in 1889 devised the first ground glass and used it to correct his own myopia of 14.00D.

Thereafter interest in contact lens began to accumulate rapidly. Artificial eye makers in Wiesbaden, Germany fitted a protective glass shell in 1887 to the eye of a patient who had a partial lid removal. In 1920, Zeiss produced a fitting set used to correct keratoconus. Probably it appears to be the first trial set of contact lenses ever produced. J Crawford and Hill of Imperial Chemical Industries invented Polymethyl Methacrylate (PMMA) in 1934 under the trade name Perpex Kevin M Tuohy in 1946 conceived the idea of making corneal lenses from PMMA. The first lens produced was approximately 11 mm in diameter and 0.4 mm thick. Tuohy's corneal contact lens design was a mono-curve which had to be fitted 1.50 D flatter than the central corneal curvature. This was improved in the concept of a multicurve design which was first described by Butterfield. The flatter posterior peripheral curves approximated the nonspherical corneal shape and thus anticipate the modern concept of fitting rigid corneal contact lenses.

In 1954, Professor Otto Wichterle and Dr Drashoslav Lim of the Institute of Macromolecular Chemistry of the Czechoslovak Academy of Sciences in Prague, suggested that a plastic which is more closely simulated living tissue would be more suitable for orbital implants than the metallic elements being considered. They discovered polyhydroxyethyl-methacrylate (PHEMA), which is a water-absorbing polymer (38.6%). They trialled their first lenses in 1956. Though it was unsuccessful due to the heavy weight and the fragility of the material, it was successfully modified by using axerogel that could be hydrated without affecting its physical properties. This resulted in the hydroxyethyl methacrylate (HEMA) contact lens processed by spin-casting.

Wichterle's lens spin-casting production technology, materials and design attracted the interest of the National Patent Development Corporation (NPDC) and Dr Robert Morrison of the United States. In 1964, they bought the patent rights and decided to commercialize the lens. In 1996, Bausch and Lomb acquired the licensing rights to manufacture the spin-cast lenses until the US Food and Drug Administration (FDA), in 1968, classified them as a 'drug' requiring government approval. The FDA granted approval to Bausch and Lomb to market the soft contact lens, Soflens™ in 1971.

By 1956, Walter E Becker had developed his silicone elastomer contact lens. He submitted a patent application in that year. In the 1970s, Ron Seger and Wayne Trombley of Dow Corning in the USA designed a new silicone elastomer lens, called Silsoft™, to be worn as a daily wear cosmetic lens and as an extended wear lens for aphakia. It was submitted to the FDA which granted market approval in 1981. This technology was bought by Bausch and Lomb in 1985.

Dr Orlando A Battista, a scientist-inventor at the Research Services Corporation in Fort Worth, Texas in the US, in 1978 is credited as having conceived the idea of a 'throw-away lens', now called the disposable soft contact lens. In the late 1980s, advanced computer technology allowed mass production of lenses without massive increases in manufacturing costs. In 1987 Vistakon released the Acuvue lens on a limited basis in the USA and in 1988 Vistakon launched Acuvue, B and L launched sequence and CIBA Vision launched NewVues.

The story of development of contact lenses has not yet been completed and much more research is required. The subject is changing rapidly and there are so many materials and designs of lenses are available. As practitioners we need to be receptive and responsive to them to explore.

Different Types of Contact Lenses

Based on wearing modalities, contact lenses can be classified as under:

Daily Disposable Lenses

Daily disposable contact lenses are used once and when they are removed from the eyes in the night before sleep, they are thrown away in the trash. When it comes to putting something into eyes, everybody would like to be conscious about his ocular health and in that respect shorter is always better. The convenience of these lenses makes them popular with lots of people.

As soon as the contact lenses are placed on the eyes, the tear deposits start building up on the lens surface. Even the best lens care system cannot remove the entire deposits from the lens surface. Over a period of time, layers of deposits build up and protein denatures. The overall effect is noticed as reduction in wettability of the lens surface which ultimately may reduce visual acuity, increase irritation and discomfort and increases the risk of infection and allergies. Daily disposable lenses allow the wearer an opportunity to replace the lens much before the likelihood of the problem arises.

In addition, the wearer of daily disposable lenses also enjoys the following benefits:
- Excellent vision throughout the day
- No ocular health compromise
- More comfort at the end of the day
- No maintenance
- Spare lenses are always available
- Eliminates the risk of potential ocular problem
- Lower incidence of visit to practitioner

Bi-weekly Disposable Lenses

Some people may find it difficult to afford the cost of daily disposable lenses. They may find it more economical to use two weeks contact lens modality instead. As the name suggests, these contact lenses are worn for two weeks before being discarded. Remember, they need to be removed each night, therefore, cleaning, rinsing and storing in solution filled case is mandatory. The wearer has to keep the track of dates on which a new pair was put on the eyes and the date on which day he has to throw away the same. The wearer of bi-weekly disposable lenses enjoys following benefits:
- Simpler lens care
- Back up lens available
- Less dryness
- Increased comfort
- Better vision
- Better overall satisfaction

Monthly Disposable Lenses

Monthly disposable modality is the most popular modality and is the first lens of choice by millions of people around the world. These contact lenses can be worn for one month or as directed by the practitioner. This means that at the end of every day, you remove your lenses, store them in solution, and clean before reinserting them.

Traditional Lenses

Contact lenses may be worn for a year or longer on daily wear basis. A traditional or conventional contact lens wearer must clean them on a daily basis and store them in proper protective lens case. Daily cleaning, rinsing, disinfection, and protein tablet deproteinizing are all very critical to ensure trouble-free wearing.

Contact lenses can also be classified on the basis of material type:

Soft hydrogel lenses

Soft contact lenses are made with a stable, solid polymer component that can absorb or bind water. Poly hydroxyethyl methacrylate (HEMA) is used to manufacture soft hydrogel lens. The lenses are made in their dry state and then hydrated in saline solution where they absorb water. The water so absorbed gives the lens its softness and makes them comfortable and pliable. Water content also increases its oxygen permeability. On an average, water content varies from 38–80%. Higher water content makes a lens less durable.

Silicone hydrogel lenses

Silicone hydrogel lens material is a combination of silicone rubber and hydrogel polymer. The silicone phase facilitates oxygen transmission and the hydrogel phase allows good lens movement and fluid transport. Silicone hydrogel lens materials are very different from other class of contact lens material and within the silicone hydrogel class itself major difference exists as well. The hydrogel lens materials are more of a single material family. They behave more homogenously and in that increased water content results in improved oxygen permeability. On the other hand, silicone hydrogel materials that have been introduced so far contain a variety of polymer chemistries, surface treatments, and material properties that result in less predictable eye-lens relationships.

Rigid Gas Permeable Lenses

Rigid gas permeable (RGP) contact lenses are made of rigid plastic material and contain no water. RGP lenses permit oxygen to pass directly through the lens to the eye. Because they transmit oxygen through the material, these lenses are referred to as gas permeable. They are more durable and resistant to deposits, and generally provide a crisper vision. They tend to be less expensive over the life of the lens as they last longer than soft contact lenses. They are easier to handle and less likely to tear. However, they are not as comfortable initially as soft contacts and it may take a few weeks to get used to wearing RGP lenses.

Color Cosmetic Contact Lenses

Colored contact lenses are used to change the eye color. One can change the color of his/her eyes to match facial make up. Sometimes they are also used for therapeutic reasons. They are available in wide range of colors, crazy patterns, and appeal. They are basically worn to cater the mood and aesthetic values. Colored contact lenses are also used for masking the corneal opacities. Patients with albinism or aniridia are fitted with pinhole contact lenses and amblyopic patients with dark pupil lenses.

Contact lenses can also be classified as under:

Daily wear

Daily wear lenses are used on daily basis during the daytime. They are removed before sleeping in the night.

Flexi wear

Flexi wear lenses are used on daily wear basis with occasional overnight wearing.

Extended wear

Extended wear lenses are worn up to 7 days and 6 nights at a stretch without being removed from the eyes.

Continuous wear

Continuous wear lenses are worn up to 30 days and 29 nights at a stretch before removal.

Manufacturing Methods of Contact Lenses

RGP and soft contact lenses are two principal types of contact lenses that are widely practice. We will discuss the manufacturing methods of both the types separately.

RGP Lens Manufacturing Methods

Lathing and molding are two primary methods used in the manufacturing of RGP contact lenses. These methods are employed to create the precise shape and optical characteristics required for RGP lenses.

Lathing

Lathing, also known as lathe-cut or lathe-turned manufacturing, is a subtractive manufacturing process. It involves the removal of material from a solid lens blank to shape it into a contact lens. A solid, transparent lens blank made from an RGP material is mounted on a lathe machine. The lathe machine uses a high-speed cutting tool to carve and shape the lens blank into the desired lens design. The tool is computer-controlled to ensure precision. As the lens blank rotates, the cutting tool removes material gradually, creating the curvature and optical features of the lens. The lathe-cut lenses are then polished to achieve a smooth and clear surface. Lathing allows for precise customization of RGP lenses to match the individual's prescription and specific requirements, making it suitable for complex prescriptions and irregular corneal shapes.

Molding

Molding is a manufacturing process in which RGP lenses are created by molding liquid lens material into a specific shape using molds. Liquid or molten RGP lens material is injected into a set of molds. These molds have two parts: one for the front surface (anterior) and one for the back surface (posterior) of the lens. The molds are closed, and the lens material is allowed to cure and solidify within the mold. Heat may be applied during curing to facilitate the polymerization of the material. After curing, the molds are opened, and the newly formed RGP lens is removed. The lens may undergo additional processes such as polishing to achieve the desired optical clarity and surface smoothness. Molding is well-suited for producing RGP lenses in large quantities with consistent quality. However, it may be less customizable compared to lathing, making it more suitable for standard prescriptions.

Both lathing and molding have their advantages and are used in the production of RGP contact lenses to meet a wide range of patient needs. The choice of manufacturing method depends on factors such as the complexity of the prescription, the level of customization required, and the production volume.

Soft Lens Manufacturing Methods

General Properties of Contact Lenses Material

Material properties together with surface properties influence the lens fitting on eye, wearing comfort, and oxygen permeability and may lead to ocular difficulties. The general properties of contact lens material are given below:

Oxygen Permeability

Corneal hypoxia has been implicated in many of the ocular complications associated with contact lens wear. In the absence of a contact lens, the oxygen required for the metabolic functioning of the cornea comes primarily from the atmosphere. The peripheral cornea may also receive some oxygen supply from the limbal vasculature, while the posterior cornea is supplied oxygen from the aqueous humor. In order to maintain normal corneal metabolism during contact lens wear and prevent hypoxia, it is necessary that any material used as a contact lens is able to allow the passage of oxygen to be maintained.

Oxygen permeability is the physical property of the material and is a measure of the oxygen performance of a lens material. However, actual amount of oxygen transmitted (**Fig. 3.89**) to the cornea after putting on the contact lenses depend also upon the lens thickness which is the important feature of finished contact lenses. Manufacturers often quote permeability values and transmissibility values separately. Transmissibility is usually based on the thickness of a –3.00 lens but lenses of different back vertex powers will have different thickness and hence transmissibility. Also, for accurate values the measurements should be edge corrected. Water contents of the lens material and dehydration during lens wear also affect the transmissibility.

Contact lens needs to provide atmospheric oxygen to the cornea. Normal concentration of oxygen in air is 20.95%. A reduction in amount of oxygen reaching cornea through lens causes several problems, for example, striae may be observed in the posterior stroma if the oxygen reaching through the lens falls below 5% or folds may be observed in the deep stroma if oxygen reaching through the lens falls below 8%.

Wettability

Wettability can be thought of as the formation of a continuous fluid film over the contact lens surface (**Fig. 3.90**). In order to achieve good vision and consistent comfort, a stable uniform

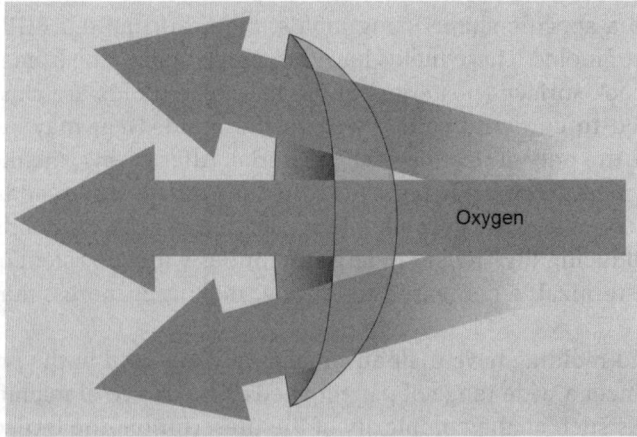

Fig. 3.89: Schematic representation of oxygen transmission through lens.

tear film must be supported over the front surface of a contact lens. A lens that does not have good wetting characteristics will result in a rapid breakup of the pre-lens tear film and a consequent reduction in vision quality. A stable pre-lens tear film provides a lubricating effect, allowing comfortable lid movement over the front surface of the lens. A wettable contact lens material is more likely to allow a continuous tear film between the back surface of the lens and the corneal epithelium, which is important consideration for biocompatibility. A contact lens surface with poor wettability has a greater tendency to attract tear-film deposits. As the tear film dries out due to evaporation between blinking, the dry spots form areas prone to deposit formation, especially protein, and this in turn further reduces surface wettability.

Traditionally, wettability can be measured by measuring the contact angles. When a drop of liquid is placed on a solid surface, an angle is formed between the surface and a tangent to the surface of the drop at the point of contact is referred to as a contact angle. The lower the angle, the more completely the liquid wets the surface (**Fig. 3.90**). An angle of 0° implies complete wettability, allowing the tear spread evenly over the lens surface to provide stable tear film. Clinically, it can be measured using subjective scales of tear break-up over a lens.

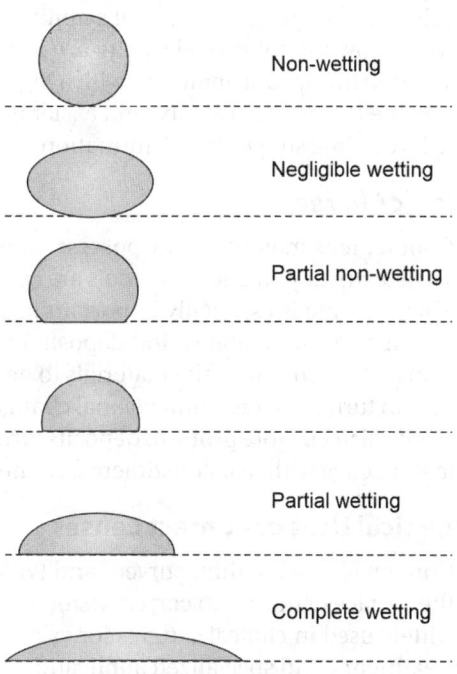

Fig. 3.90: From non-wetting to complete wetting of contact lens surface.

Biocompatibility

Since lenses come in contact with the eye, they should be considered as biomaterials, which must fulfill most of the general biological requirements of all other biomedical polymers. Specific toxicity, carcinogenicity, and sterility tests for the evaluation of biomaterials in general have been recommended.

Water Content

Water content of a lens material is the amount of the fluid taken up by the contact lens material. Most contact lens materials, both hard and soft, absorb some water. The amount absorbed is usually expressed as a percentage of total weight. Most of the material used today have water content which ranges from 38% to 79%. Contact lens with water content less than 50% is called low water content and contact lens with more than 50% water content are called high water content lenses. When a material absorbs water, it swells which makes high water content lens thicker. Higher water content materials allow more oxygen through them than the low water materials. Materials that absorb less than 4% water by weight are referred as hydrophobic and those that absorb 4% or more water are termed as hydrophilic. With hydrophilic polymers, increasing the water content generally increases the oxygen transmissibility. However, this often increases lens fragility and may make materials more prone to deposit formation.

Modulus of Elasticity

A contact lens is subject to stress because of external forces on the eye by the lids, during handling and also during the manufacturing process. The modulus of elasticity is a constant value that expresses a material's ability to keep its shape when subjected to stress. Materials with a low modulus of elasticity are less resistant to stress and they quickly conform to the shape of the eye and materials with a high modulus resist stress, hold their shape better, tend to provide better visual acuity, and easier handling. A truly elastic material is one that will return to its original shape after deformation, once the load has been removed.

Ionic Charge

Contact lens materials may possess an electrical charge or they may be electrically neutral. The electrically charged materials are called ionic and no charge materials are called nonionic. This attribute is especially important in soft hydrogel lens materials, as it affects factors such as solution compatibility and deposit formation. In most cases, contact lenses are negatively charged which causes the materials to be more reactive, especially in solutions that are acidic. This in turn can cause dimensional changes and even material degradation. It may also cause a material to be more prone to deposits formation. Nonionic materials tend to be more inert and less reactive with tear constituents, so they also tend to be more deposit resistant.

Clinical Uses of Contact Lenses

Contact lenses are thin, curved, and typically transparent devices that are placed directly on the surface of the eye to correct vision problems or serve other therapeutic purposes. They are widely used in clinical settings for various purposes, including vision correction, therapeutic treatments, and specialized applications.

Myopia

Contact lenses find their most widespread clinical application in the correction of myopia. In low myopia, the main advantages of using contact lenses are cosmetics as spectacles are avoided and the appearance of small eyes produced by myopic spectacles is also avoided and a large and attractive globe is seen. To this are the added advantages of the increased size of retinal image, an effectively wider field of clear vision and elimination of distortion experienced when looking through an eccentric portion of the lens. However, the use of contact lens requires greater use of accommodation and convergence which may not be of any issue in young population but is important in presbyopic patients in which difficulties in near vision may be precipitated.

    Contact lenses are very useful for moderate degree of myopia and a variety of contact lenses are available, the choice of which depends on the personal fancy and experience of the individual practitioner. In the higher degree, the optical advantages are correspondingly increased but care must be taken while fitting. These lenses are a little heavier and every effort is made to make them thinner. The inevitable thickness of lens edges leads to difficulties with upper eyelid since its movement over the edge may be partially obstructed. This difficulty may be overcome by beveling the peripheral portion of the lenses, an experiment which effectively reduces the optical zone. Reducing the diameter of the lenses is another way to reduce the lens weight in high lens prescription.

Hypermetropia

The incentive to wear contact lens is much less in the hypermetropia than in myopia as most young patient do not need constant optical correction and older patients are not so concerned about cosmetic considerations. The optical advantages of using contact lenses are relatively less. However, there may be reduced requirements for accommodation and convergence as well as the avoidance of prismatic effect of strong convex lenses. The size of the retinal image is smaller in hypermetropia with contact lenses than spectacle lenses.

Aphakia

The aphakia patients are corrected with high convex lens and when spectacle lenses are worn the size of the retinal image is one-third larger than in the phakic eye which causes intolerable aniseikonia, peripheral vision accompanied by distortion due to oblique astigmatic effects and other aberrations. The prismatic effect of the edge of the lens leads to a roving ring scotoma in the field of vision which in any event is restricted. Many of these undesirable effects can be eliminated by wearing contact lenses.

The fitting of contact lenses in such cases poses special problems:
- The lenses are excessively heavy. A lenticular design is widely used but it must be of high quality.
- If the patient has complete iridectomy, corneal lens may give rise to considerable flare arising from the non-optical peripheral portion of the anterior surface.
- Decentration of lens may also result.
- The period after surgery when fitting of lenses should be first attempted is a matter of debate. There are opinion that says that hydrophilic lenses can be fitted after five days of cataract surgery.
- The atonic lids of these patients often add to the difficulties.
- Interestingly, many aphakic patients are wearing contact lenses for distance vision with able to see sufficiently well to read without the need for near addition.

Astigmatism

Total astigmatism is defined as an uncorrected eye's manifest ocular astigmatism. It is the summation of all the astigmata present in that eye. The various astigmata present may be additive or subtractive. The primary contributing organ is the cornea. The cornea is seldom truly spherical even in the immediate vicinity of the eye's optical axis. As the cornea accounts for approximately two-thirds of the total refractive power of the eye, any corneal astigmatism can be visually significant. The term corneal astigmatism is usually applied to anterior surface astigmatism. True corneal astigmatism should take into account the refractive effects of the posterior cornea as well as any refractive index anomalies in the cornea as a whole. However, the posterior corneal curvature is not easily measured with current instrumentation. Further, the optical effectiveness of the posterior corneal interface is low because of the small refractive index differences at the cornea/anterior chamber interface. Meridional differences in refractive power of the crystalline lens are an obvious internal source of ocular astigmatism. A tilted and/or decentered crystalline lens can also induce significant astigmatism. Apart from corneal and lenticular astigmata, the other main ocular factor is the posterior pole.

Residual astigmatism is a term used to describe the remaining or uncorrected astigmatism that may still exist after the patient has been refracted and prescribed with contact lenses or eyeglasses. When we talk about contact lenses it is made up of two elements—the true residual astigmatism of the eye itself and the residual astigmatism induced by the tear film beneath contact lens. The true residual astigmatism is inherent to the patient's eye, which remains uncorrected even with the best-fitting contact lenses. The induced residual astigmatism is due to poor fitting of contact lenses. This induced astigmatism can add to the patient's true residual astigmatism, making the overall residual astigmatism worse. If the residual astigmatism reduces the visual acuity significantly with spherical lenses, a toric lenses may be indicated or a scleral lens may be indicated if the residual astigmatism very high. A posterior surface toric is also useful in some cases especially when corneal astigmatism is present. Another type of lens with spherical central optic zone with toroidal peripheral zone may also be used in cases where peripheral cornea may demonstrate a different toroidicity from that of an apical zone. In extreme cases, if the back central optic curvature is toroidal and this itself induces significant degree of residual astigmatism, in such case, a toric curvature may be generated on anterior optical surface also, making a bitoric lenses.

Keratoconus

Keratoconus is a condition where contact lens plays a significant role in its optical treatment. There are, however, several contentious aspects of their application particularly in relation to the type of lens and the manner in which they are fitted and their therapeutic effects. The earliest successes that have been reported were with scleral lenses which are continued to be used successfully today. At the same, time there were many reports of fitting corneal lenses successfully. However, there were debate on their designing element and the manner in which they were fitted. Also, overall size of the lens has also given rise to some debate. Attempts have been made to contour the apex and remainder of the cornea, a procedure that requires multi-curve lens design with relatively small zone and progressively flattening zones. It has also been claimed that smaller lenses may be satisfactory in the early stages of the condition. Fitting technique has also been a matter of debate. Classic keratometry is often unreliable. Eccentric keratometry or specific keratometry of Bonnet may be required, while photokeratoscopy may provide added information. But none of these procedures give perfect guidance in deciding the optimum shape of the lens. Trial lens of corneal lenses of bicurve, tricurve and multicurve designs specially made for keratoconus are available, which looks like more reliable. But the vagaries of shape of the cornea are numerous in this disease. Close observation and further modification of the lenses as required must form the part of the follow-up of all such patients.

Anisometropia

Contact lenses are of value in this condition because they abolish the prismatic effects obtained with spectacle lenses when eyes look through parts of the lenses other than their optical centers. However, there are some differing opinions as well. The use of contact lenses in all types of anisometropia works of not. Theoretically, the advantages of contact lenses over spectacle should be most marked in refractive anisometropia rather than axial anisometropia. The problem is it is not possible to determine clinically whether the eyes of an individual subject is having refractive anisometropia or axial anisometropia. It is likely many of such cases may have the components of both. It is, therefore, good to try contact lenses in case where spectacle is not acceptable.

Presbyopia

Several choices are available for a presbyopic patient who wants to sue contact lenses. The simplest expedient is to use a spectacle correction for near work on top of distance correction with contact lenses. Alternatively dissimilar contact lenses can be used—one eye for distance vision and another for close work. They work surprisingly with little disturbances of binocularity. A third possibility is the use of bifocal contact lenses in which the choices are little limited and the results are not entirely satisfactory. The two principal types of bifocal corneal contact lenses the rotating and segment type. The rotating type, also known as annular type the optical centers of the distance and near corrections are same and two are thus concentric with the latter in an annulus round the periphery. The lens rotates freely and a change from distance vision to near vision is effected by the relative vertical movement of the eye and the lens. The segment type bifocal contact lenses incorporate a feature designed to prevent lens rotation on eye, thus maintaining the segment position in an inferior orientation. Several options may be applied to achieve the desired orientation. Prisms, metallic ballast, truncations of various types as well as unusual shapes of the whole contact lenses have all been applied. The fitting of such contact lenses is directed to producing alternating vision wherein the lower segment comes opposite the pupil only on downward gaze.

LOW VISION AIDS

INTRODUCTION

When the defective vision is due to some cause other than an optical anomaly of the eye, the first therapeutic consideration is medical or surgical treatment and when the improvement is not possible, or perhaps because of fear or ignorance, when such treatment is refused, optical devices may alleviate the patient's visual disability to some extent. The devices used in such cases are known as visual aids. Since they are used by individuals having low vision, the term is always coined with low vision aids. The benefits of low vision aids are many which can be generalized as below:

Benefits of Low Vision Aids

- **Low vision aids** assist individuals with visual impairments or low vision in performing daily tasks and activities.
- **Low vision aids** can help enhance the remaining vision of people with conditions such as macular degeneration, glaucoma, diabetic retinopathy, and other eye disorders that cause vision loss.
- **Low vision aids** aim to maximize a person's independence and quality of life by making it easier to read, write, navigate, and perform other essential tasks.

Vision loss may be due to:
- Decreased visual acuity
- Visual field defect
- Decreased contrast sensitivity
- Loss of color perception

Low vision has been defined in several ways. Some practitioners define low vision as a visual acuity of up to 6/24 or worse in the better eye using the best corrected spectacle correction or visual field of 20 degree or less. However, a more functional definition is that low vision comprises bilateral vision loss that adversely affects the performance of daily activities. The patient has either poor Snellen's acuity or poor field of vision or both. With such subnormal vision, the subjects are unable to perform their task.

Types of Low Vision Aids

Magnifiers

- **Handheld magnifiers:** These are portable magnifying lenses that can be used for reading and examining objects up close.
- **Stand magnifiers:** They can be placed on a flat surface and offer hands-free magnification for reading or other tasks.

- **Pocket magnifiers:** Compact magnifiers that can fit in a pocket or purse for on-the-go use.
- **Electronic magnifiers:** These digital devices have a camera that captures an image and displays it on a screen with adjustable magnification levels.

Spectacle-mounted Magnifiers

These are special eyeglasses with built-in magnifying lenses that allow users to see objects clearly at a close distance.

Telescopic Lenses

Telescopic glasses or monoculars can help individuals see objects at a distance by magnifying them.

Closed-circuit Television

Closed-circuit television (CCTV) system uses a camera to project a magnified image of printed material or objects onto a screen, making it easier for users to read and perform tasks.

Large Print and High-contrast Materials

Books, newspapers, and other reading materials are available in large print formats with high-contrast text to improve readability.

Audiobooks and Voice-controlled Devices

Audiobooks and devices like smart speakers can provide access to written content through spoken text.

Screen Magnification Software

Computer software and mobile apps can magnify on-screen content and provide customizable color contrasts for easier reading and navigation.

Braille Devices

Braille displays and notetakers enable individuals with visual impairments to read and write in Braille.

Tactile Markings and Labeling

Raised dots, textures, or color-coding can help individuals identify and organize items in their environment.

Mobility Aids

White canes and guide dogs assist with safe navigation in outdoor and indoor environments. Low vision aids should be tailored to the individual's specific needs and preferences. An eye care professional or low vision specialist can assess a person's vision and recommend appropriate aids and training to maximize their independence and quality of life.

The management of low vision patient is really challenging as it requires patient's cooperation, adaptability and motivation so that he is ready to use the device. It also requires practitioner's enthusiasm and readiness to spend time with patient to bring him out of the psychological barrier. There are prevailing notions regarding reading at a very short distance or assuming unusual postures for reading. Such notions need to be handled tactfully. Moreover, patient with less than 3/60 vision can hardly get any benefit. The precise pathology and the lesion are also important to understand as it may affect the type of visual aid which is appropriate.

Low vision care can be considered as a philosophy and vision rehabilitation as the service. The philosophy combined with service work together to make the visual impaired aware of their remaining visual capabilities so that they do not dwell on their impairment. It offers the patient a real opportunity to regain his visual independence. In practice, it has been observed that more than 95% of people with low vision have some level of useful vision and more than 90% among them requires reading aids.

The basic principle of low vision practice is magnification, illumination and contrast. Low vision patients do not recognize small and far off targets. When targets are magnified, their image covers more retinal areas, which may have more responsive visual receptors. Thus a low vision patient is assisted to use his remaining vision. The understanding is that in order for magnification to work for a low vision patient there must be some areas of the central retina that should function.

Illumination control is essential for low vision patient. A good rule is to give the patient as much light as they can manage without glare. Good room light may yield optimal visual performance for a normal person, but that's not true for eyes with pathology. Most people with low vision have significantly worse function in normal room light condition and encounter difficulty at light levels that a normal individual find acceptable. This is particularly true for patients with photoreceptor dysfunction.

Contrast management is the third important pillar of the low vision practice. Bigger is not always better. Often increasing the contrast of the text is more effective than increasing the size of the text for a low vision patient. People with low vision normally have difficulty seeing objects or print that has poor contrast. A clear explanation regarding illumination and contrast to the patient can help maximize the function of residual vision.

The service is geared to help patients to maximize the use of residual vision with the help of various optical and non-optical devices. It does not help the patient to see better in general. It only means helping the patient function better for certain task so that the patient is visually independent. The practitioner makes a list of all the tasks that frustrate the patient in his day-to-day life and work with him to see how can they be managed with the help of various aids. There is no "quick fix" method or "single magic pair of glass" that will do it for all. Instead, depending on the severity of the vision loss, a typical low vision patient may need 3 or 4 different aids to help him manage his various visual tasks.

Another way to understand low vision service is that low vision service cannot "help the bad eye". It helps maximize the use of residual vision in the better eye to accomplish the task. Low vision is not medical service, so going for low vision does not mean that the patient will get treatment to fix his vision. In fact, low vision specialist will not be doing things for you. They will accurately describe their role as someone who can work together with you and guide you on your work. It is a beginning of a lifelong process that continues for the rest of patient's life. As people's needs and vision change, low vision rehabilitation will also change to help adapt and make improvements so that they can maintain their "quality of life" as possible.

Unlike other eye examination, the low vision process can take many hours of directions and hard work—not only during examination but also afterwards. The patient has to be motivated to take the responsibility for whatever may be asked to get the maximum improvement. You just cannot "sit back" and expect the doctors to do it all.

There has been a dramatic change in the management of low vision patients during last decade. A shift has been noticed from optics and low vision devices towards visual functions. With this new approach, the management of low vision patients is now thought of as a continuing process, beginning with surgical and medical intervention and proceeding through to the prescription of low vision devices and necessary rehabilitative services. In a tertiary care center, it may also include training by an orientation and mobility instructor. The ultimate objective is to enhance the patient's ability to function as close to the norm as possible, using a variety of strategies.

MAGNIFICATIONS OF LENSES

INTRODUCTION

The magnification of a lens is defined as the ratio of the height of an image to the height of an object. It is given by following equation:

$$m = \frac{h'}{h}$$

Where,
m = Magnification
h' = Height of the image
h = Height of an object

It is also given in terms of image distance and object distance and is given by following equation:

$$m = \frac{v}{u}$$

Where v is the image distance and u is the object distance.
Therefore, lens magnification formula may be given as:

$$m = \frac{h'}{h} = \frac{v}{u}$$

Let's take an example:

A mango is 9 cm in front of a lens. If the image of the mango is made at a distance of 15 cm behind the lens, what is the magnification index of the lens?

Let us take the magnification formula in terms of object distance and image distance.

$$m = \frac{v}{u}$$

In our sum object distance is given to be 9 cm and image distance is given to be 15 cm. Using the Cartesian sign convention, the distance between mango and the lens is negative and distance between image and lens is positive. Accordingly, v will be 15 cm and u will be – 9 cm.

Sign convention: The Cartesian sign convention for lenses states that heights of upright objects and images are positive, heights of inverted objects and distances are negative, and distances to the left of a lens (in front of the lens) are negative whereas distances to the right of a lens (behind the lens) are positive.

Substituting the values, we get

$$m = \frac{15}{-9}$$

$$\text{or, } m = \frac{-5}{3}$$

Which is equivalent to –1.67 cm, since the magnification index is approximately –1.67, which is negative, the image is real. And the image size is larger than 1 (m> 1), the image formed is larger than object size.

Let's take another example:
A cylinder having a height of 3 cm is placed in front of a lens. If the image of the cylinder is upright and 1.5 cm tall, what is the magnification index of the lens?

In this problem, object distance and image distance are not given, instead the height of the object and image are given as 3 cm and 1.5 cm.

Using the Cartesian sign convention, the heights of both will be positive, since they are both upright.

We take the magnification formula in terms of height of the object and height of the image.

$$m = \frac{h'}{h}$$

Substituting the values:

$m = \frac{1.5}{3}$, which is equal to 0.5.

Since the magnification index is 0.5, which is positive, the image is a virtual image. Also since m <1, the image is smaller than the object.

Magnification Produced by Convex Lens

A convex lens can produce both real and virtual image, depending on the placement of the object relative to the lens. Real images are inverted, while virtual images are erect. Based on the position of the object, the image can be diminished, enlarged or the same size. The same can also be interpreted as given below:
* If the magnification index is less than one (m <1), it means the image is smaller than the object, the image is diminished.
* If the magnification index is greater than one (m> 1), then the image is larger than the object, the image is magnified.
* If the magnification index is one (m = 1), then the image is the same size as an object.

We can also study the nature, position and relative size of the image formed by a convex lens for various position of the object using a convex lens having a focal length of 15 cm.

Cases 1: The object AB is placed at a distance which is more than twice the focal length of the convex lens **(Fig. 3.91)**.

In the above diagram, the object AB is place at the point B which lies away from point $2F_1$, i.e., twice the focal length of the lens, say at 40 cm. Observe the optical axis passing through the optical center of the convex lens. A parallel ray coming from top of the object, i.e., point A will pass through the point of the lens F_2. Another ray passing from the same point A will pass through the optical center without deviation and will meet the previous ray at point A'. An inverted image is formed as B 'A', where these two rays intersect at point A' and on optical axis at point B'. Since the image is below the optical axis, it is inverted.
Image is real, inverted and diminished.

Case 2: Object is placed at a distance which is twice the focal length of the lens, i.e., 30 cm at point $2F_2$ **(Fig. 3.92)**.

In this case, the object is placed at point $2F_1$. Notice the position of the object which is moved closer to the lens and the image is shifted away from the lenses at point $2F_2$. In this case, the image formed is real, inverted and of the same size and magnification is equal to 1.

Case 3: Object is place between F_1 and $2F_1$ **(Fig. 3.93)**.

We know that the f is equal to 15 cm and 2f is equal to 30 cm. Now let us keep the object distance to be right at midway, i.e., 20 cm. Notice the image will be shifted further and will be formed beyond $2F_2$. A real, inverted and enlarged image is formed.

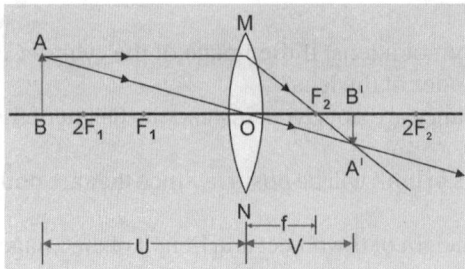

Fig. 3.91: Magnification of Cx lens when the object is placed at a distance which is away from twice the focal length of the lens.

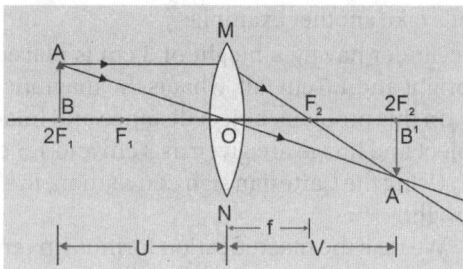

Fig. 3.92: Magnification of the lens when the object is placed at distance which is twice the focal length of the lens.

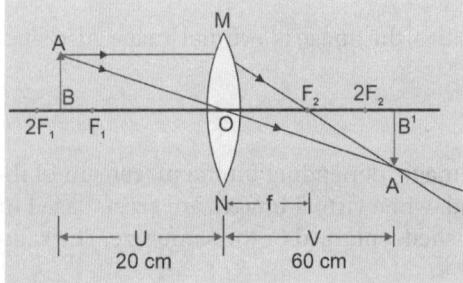

Fig. 3.93: Magnification of the lens when the object is placed at a distance which is just between F_1 and $2F_2$.

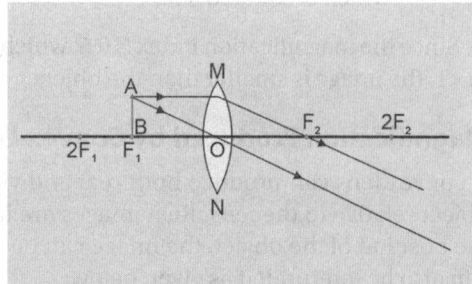

Fig. 3.94: No image is formed when the object is placed at F_1.

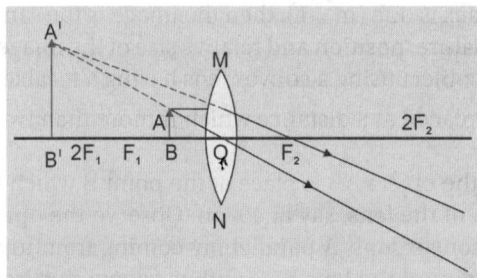

Fig. 3.95: Virtual image is formed when the object is placed in between F_1 and O.

Case 4: Object is placed at F_1 which is 15 cm from the lens, i.e., same as the focal length of the lens **(Fig. 3.94)**.

Notice in this case, rays of light after passing through the lens do not intercept and pass parallel. Clear image, in this case, is formed only at infinity.

Case 5: Object is placed between F_1 and O, i.e., a distance shorter than the focal length of the lens. Let us keep it at 9 cm. You will notice that no image will be formed in this case **(Fig. 3.95)**.

Magnification Produced by Concave Lens

A concave lens always produces a virtual, upright and reduced image. Therefore, the magnification is always positive and the produced image is smaller than the object (m<1).

Spectacle lenses used for vision correction can bring in magnification of the retinal image. Most individual adapt to such magnification and do not report any symptoms. However, in some cases, the magnification so produced can be annoying to an individual or problematic for the following reasons:

Visual Distortion

The magnification caused by spectacle lenses can lead to visual distortion, especially when the magnification is significantly different between the two eyes. For example, if one eye has a stronger prescription than the other, the difference in magnification can cause an unbalanced or distorted perception of the world, making objects appear larger or smaller than they should be.

Perceived Changes in Object Size

Objects viewed through the lenses may appear larger or smaller than they do without glasses. This can be disorienting, as individuals may have difficulty judging the true size and distance of objects, especially when switching between wearing glasses and not wearing them.

Peripheral Vision Changes

Spectacle lenses can also affect peripheral vision, as objects in the periphery may appear to be distorted or magnified. This can be annoying and take some time for individuals to adapt to, particularly if they are not used to wearing glasses.

Distorted Depth Perception

The change in magnification can impact depth perception. When objects are viewed through the lenses, they may appear closer or farther away than they actually are, leading to difficulties with tasks that require accurate depth perception, such as sports or driving.

Motion Sickness

Some individuals may experience motion sickness or dizziness when wearing glasses with significant magnification. The altered visual input can be disorienting and lead to discomfort, especially when in motion, such as when walking or driving.

Cosmetic Concerns

High levels of magnification can also affect the appearance of the eyes. For instance, strong prescription lenses may cause the eyes to appear larger or smaller than they are which can be a cosmetic concern for some individuals.

Adaptation Time

It takes time for the brain to adapt to changes in magnification caused by new glasses. During this adaptation period, individuals may experience some discomfort or annoyance as they adjust to the altered visual input.

In cases where the magnification produced by spectacle lenses becomes annoying or problematic, it is essential for individuals to communicate their concerns to their optometrist or ophthalmologist. These eye care professionals can make adjustments to the prescription, lens design, or frame selection to minimize the annoyance and discomfort while still providing the necessary vision correction. Properly fitted and customized glasses can help individuals achieve both clear vision and visual comfort.

The magnification caused by spectacle lenses is influenced by several factors, including lens power, lens form, lens thickness, and vertex distance. These factors can affect the perceived size and shape of objects when viewed through the lenses.

Factors Affecting Magnification

Lens Power

Lens power, measured in diopters (D), is one of the primary determinants of magnification in spectacle lenses. It is related to the curvature of the lens surfaces and indicates how much the lens bends light. Concave (minus) lenses diverge light and result in a reduced image size on the retina, causing a minification effect (objects appear smaller). Convex (plus) lenses have positive powers and they converge light and result in an increased image size on the retina, causing a magnification effect (objects appear larger). Astigmatism which is corrected by cylinder lenses creates differences in focal lengths along different meridians. Light focused along the steeper meridian will converge or diverge more than light focused along the flatter meridian. Because the light rays along the steep and flat meridians are bent differently, they can create perceived magnification effects. Objects oriented along the steeper meridian may appear larger, while those along the flatter meridian may appear smaller. This can also cause distortion of shapes. For example, a circular object may appear elliptical, with the degree of elongation and orientation of the ellipse depending on the orientation of the astigmatism.

Lens Form

The curvature and design of the lens surfaces play a crucial role in magnification. Spherical lenses have a consistent curvature across their entire surface and produce magnification effects that are uniform across the field of view. Aspheric lenses have varying curvatures across the lens surface, reducing spherical aberrations and minimizing distortions in peripheral vision. They may have a different magnification profile compared to purely spherical lenses which is seen has reduced magnitude of magnification.

Base Curve and Front Curve

The base curve of a lens refers to its curvature on the front surface. A flatter base curve can lead to less magnification, while a steeper base curve can result in more magnification. This can be important when fitting contact lenses or choosing specific lens designs for high prescriptions.

Lens Thickness

Lens thickness can influence magnification. Thicker edges can cause prismatic effects. Prismatic effects occur when the lens bends light differently at different points, causing a shift in the apparent position of objects and creating perceived magnification or minification. High-index lenses, which are thinner for a given prescription, can reduce the thickness-related prismatic effects.

Vertex Distance

The vertex distance is the distance between the back surface of the lens and the front surface of the eye (the cornea). It can vary depending on the frame and how the glasses are fitted. A shorter vertex distance (lens closer to the eye) can result in increased magnification because the lens is brought closer to the focal point of the eye. A longer vertex distance (lens farther from the eye) can lead to decreased magnification because the lens is moved away from the focal point of the eye.

It is important to note that while these factors influence magnification, they are also interrelated. For example, changes in lens power can affect lens thickness, and different lens designs may be used to minimize aberrations or optimize visual comfort.

Instruments and Equipment used in Eye

CHAPTER 4

Ajay Kumar Bhootra, Sumitra Agarwal

REFRACTOMETER

INTRODUCTION

A refractometer operates on the principle that the speed of light changes as it passes through different mediums. By measuring the angle at which light is bent, the refractive index of a substance can be determined. In the field of ophthalmology, a refractometer can also refer to an instrument used to measure the refractive error of the eye, providing information about the need for corrective lenses. We will discuss the refractometer that is used to measure the refractive error of the eyes. There are two types of refractometer—manual refractometer and auto refractometer.

Manual Refractometer

Manual refractometers are also known as phoropter. A manual refractor, or phoropter, requires the eye care professional to manually adjust lenses and settings based on the patient's responses. The phoropter is a key tool in the subjective refraction process. The patient provides feedback on the clarity of vision, and the eye care professional refines the prescription accordingly. The manual refractometer allows for a more customized and patient-specific approach. It takes into account not only objective measurements but also the individual's subjective experience and preferences. They are often used for a more detailed examination, especially when fine-tuning the prescription for factors like astigmatism or presbyopia.

Auto Refractometer

The advent of auto refractometer **(Fig. 4.1)** has changed the scenario of eye examination procedure. Today many practitioners have started relying more on auto refractometer for its speed and accuracy. Auto refractometer uses infrared light to determine the refractive status of the eye. Multiple readings are taken and the system computes the amount of refractive error on the basis of different reading taken and gives a print out of the results. The human observation and judgment involved during retinoscopy are being replaced by the logic function of the computer from the beginning till the endpoint, making the examiner more machines dependent rather than relying on his own judgment.

Auto refractometers have made the objective method of refraction automated, more repeatable, reproducible, faster, user friendly and also patient friendly. The examiner takes several measurements of a patient and each measurement is assigned with reliable co-efficient in the form a single digit number which helps the examiner judge the accuracy of the measurement.

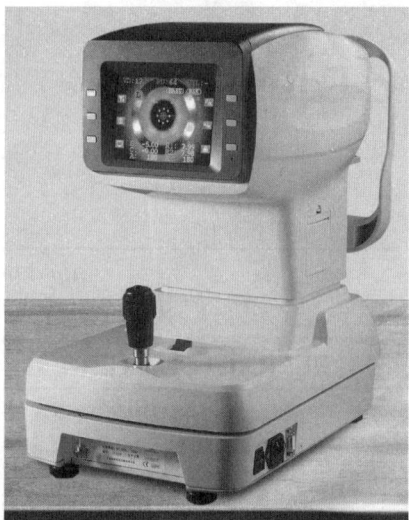

Fig. 4.1: Auto refractometer.

Calculation of Refractive Error

The refractive error is calculated by analyzing how the patient's eye influences the infrared rays. The following design principles are commonly used in most auto refractometer for analysis:
- Scheiner disc principle
- Retinoscopic principle
- Best focus principle
- Knife-edge principle
- Ray-deflection principle
- Image size principle

Most commercially auto refractometers that are available either uses Scheiner disc principle or retinoscope principle coupled with automated Badal Optometer. Each auto refractometer design is programmed to calculate the refractive error on the basis of an empirical calibration found by the clinical refraction of the patient extending over the instrument's dioptric range. Accommodative fluctuations may affect spherical more than cylinder power. The resolution of the cylinder power is the function of the automated refractor's measurement system and it is essentially fixed. The resolution of axis of cylinder power, however, depends on the magnitude of cylinder. As cylinder power increases, the ability to determine the cylinder axis is enhanced.

Auto refractometers are designed to calculate the refractive state of the eye at the plane of the cornea. The desired refraction at spectacle plane is calculated by vertex distance compensation range provided by the individual auto refractometer.

Clinical use of Auto Refractometer

The following steps in the given order may be followed for the effective use of auto refractometer:
- Make the patient sit comfortably on patient chair
- Ask him to put the chin on chin rest and head against forehead rest
- Instruct him to keep the head as still as possible and to keep the eyes open between blinks. Most auto refractometer automatically discard readings that is obstructed by blink.
- The patient should be relaxed and should be fixating at the target of the eye being tested even when the target is blurred.

- The examiner, then aligns the instrument on the center of the entrance pupil with the help of joystick and actuate the button to capture the reading.
- Usually, auto refractometer takes a few seconds to capture the reading.
- It may be necessary for the examiner to track the eye with joystick after actuating the button in case the patient is unable to maintain fixation.
- When the examination is completed for one eye, similar process is repeated for the other eye.

Limitations of Objective Auto Refractometer

Although auto refractometers are very useful in most situations, there are certain situations where it fails to provide reliable measurement of refractive error. It must be remembered that results of objective auto refractometer should not be used as the final refractive correction without further confirmation. They should only be used to determine an initial objective refraction before the performance of subjective refraction. The practitioner must keep in mind the various limitations of auto refractometers and be wary of conditions that may produce invalid results, for example:
- Ametropia outside the range of auto refractometer.
- Auto refractometer often fails with small pupil below the minimum size.
- Often auto refractometer fails to control accommodation adequately.
- Anterior segment abnormalities resulting in opacities, cloudy ocular media, distorted pupil and irregular astigmatism caused by corneal irregularities such as keratoconus, corneal trauma and post refractive surgical corneas are the cases where the measurements are not reliable.
- Posterior segment abnormalities resulting in a poor fundus reflex, such as retinal detachment, staphyloma and retinopathies.
- Young patients with active accommodative system may produce more minus than revealed in retinoscopy or subjective refraction.
- Certain geriatric and pediatric patients are difficult to measure with auto refractometer because of inability to keep the head in position and the eyes fixated.
- During the automated objective refraction, the clinician will not be able to identify latent hypermetropia, pseudomyopia and various other accommodative abnormalities, nor will the clinician be able to reasonably estimate the extent to which the accommodative system has altered the spherical portion of the refractive end point.

TONOMETER

INTRODUCTION

A tonometer is a medical device used to measure intraocular pressure (IOP) inside the eye. Intraocular pressure is the pressure of the fluid in the eye, which can be important in the diagnosis and management of conditions such as glaucoma.

Intraocular pressure refers to the fluid pressure inside the eye. The eye is filled with a clear, watery fluid called aqueous humor, which is produced by the ciliary body and circulates through the anterior chamber before draining out of the eye through a network of channels called the trabecular meshwork. The balance between the production and drainage of this fluid helps maintain a stable intraocular pressure. Measuring intraocular pressure is an important aspect of eye examinations because abnormal pressure levels can be associated with certain eye conditions, most notably glaucoma. Glaucoma is a group of eye diseases characterized by damage to the optic nerve, often caused by increased intraocular pressure. Elevated intraocular pressure can put stress on the optic nerve, leading to progressive vision loss if not properly managed.

Normal intraocular pressure typically falls within a range of 10 to 21 millimeters of mercury (mm Hg). However, it is essential to recognize that normal pressure can vary among individuals, and a person with an intraocular pressure within the normal range can still develop glaucoma. Conversely, some individuals may have elevated intraocular pressure without developing glaucoma. Regular eye examinations, including the measurement of intraocular pressure, are crucial for monitoring eye health and detecting conditions such as glaucoma early on. Tonometers are used to measure intraocular pressure. There are different types of tonometers, and they can be classified into two main categories:
1. Contact tonometer
2. Non-contact tonometer

Goldmann Applanation Tonometer

The Goldmann applanation tonometer (GAT) **(Fig. 4.2)** is a widely used instrument for measuring IOP in the eye. It was developed by Swiss ophthalmologist Hans Goldmann.

Principle of Measurement

The Goldmann tonometer measures intraocular pressure by applanating (flattening) a small area of the cornea. The applanation area is a circle of approximately 3.06 mm in diameter. The tonometer is mounted on a slit lamp, a specialized microscope used in eye examinations.

Set-up

- Disinfect the forehead and chinrest of the slit lamp biomicroscope
- Disinfect the tonometer prism
- Adjust the papillary distance and focus the oculars.
- Set the magnification on low (10X) to medium (16X)
- Insert the cobalt blue filter
- Instil one drop of anesthetic drop

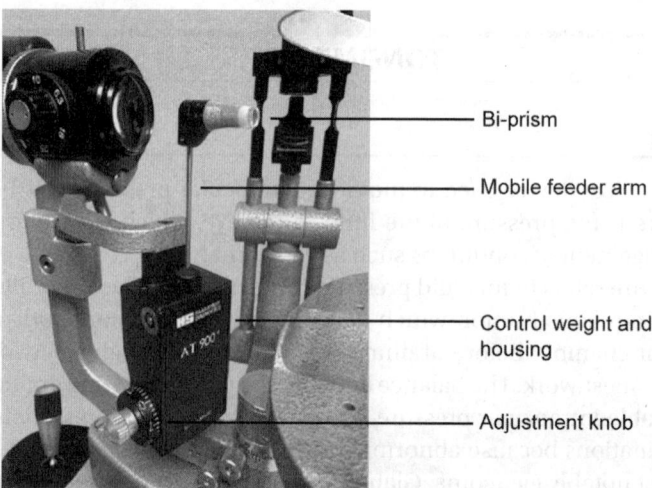

Fig. 4.2: Goldmann applanation tonometer.

Chapter 4: Instruments and Equipment used in Eye

❖ Wet the fluorescein strip with a sterile saline and touch the moistened strip to the temporal bulbar or inferior palpebral conjunctiva.

Procedure

❖ Ask the patient to put the chin on chinrest, keep both the eyes open and look straight ahead.
❖ The practitioner should hold the upper lid firm against the patient's orbital rim.
❖ Now move the tonometer prism positioned slightly inferior to the visual axis toward the cornea. When the prism is 2–3 mm away from cornea, elevate the tonometer to align the prism with corneal apex and slowly touch the corneal apex.
❖ When the prism is in contact with cornea, look through the left ocular. This is because tonometer prism is properly aligned with left ocular only.
❖ As the prism touches the cornea a circular ring broken into two semi-circles as shown in **Figures 4.3A to C** will be visible.
❖ The adjustment knob is then rotated so as to achieve the image. Care should be taken to ensure that:
  • The size of the semi-circle is same.
  • The mire should not be very thick or thin. Usually, the thickness of 0.50 mm is considered ideal.
  • The edge should be sharp.
❖ As soon as you obtain the correct reading of the IOP, withdraw the tonometer prism from cornea.
❖ Wipe the prism tip with tissue to remove any fluorescein.

Limitations of Applanation System

The applanation results may be erroneous in the following cases:
❖ Irregular cornea
❖ High astigmatic cornea

Non-contact Tonometer

The non-contact tonometer (NCT) **(Fig. 4.4)** is a device that measures IOP without direct contact between the eye and the instrument. In this procedure, a quick puff of air is directed

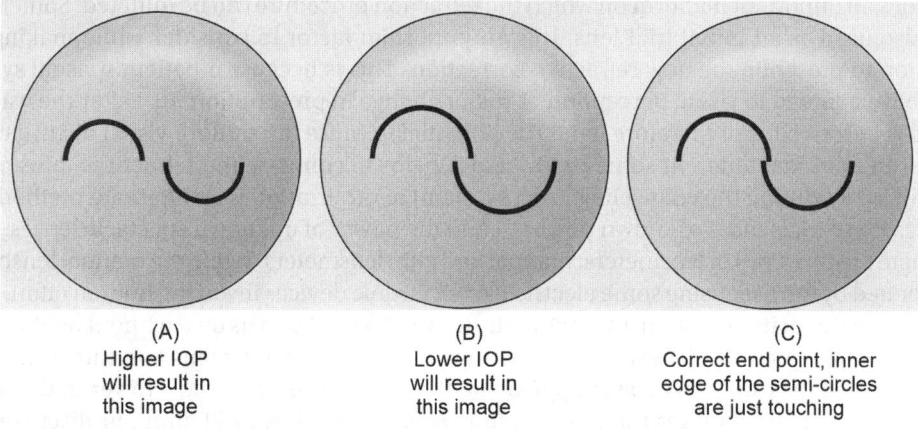

(A) Higher IOP will result in this image

(B) Lower IOP will result in this image

(C) Correct end point, inner edge of the semi-circles are just touching

Figs. 4.3A to C: Applanation tonometry semi-circles viewed through the Goldmann prism.

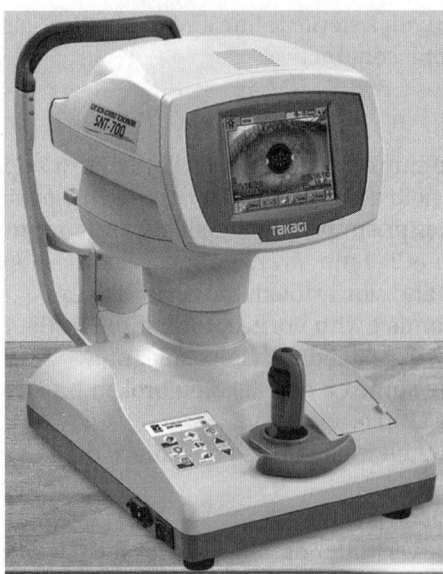

Fig. 4.4: Non-contact tonometer.

at the cornea, causing a slight deformation. The instrument then gauges the eye's resistance to this deformation to estimate intraocular pressure. Unlike contact tonometers, numbing drops are typically not used with the non-contact method. The procedure is swift and generally well-tolerated. However, it is crucial to communicate any concerns or discomfort to your eye care professional during the examination to ensure a comfortable experience.

LENSMETRY

INTRODUCTION

If the patient is already a user of spectacles, the lens power of the old spectacles should be found out using electronic equipment known as a lensmeter. The power of the old spectacle lens provides an important platform on which the refraction procedure can be initiated. Sometimes it is also used as an initial trial lens. It is an important factor to consider while making the decision to prescribe the new refractive correction. This is because a patient's visual system may have adapted to visual perception. A major change in prescription may alter the way the world is perceived, and therefore it has the potential to cause discomfort, visual disturbances, and even non-adaptation in some cases. It also helps to compare the refractive status of the patient's eyes during the counseling process. Hand neutralization is an alternate method that utilizes loose trial lenses of known power to find the power of unknown spectacle lenses.

There are two types of lensmeters: manual and auto lensmeters. While the manual lensmeter is operated by the user using some electrical or electronic devices involving human effort, skill, and knowledge of its operation, the automatic lensmeter works on its own without deliberation and connotes a predictable response. You simply put the lens on the lens aperture, center the lens well, and the exact lens power appears on the digital display screen. However, the use of a manual lensmeter requires training or a little experience. So we will limit our discussion to manual lensmeter only.

Manual Lensmeter

Like auto lensmeter manual lensmeter (**Fig. 4.5**) is used to ascertain the spheric, cylinder and axis of an ophthalmic lens. It is also used to locate the optical center of the lens, determine the prism diopter in terms of base direction and the amount of prism present.

Targets

Reticle inside the lensmeter is used for focusing the instrument with the help of eyepiece and to determine the prism power. The reticle is a permanently etched series of concentric rings. It also contains orientation lines for each lens meridian and a protractor scale. Each ring denotes one prism diopter.

The target consists of two sets of illuminated lines perpendicular to one another for reading the power of the lens. These lines are focused by the power wheel. They are a little thicker and closely spaced lines. Target types vary with different brands and different models of lensmeter. Three common types of targets that are most commonly found in different brands of lensmeter are given in **Flowchart 4.1**.

Figure 4.6 shows the pictorial representation of different types of targets.

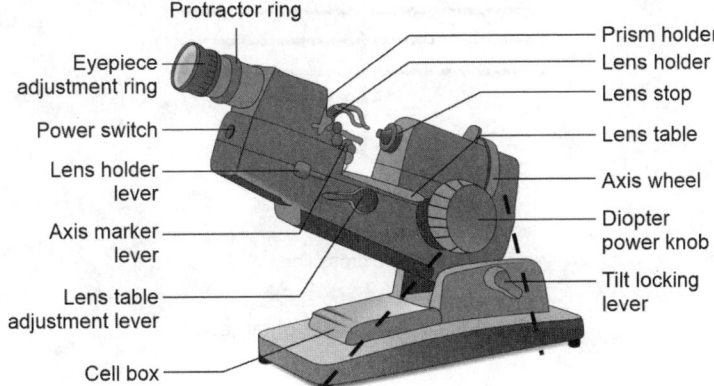

Fig. 4.5: Manual lensmeter.

Flowchart 4.1: Common types of targets found in lensmeter.

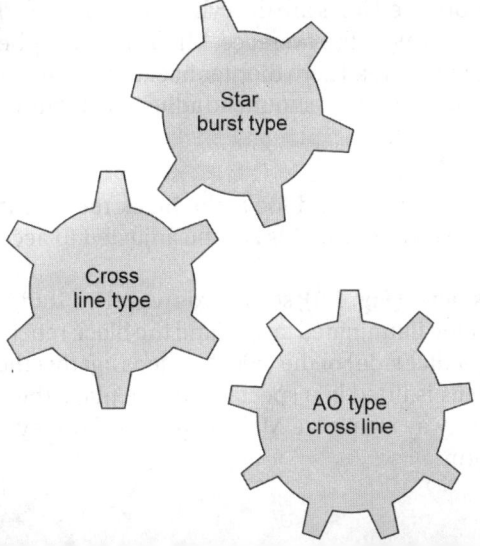

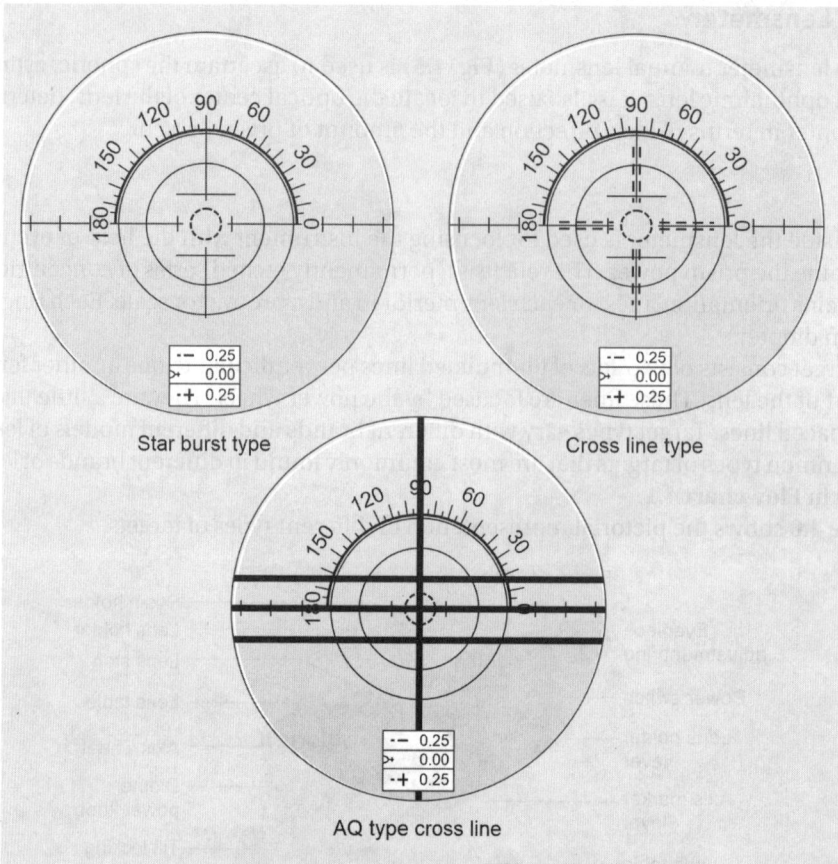

Fig. 4.6: Different types of targets.

Critical Factor

Lensmeter does not read lens prescription; it measures the powers of the lens in each meridian. In order to distinguish the sphere and cylinder lines for a particular lensmeter, with no lenses in place set the axis wheel at 180° and focus the lines. The vertically oriented lines are the sphere lines and the horizontally oriented lines are the cylinder lines. Keep the lensmeter in switch off condition and focus the reticle with the eyepiece. Then switch on the instrument. At this time, the power wheel should actually read zero diopter because there is only air in place. But often a small offset may be detected. Findings should be adjusted for any offset observed at this time.

Step-by-Step Procedure

- ❖ Sit right in front of the lensmeter and focus the black reticle with eyepiece. If it is not in focus, the reading will be erroneous. This is to be adjusted to accommodate the user's own refractive error **(Fig. 4.7)**.
- ❖ Now switch on the lensmeter **(Fig. 4.8)**, set the axis wheel on 180° and bring the reading scale to zero and see whether the illuminated targets and the black reticle both are sharply in focus.
- ❖ Place the back vertex (ocular side) of the **(Fig. 4.9)** lens against the stop of the lensmeter on the platform or if the lens is fitted in a spectacle frame place the spectacle lens so that, the temples of the frame is away from you. Make sure both front eye rims-right and left are in contact with the platform.

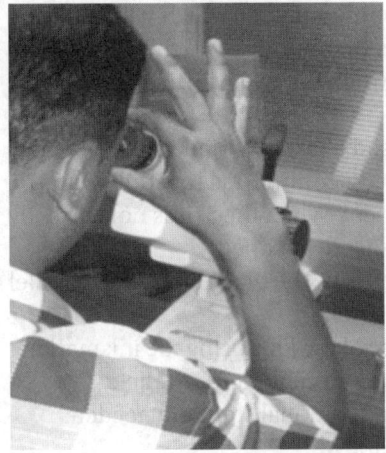

Fig. 4.7: Adjusting the eye piece of the lensmeter.

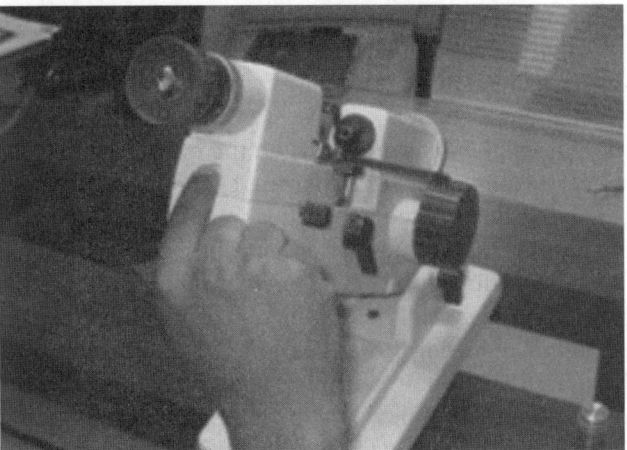

Fig. 4.8: Switching on the lensmeter.

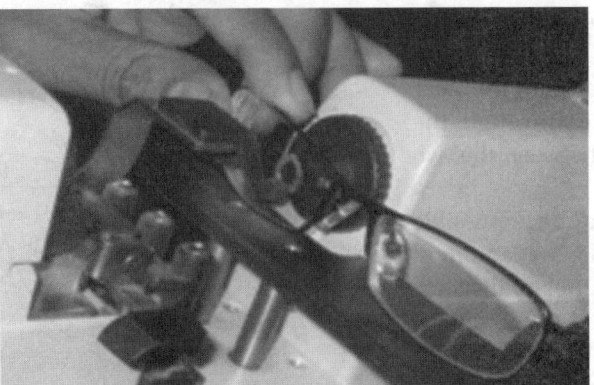

Fig. 4.9: Placing spectacle lens onto the platform.

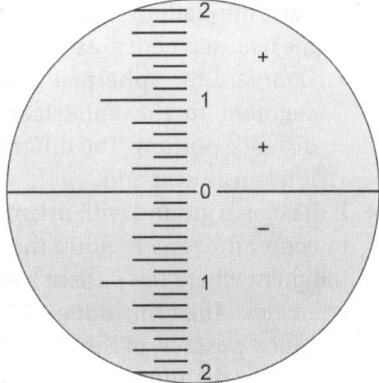

Fig. 4.10: Power reading scale inside the lensmeter.

- Center the lens by moving it on the platform so that the illuminated target is aligned to the centre of the reticle by moving the lens side to side or by moving platform up and down. If the lens also has prism correction, it will be difficult to align.
- Rotate the power wheel to focus the targets sharply and observe the two illuminated lines which are perpendicular to each other. If both the lines are in focus together, the lens is said to have only spherical power. The star burst ring is seen as a well-defined circular ring made of identifiable dots. The amount of spherical can be read on the power reading scale **(Fig. 4.10)**. Red letter shows minus power and the other shows plus power.
- If only one set of lines is in focus and the other is blurred, the lens is said to have cylindrical power. Since cylinder lens forms the line image, the circular star burst ring made of dots is seen as oblong shape image made of well-defined lines which are focused twice on two principal meridians.
- Cylinder power may either be plano-cylinder or sphero-cylinder. In case of plano-cylinder, the spherical line will be focused when the power scale reads zero and cylinder line at some number which will show the amount of cylinder present in the lens. In case of sphero-

cylinder lens, the spherical line will be focused first at some number which will show the spherical component and then the cylinder line at some other number which will show the summation of spherical and cylinder. The difference between the two will give the cylinder element.

- ❖ Axis will be determined when the cylinder line is focused sharply. Orient the axis wheel of the lensmeter such that the cylinder lines are perfectly continuous together with the oblong illuminated image. Read the axis from the axis wheel. When the axis is not correctly positioned, the lines will appear "broken" or as if a "gates were left open."
- ❖ Axis can directly be determined by rotating the protractor ring. The black line when parallel to focused cylinder line will point at the axis on the protractor.
- ❖ Before removing the lens, put the dot on the optical center of the lens using the ink marking device. While doing so, make sure target should be right at the center of the reticle.
- ❖ To ascertain the power of the multifocal lenses, following additional steps are needed:
  - Read and record the power of the distance portion as above.
  - Turn the lens around so that the ocular surface faces you. The bifocal segment power is measured with temples pointing towards you (FVP) when the lenses are fitted in the spectacle frame.
  - Raise the platform up and check the power through the near segment area.
  - Compare the spherical power through the near segment to the spherical power through the distance portion. The difference between the two is taken as near add.
- ❖ If the lens is ground with prism, it may be impossible to center the target within the reticle. Mark a dot at the point where the patient's interpupillary distance coincides. Align this dot at the center of the reticle. Read the position of the star burst circular ring with respect to the number of circle in the reticle. Each circle denotes one diopter of prism **(Fig. 4.11)**.
- ❖ Record the reading so derived.

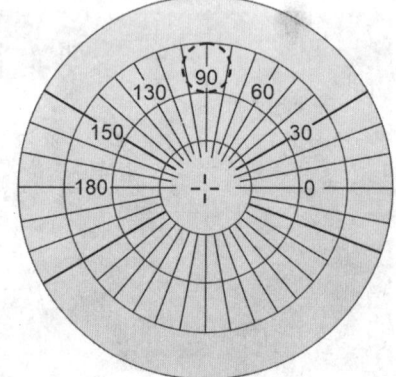

Fig. 4.11: Prism shifts the star burst circular ring position.

OPHTHALMOSCOPE

An ophthalmoscope is used to examine the interior structures of the eye. It allows for the visualization of the retina, optic disc, blood vessels, and other important structures. The key components of an ophthalmoscope include:

Light Source

Ophthalmoscopes have a built-in light source, usually an adjustable bulb or LED, to illuminate the interior of the eye.

Aperture

The aperture is an opening through which light passes. It can be adjusted to vary the size and shape of the light beam entering the eye.

Lenses

Ophthalmoscopes typically have multiple lenses that can be rotated into place to change the focus and magnification of the viewed structures.

Mirror or Prism

Ophthalmoscopes often have a mirror or prism to direct the light into the eye and to enable the healthcare professional to visualize different parts of the retina. The main types of ophthalmoscopes are as follows:

Direct Ophthalmoscope

This type allows for a direct view of the retina and is commonly used in routine eye examinations. The practitioner looks through the device to directly observe the patient's eye **(Fig. 4.12)**.

Indirect Ophthalmoscope

In this type **(Fig. 4.13)**, the practitioner uses a separate light source and holds the ophthalmoscope at a distance from the patient's eye. The light is directed into the eye, and the examiner wears a head-mounted lens to view the enlarged and illuminated image of the retina.

Application

The primary purpose of an ophthalmoscope is to enable eye specialists to examine the interior structures of the eye.

Retinal Examination

Ophthalmoscopy allows for the direct visualization of the retina, including the optic nerve, blood vessels, and the macula. This is crucial for detecting abnormalities such as signs of diabetes, hypertension, retinal detachment, and other retinal disorders.

Diagnosis of Eye Diseases

Ophthalmoscopy is a key diagnostic tool for identifying various eye conditions and diseases. It helps in the early detection of conditions such as macular degeneration, glaucoma, diabetic retinopathy, and hypertensive retinopathy.

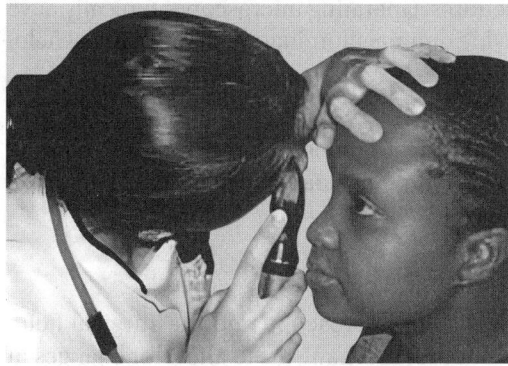

Fig. 4.12: Direct ophthalmoscope.

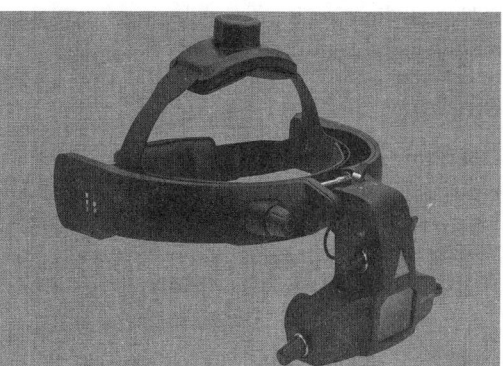

Fig. 4.13: Indirect ophthalmoscope.

Assessment of Optic Nerve

The optic nerve, which carries visual information from the eye to the brain, can be examined using an ophthalmoscope. Changes in the appearance of the optic nerve head may indicate conditions like optic neuritis or glaucoma.

Monitoring Eye Health

Ophthalmoscopy is used for routine eye examinations to monitor and assess overall eye health. Regular examinations can help detect issues before they progress to more serious conditions.

Evaluation of the Vitreous Humor

The ophthalmoscope allows for the assessment of the vitreous humor, the gel-like substance that fills the space between the lens and the retina. Changes in the vitreous humor may be indicative of certain eye conditions.

Overall, the ophthalmoscope plays a critical role in comprehensive eye care, aiding in the early detection, diagnosis, and management of various eye disorders. Regular eye exams using this instrument are essential for maintaining optimal eye health and preventing vision loss.

OPERATING MICROSCOPE

INTRODUCTION

An operating microscope is a specialized optical instrument designed for use in surgical and medical procedures. It provides a high level of magnification and illumination, allowing surgeons and medical professionals to perform precise and delicate tasks. These microscopes are commonly used in various medical fields, including ophthalmology, neurosurgery, otolaryngology (ENT), and other surgical specialties. The key features of an operating microscope include:

Magnification

Operating microscopes offer variable levels of magnification to provide a detailed view of the surgical site. Magnification ranges can vary depending on the specific microscope model and the intended use.

Illumination

Adequate lighting is crucial during surgical procedures. Operating microscopes typically have a built-in light source that can be adjusted to provide optimal illumination of the surgical field.

Binocular Vision

Operating microscopes provide a binocular view, allowing surgeons to perceive depth and work with precision. The binocular vision is often achieved through a pair of eyepieces that provide a three-dimensional view.

Adjustable Working Distance

Surgeons may need to adjust the distance between the microscope and the surgical field. Operating microscopes often have a flexible arm or other mechanisms to allow for changes in the working distance.

Fine Focus Control

Precision is essential in surgery, and operating microscopes usually feature fine focus controls to ensure a sharp and clear image.

Ergonomics

Comfort is crucial during long surgical procedures. Operating microscopes are designed with adjustable features to accommodate the comfort of the surgeon and the surgical team. These microscopes are commonly used in procedures such as:
- **Eye surgery:** In ophthalmology, operating microscopes are used for procedures like cataract surgery, corneal transplant, and retinal surgery.
- **Neurosurgery:** Operating microscopes are employed in various neurosurgical procedures, including brain and spinal surgeries.
- **ENT surgery:** Ear, nose, and throat surgeons use operating microscopes for procedures like ear surgery, sinus surgery, and vocal cord surgery.
- **Plastic surgery:** Microsurgery, which involves intricate procedures on small structures, often requires the use of an operating microscope.

SLIT LAMP BIOMICROSCOPE

INTRODUCTION

The slit lamp biomicroscope was pioneered by Alvar Gullstrand, who introduced an initial model on August 3, 1911. This instrument, initially manufactured by Zeiss and known as the large Ophthalmoscope, earned the name "Slit lamp" due to its illumination system's ability to emit a slit beam. The term "Biomicroscope" is aptly applied because this instrument enables binocular vision with variable magnification and controlled illumination.

In contemporary usage, the slit lamp stands as the most widely employed instrument for eye examinations across various levels of eye clinics. Its versatility allows comprehensive examination from the anterior to the posterior segment of the eye. While it is proficient in examining various aspects of ocular health, its primary application lies in scrutinizing the anterior segment, including the crystalline lens. The instrument's adaptability is further enhanced by additional optics and lenses that enable observation of the posterior segment.

Over time, numerous add-on devices have been developed to broaden the slit lamp's utility and applications. These advancements have expanded its capabilities, making it an indispensable tool in ophthalmic diagnostics and patient care.

Principles of Slit Lamp

The illumination system is meticulously designed to produce a brilliantly illuminated slit image by employing Köhler illumination. In this method, the condenser lens system collects light from the source, precisely focusing the image of the light source onto the projection lens. Subsequently, the projection lens directs the slit image onto the subject's eyes **(Fig. 4.14)**.

To ensure consistent focus, the illumination and observation systems are intricately synchronized around a shared center of rotation, aligning with the point where the slit beam is directed. The linkage between the light source and the microscope is purposefully configured for "parfocality," ensuring that the focal points of both the light source and the microscope coincide. This alignment facilitates the rotation of both the slit and the microscope around the focal point, centred on the eye **(Fig. 4.15)**.

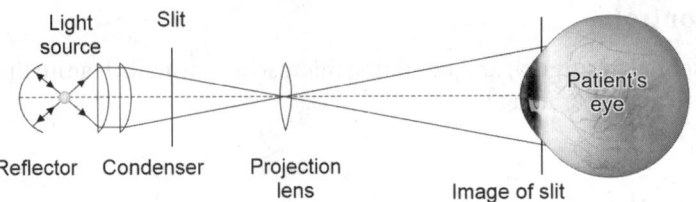

Fig. 4.14: Schematic of slit lamp illumination using Köhler's principle of illumination.

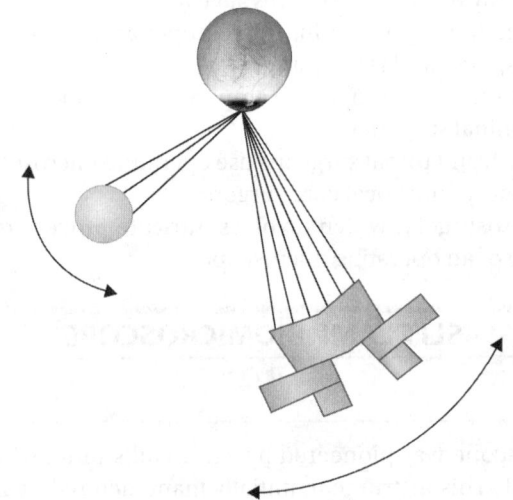

Fig. 4.15: Parfocality of illumination and observation systems.

Nevertheless, certain situations demand the temporary disengagement of parfocality. This is particularly essential for specific techniques, including:
- Sclerotic scatter
- Indirect illumination
- Retro illumination

Types of Slit Lamp

Modern slit lamps can be categorized into two types based on the position of the illumination system:

Haag-Streit Type Illumination System

The Haag-Streit slit lamp **(Fig. 4.16)** employs converging optics and features a flip lever for changing magnification. Its design incorporates a tower system with the light source positioned at the top, while filters and related components are situated below. This arrangement allows for the tilting of the slit or light, enhancing diagnostic capabilities.

Zeiss Type Illumination System

The Zeiss type slit lamp **(Fig. 4.17)** utilizes parallel optics and is equipped with a drum magnification change wheel or knob. In contrast to the Haag-Streit type, the Zeiss illumination system has the light source positioned at the bottom of the optics, along with the filter system. However, this design is less flexible for tilting compared to the Haag-Streit type.

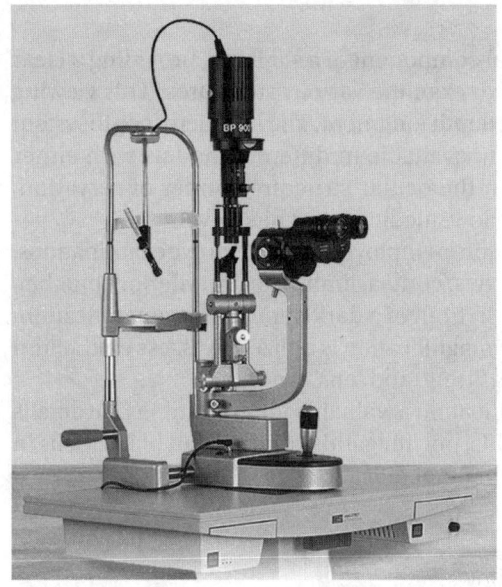
Fig. 4.16: Haag-Streit type slit lamp.

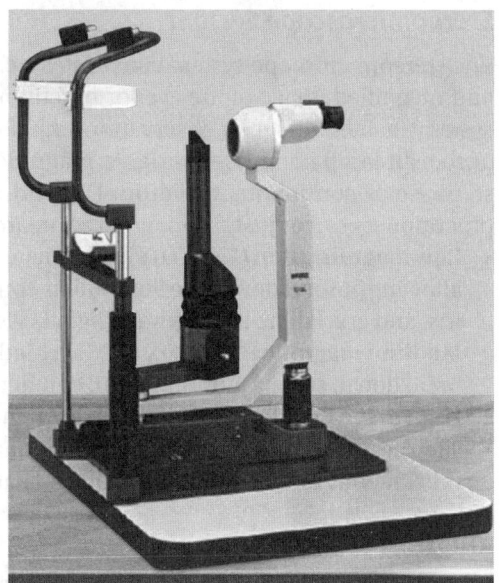
Fig. 4.17: Zeiss type slit lamp.

These distinctions in design and functionality cater to different preferences and diagnostic needs, offering practitioners options based on their specific requirements during eye examinations.

Basic Parts of Slit Lamp

The standard slit lamp is comprised of three parts as shown in **Figure 4.18**.

Slit Illumination System

Many slit lamps utilize halogen bulbs to generate high-intensity light with shorter wavelengths, offering improved visualization of smaller eye structures compared to tungsten bulbs, which emit longer wavelengths of light. The focused light source creates a thin sheet of light directed into the eye, enabling examination of ocular structures. This examination is facilitated by adjusting the:

* **Light intensity:** The intensity of the light source can be varied to optimize illumination during the examination.
* **Light height:** Adjustment of the light height allows for proper positioning and illumination of specific areas within the eye.
* **Light width:** Altering the width of the light source enables clinicians to control the extent of illumination, enhancing the examination of different ocular structures.

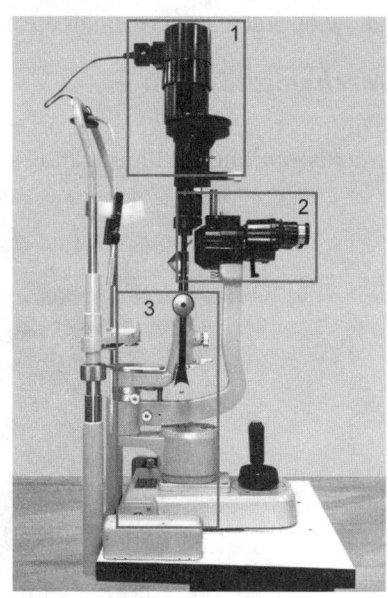
Fig. 4.18: Three parts of slit lamp: (1) Slit illumination unit, (2) Stereomicroscope system, (3) Mechanical system.

Stereomicroscope System

The stereomicroscope system constitutes a crucial component of a slit lamp, providing a clear and magnified image of the eye for practitioners to examine various structures. This viewing system enables binocular observation, enhancing depth judgment. The biomicroscopic system of the slit lamp comprises variable magnification, available in different models with either stepwise or continuous variation. Depending on the ocular structures under observation, practitioners can adjust the magnification among low, medium, and high levels.

- **Low magnification (7X to 10X):** Low magnification is employed for general eye examinations, allowing observation of the lids, bulbar conjunctiva, cornea, limbus, tears, anterior chamber, iris, and crystalline lens. Tyndall light is visible in front of a dark pupil at this magnification.
- **Medium magnification (20X to 25X):** Medium magnification is utilized to assess epithelium breakdown, stroma, endothelium, contact lens fitting, and lens condition.
- **High magnification (30X to 40X):** High magnification is valuable for examining fine details such as vacuoles, microcysts, stromal striae, folds, polymegathism, gutta, and blebs. Cells in the aqueous humor become visible only at higher magnifications.

Biomicroscopes

These essentially of two types, are classified as follows:
1. **Grenough type:** In the Grenough type biomicroscope, a flip lever is utilized to modify the degree of magnification. This design offers a convenient way to switch between different magnifications levels for precise observation **(Fig. 4.19)**.
2. **Galilean type:** The Galilean type biomicroscope employs a knob for seamless and continuous adjustment of magnification. This design allows practitioners to smoothly transition between magnification levels, providing flexibility during examinations **(Fig. 4.20)**

Additionally, it is worth noting that magnification adjustments can also be achieved by changing the eyepiece power. This added feature enhances the versatility of the biomicroscope, allowing practitioners to tailor the magnification to the specific requirements of the observation.

Mechanical System

The mechanical system serves a crucial role in facilitating the connection between the microscope and the illuminating system, a vital aspect for altering the viewing angle between

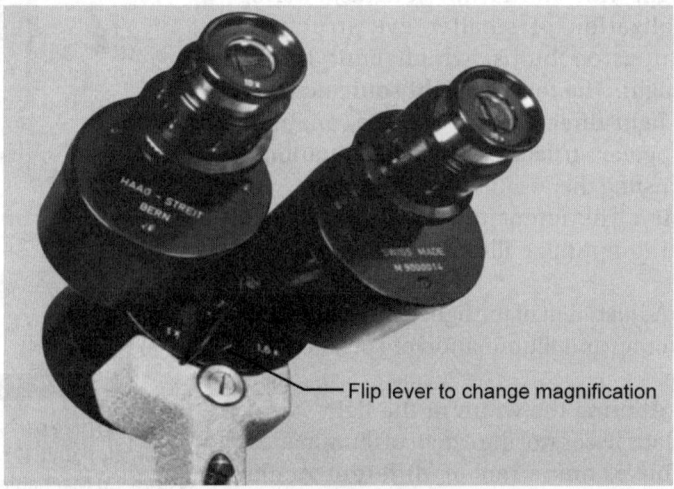

Fig. 4.19: Grenough type biomicroscope.

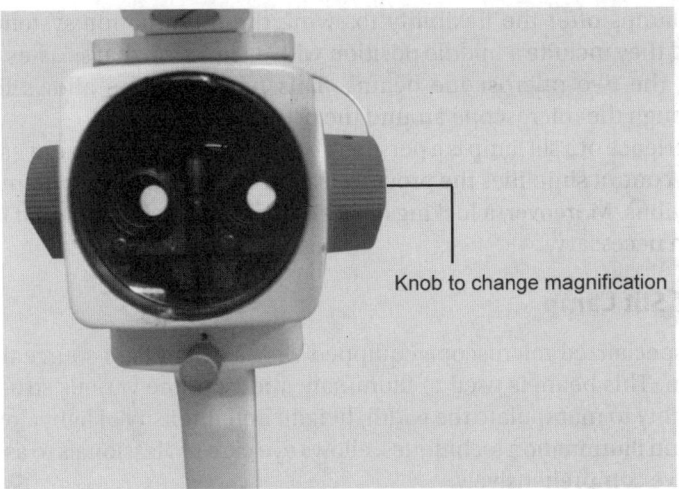

Fig. 4.20: Galilean type biomicroscope.

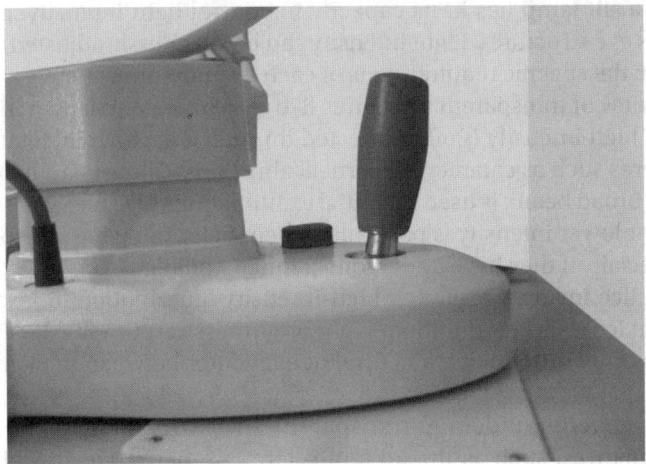

Fig. 4.21: Base of slit lamp.

illumination and observation systems in order to examine various lesions. This comprehensive setup includes a forehead rest, chin rest, fixation target, power supply unit, and locking controls, all contributing to the patient's comfort and maintaining a stable posture during examinations.

Both the illumination system and the microscope can be independently swung about a common vertical axis. During examinations, this axis of rotation is adjusted to the position of the object under observation. This movement is achieved through a mechanical instrument base equipped with a cross-slide system, carrying the mechanical support axis for both the illumination system and the microscope.

The slit lamp and the biomicroscope are maneuvered together on a cross slide using a joystick **(Fig. 4.21)**. A single control element, the joystick, facilitates horizontal movement of the instrument base. Additionally, the instrument base incorporates a vertical control mechanism, typically integrated into the joystick, allowing for vertical adjustments of the slit and the viewing axis. This enables the operator to precisely align the instrument with the object in all three spatial coordinates.

Modern slit lamps offer the flexibility to swing the illumination system in front of the microscope, and they include a middle position with a click stop that situates the illuminating prism between the two microscope beams. This narrow prism allows for stereoscopic observation through the microscope around the prism.

The user experience of a slit lamp is a personal aspect, emphasizing ease of use and operation. A single joystick control simplifies the process, leaving one hand free for manipulating the eye during examinations. Moreover, a locking device is incorporated into the slit lamp to secure it in position when necessary.

Clinical use of Slit Lamp

A slit lamp is a specialized microscope equipped with a bright light source that emits a thin, slit-shaped beam. This beam is used to illuminate and examine various structures of the eye in detail. The ability to manipulate the width, height, and intensity of light along with utilizing different filters and illumination techniques, allows eye care professionals to assess the anterior segment of the eye comprehensively.

Changing Light Intensity

The versatility of a slit lamp lies in its capacity to control light intensity, a crucial factor in examining various eye structures. Light intensity can be seamlessly adjusted, ranging from low to high, catering to the specific requirements of each examination.

For a detailed view of transparent structures like the cornea and lens, a high-intensity light is employed. This high intensity is often directed through a narrow slit, focused on the eye to illuminate structures such as cataracts or corneal abrasions. Conversely, a low-intensity light, emanating from a broad beam, is used for initial examinations of external tissues. Initiating the examination under lower intensity is particularly beneficial, allowing patients to adapt to the illumination, especially if they have undergone papillary dilation.

A prudent practice involves reserving high-intensity illumination for examining intricate details and using it for a shorter duration. Light brightness can be effortlessly regulated using the rheostat knob or by introducing a neutral density filter between the light source and the patient's eyes.

Adhering to a general guideline, transparent structures benefit from brighter light, while opaque structures, such as the lid and sclera, are better viewed with dimmer light. It is noteworthy that novice users may tend to default to the highest illumination intensity throughout the examination. However, a more effective approach involves returning to the lowest intensity after the examination. This not only enhances the longevity of the light bulb but also reduces photosensitivity for subsequent patients, ensuring a more comfortable and efficient examination process.

Changing the Light Height

A notable feature of the slit lamp is the flexibility to modify the height of the light beam, ranging from 1 mm to 14 mm. At its maximum height of 14 mm, the slit transforms into a circular shape **(Fig. 4.22)**.

This dynamic adjustment plays a pivotal role in enhancing the examination experience. Reducing the height of the slit beam, especially during higher illumination levels, contributes to increased patient comfort. Additionally, it facilitates more localized and focused examinations, allowing for precise scrutiny of specific areas.

A dedicated control knob is provided to effortlessly manipulate the height of the light beam. By turning the knob in one direction, the slit elongates, while turning it in the opposite direction

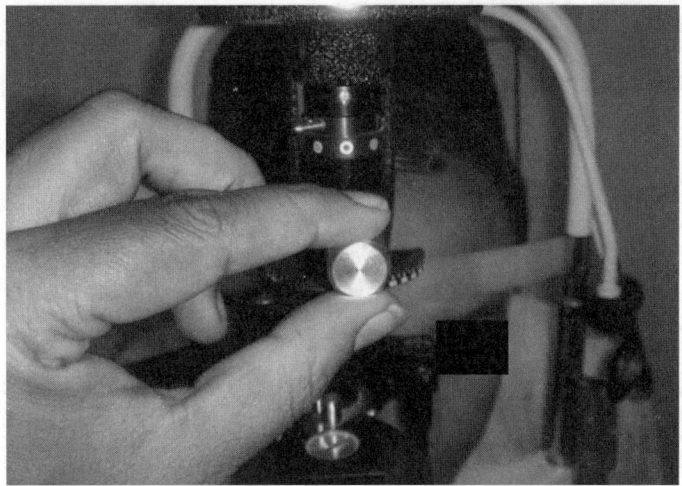

Fig. 4.22: Control knob to change the light height.

Flowchart 4.2: Different light widths for slit lamp examination.

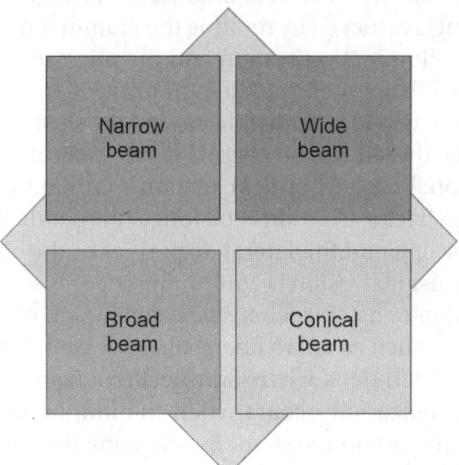

shortens the slit. This straightforward control mechanism empowers the practitioner to tailor the examination conditions to meet the specific requirements of each patient and clinical scenario. Such adaptability ensures not only optimal diagnostic precision but also a patient-friendly experience during slit lamp examinations.

Changing the Light Width

Changing the slit beam width is perhaps the most important aspect of the slit lamp examination. There are basically four most common light widths used for various illumination techniques as shown in **Flowchart 4.2**.

Narrow beam

The slit lamp is specifically configured for precise observation using a narrow beam of light, referred to as an optical section. This optical section **(Fig. 4.23)** is created by a narrow slit,

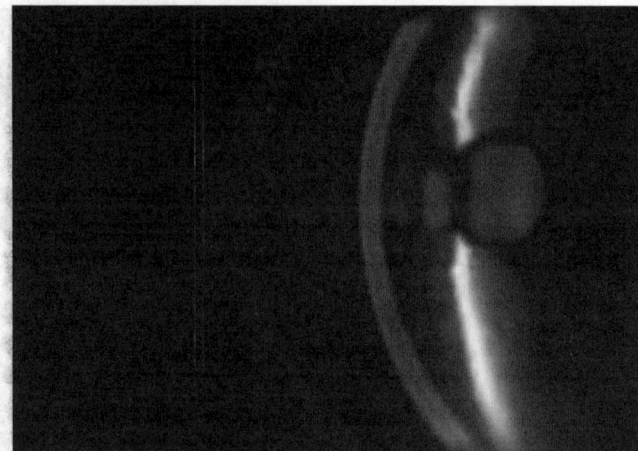

Fig. 4.23: Optical section.

typically ranging from 0.1 mm to 0.2 mm in width. The optimal angle between the illuminating system and the microscope is set between 45 to 60 degrees, allowing the light to cut through the cornea like a knife. To enhance the cross-sectional view, the angle can be further increased to 90 degrees. This adjustment is achieved by rotating the illumination system alone or, in certain cases, by rotating both the illumination system and the microscopic system. Ideally, a larger angle and a narrower slit width are preferred to minimize patient dazzling.

The optical section is designed to be rotatable around the slit axis, providing flexibility in the examination process. While the slit can be aligned either vertically or horizontally, horizontal positioning is an exceptional case in optical section examinations. Horizontal alignment restricts stereoscopic vision because the slit is no longer perpendicular to the plane where the viewing axes of the microscope and the lateral disparities of the observer lie. As a result, the effectiveness of three-dimensional vision is compromised.

The optical section facilitates a comprehensive examination of corneal layers and enables the localization of structures such as nerve fibers, blood vessels, infiltrates, and cataracts. It is particularly viewing the crystalline lens, where narrow slit configurations make the discontinuity zones visible. Optimal visualization occurs when the illumination system is aligned at a 15-degree angle with the microscopic system. By adjusting the slit width and magnification, the optical section technique produces brilliant images ranging from the cornea to the rear face of the crystalline lens. This versatile approach enhances the detailed assessment of ocular structures and pathological features.

The optical section serves as a valuable tool for pinpointing pathological changes within the corneal layers. A proficient corneal section reveals a minimum of four distinct layers: tears (outer layer), epithelium (including Bowman's membrane), stroma portrayed as the central grey granular area, and a fainter back line representing the endothelium (along with Descemet's membrane). To enhance the visibility of these layers, the angle between the illumination and magnification systems can be increased. This can be achieved by displacing the observation arm from its central position to a more nasal location while extending the illumination column more temporally. Such adjustments amplify the view of individual layers in the cornea or lens, facilitating a more accurate determination of lesion depth.

An additional application of the optical section is the assessment of the anterior chamber angle's degree of openness. Utilizing low magnification (6x or 10x) for an adequate field of view, set the beam 60 degrees to the side of the microscope. Place a narrow slit as close to the limbus

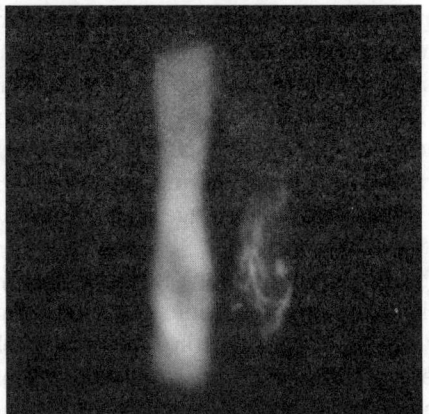
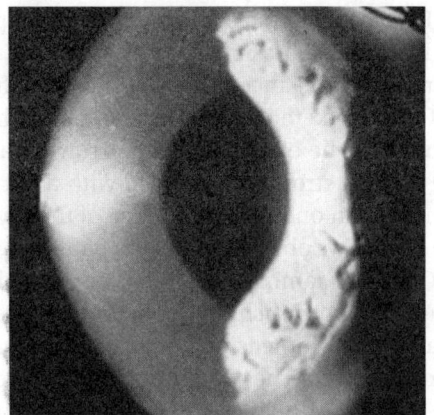

Corneal scarring observed with parallelepiped   Fleischer's ring noted with parallelepiped

Fig. 4.24: Wide beam.

as possible and normal to the cornea. To evaluate anterior chamber depth, compare the width of the cornea observed through the optical section with the dark section seen between the front surface of the iris and the back of the cornea. Concern arises when chamber depths are less than or equal to a quarter of the corneal thickness. To enhance resolution, minimize the slit width and improve clarity by increasing magnification.

This technique is employed specifically for investigative purposes, not for routine searches for abnormalities. However, once an abnormality is identified, determining its precise depth becomes more accessible using the optical section. Pay close attention to variations in corneal curvatures, corneal thickness, and the depth of visible features within the cornea during the examination process. This refined approach ensures a thorough and detailed assessment of the anterior chamber angle and related ocular features.

Wide beam

A wide slit **(Fig. 4.24)** also known as parallelepiped allows clearer observation of corneal and its layers. A 3-dimensional block of cornea can be observed. It allows a wider field for observation and more extensive examination of the cornea layer. Generally, a very wide beam is used for surface study, whilst a very narrow one is used for sections. A useful combination of the two is the parallelepiped section of the cornea, which uses a 2 mm to 3 mm slit width enabling corneal surface as well as stroma to be studied. While layers of cornea:

- Corneal epithelium is seen as very thin blue streak at the onset
- Then Bowman is seen as white band
- The grey granular portion is stroma
- Followed by again whitish layer of Desmets
- Last is endothelium

Slit lamp is set up for parallelepiped observation with following adjustments in set up:
- Vertical beam 2–4 mm wide
- High intensity
- 40–70 degree angle
- Med-high magnification
- Direct illumination
- Instrument coupled

This also allows us to ascertain the depth of any interesting feature, for example, foreign body, corneal abrasion, etc. It is, therefore, useful to vary the slit width during examination. To increase the distance between layers even further, make the illumination arm angle even larger.

Punctate keratitis can be seen using medium magnification, corneal nerve fibers in the stroma can be observed with narrow parallelepiped and high magnification. Nerve fibers in the corneal stroma is observed with a narrow parallelepiped and high magnification. Direct illumination on the front surface of the crystalline lens reveals the 'orange peel' effect and on the iris allows observation of iris pattern.

Corneal examination should be carried out with direct illumination and a parallelepiped setup. The cornea should be scanned systematically using this technique. This allows a good quality three-dimensional image of the corneal layers—epithelium, stroma and endothelium—to be viewed. The wider the angle, the greater the separation of the structures and, therefore, the easier it is to differentiate them. The initial magnification should be medium, and then if necessary increase it to closely examine any areas requiring further investigation.

Conical beam

Conical beam illumination is a crucial technique in ophthalmology, specifically for examining the anterior chamber to detect conditions such as flare, pigmentation, or cell debris **(Fig. 4.25)**. To optimize this method, a slit lamp is set up with meticulous adjustments:

- Ensure a completely darkened room to enhance sensitivity to subtle changes in the anterior chamber.
- Set the microscope to medium to high magnification for detailed observation.
- Use high illumination to maximize visibility of anterior chamber details.
- Employ a narrow circular beam to focus on specific areas.
- Set the angle of the beam between 40 to 50 degrees for optimal illumination.
- Position the observation system in front of the eye to align with the conical beam.
- Align the biomicroscope directly in front of the patient's eye with the brightest illumination tolerated by the patient.
- Focus the conical beam between the cornea and the anterior lens surface.
- Concentrate observation on the dark zone between the out-of-focus cornea and lens, normally appearing optically empty and totally black.

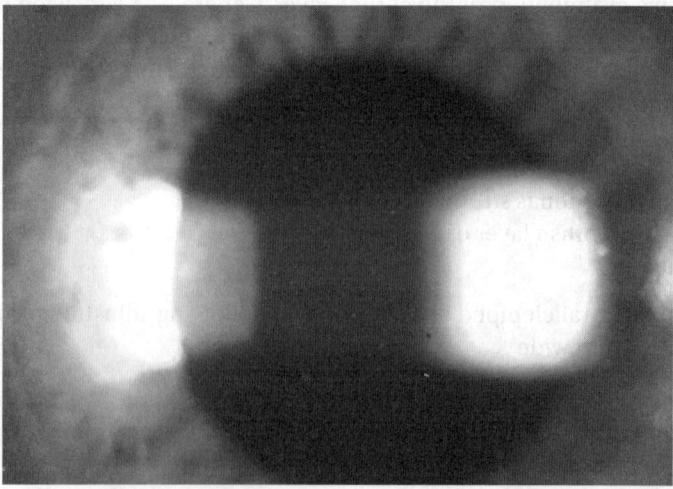

Fig. 4.25: Aqueous flare—Tyndall's phenomenon.

Conical beam examination procedure

- Perform examination for cells or flare before dilation or tonometry, as these procedures may alter the observed conditions.
- Allow both the examiner and the patient a period of time to adapt to the dark environment.
- Use the conical beam to detect floating aqueous cells and flare through the Tyndall effect, similar to observing dust in sunlight.
- Reduce the beam to a small circular pattern.
- Position the light source 45 to 60 degrees temporally, directed into the pupil.

Identification of flare and cells

Flare (protein escaping from dilated vessels) manifests as a gray or milky appearance in the normally empty zone. Cells (white blood cells escaping from dilated vessels) reflect light, appearing as white dots.

Conical beam examination is essential for diagnosing inflammation based on the presence of cells and flare in the anterior chamber. This meticulous approach ensures accurate observation and grading of ocular conditions.

Broad beam

Broad beam **(Fig. 4.26)** is the first illumination technique applied for examination of ocular structures with slit lamp. Usually, the slit lamp examination starts with broad beam with low illumination intensity. It may be applied with low illumination or with high illumination.

Broad beam: Set-up

- Low to high magnification can be used.
- However, only low magnification can take the full advantage of the broad beam field of illumination since a wider field of view and high magnification are mutually exclusive.
- The use of different filters reduces glare, widens the field of vision and distributes the light uniformly.

Broad beam: Application

This is helpful to have overall view of the anterior structure of the eye: lids, lashes, conjunctiva, cornea, sclera, iris, pupil.

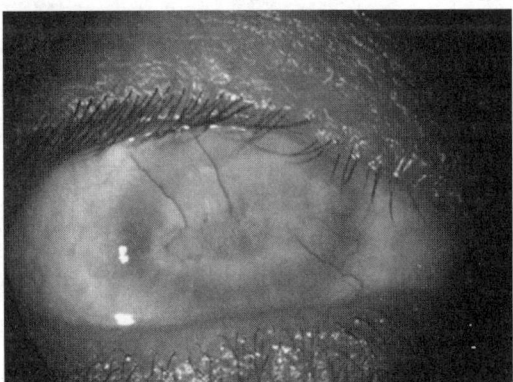 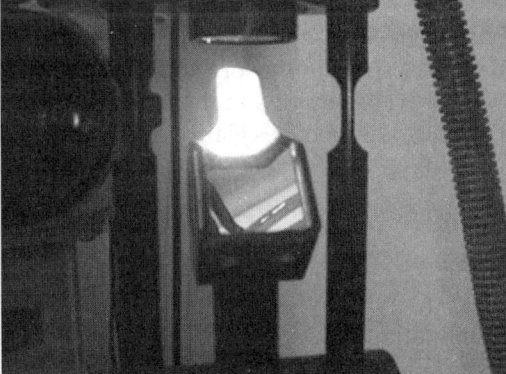

Fig. 4.26: Broad beam.

Broad beam: Procedure
- The practitioner should carry out several sweeps across the anterior segment and adnexa with a broad beam and low magnification.
- Starting with the lids closed, the lid margins and lashes should be examined for signs of marginal blepharitis or styes.
- Next, the patient should be asked to open his or her eyes, and the lid margin be examined for patency of the tear ducts and meibomian glands.
- Once upper and lower margins have been examined, the practitioner should look at the bulbar conjunctiva to assess hyperaemia and the possible presence of a pingueculum or pterygium.
- This illumination should also be used to view the superior and inferior palpebral conjunctiva for hyperemia, follicles and papillae.
- This illumination would also be used to give an assessment of soft lens fit in terms of centration, movement and tightness.
- Diffuse illumination may also be used to assess lens spoliation by dark-field illumination. For this, the lens should be removed from the eye, held in the slit beam in the plane of the headrest and viewed under magnification through the eyepieces.

Types of Illuminating Techniques

In slit lamp examination, various illuminating techniques are employed to visualize and assess different structures of the eye in detail. Each illuminating technique serves a specific purpose and allows the examiner to systematically evaluate different aspects of ocular health during a slit lamp examination. The choice of technique depends on the structures being examined and the information needed for diagnosis and treatment. Some common types of illuminating techniques used in slit lamp examination:
- Diffuse illumination
- Direct illumination
- Indirect illumination
- Retro-illumination
- Specular illumination
- Sclerotic illumination
- Tangential illumination

Diffuse Illumination

Broad beam of light is spread and diffusing filter is established by inserting a ground glass screen or diffuser in the illuminating path **(Fig. 4.27)**.

Significance

If media, especially that of the cornea, are opaque, optical section images are often impossible depending on severity. In these cases, direct diffuse illumination may be used to advantage. Diffusing filter reduces glare, widens the field of illumination and distributes the light more uniformly.

Application

General view of the anterior eye including palpebral conjunctiva, lids, lashes, cornea, sclera, iris, pupil and contact lens fitting characteristics, e.g., centration, movement.

Illumination settings
- Slit fully opened
- Inserted diffuser

Chapter 4: Instruments and Equipment used in Eye

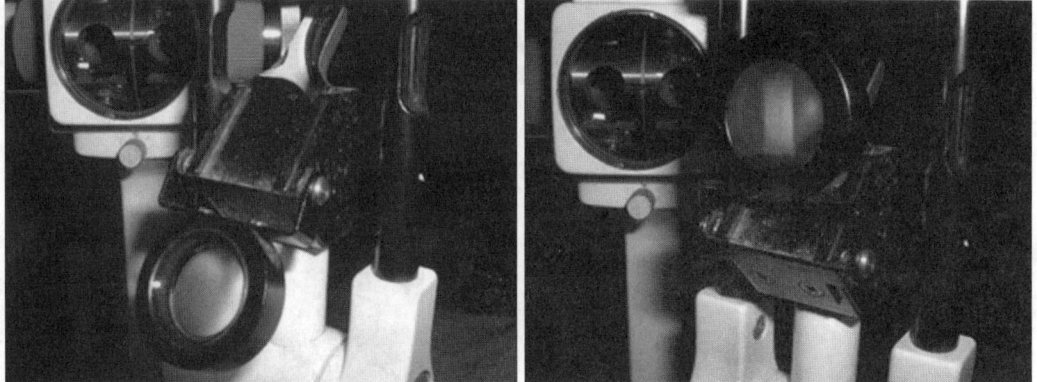

Fig. 4.27: Diffuse illumination set up.

- Microscope positioned at 0°
- Angle of slit illumination system approx. 30°–50°

Magnification

Low to medium magnifications

Procedure

- Instruct the patient to close the eyes, scan across the upper lid and lashes starting from temporal canthus.
- Ask the patient to open the eyes and scan across the lower lid and lashes, observe tear meniscus, the lid apposition to globe, opening of meibomian glands.
- Apply a little pressure around the punta and observe it for clearance or occlusions.
- Scan across the entire eye from temporal canthus to nasal canthus to have overall view of anterior of the eye.

Direct Illumination (Fig. 4.28)

The slit beam, i.e., illumination and observation system, i.e., microscope both are focused on the same point.

Significance

Direct focal illumination refers to projecting the light on the subject at the plane of focus. Unlike diffused light concentrated light penetrates transparent structures.

Application

Use narrow slit beam to observe variation in corneal curvature, corneal thickness and depth of foreign body. Use parallelepiped wider beam of 2 to 3 mm to observe corneal stroma, epithelium breakdown, lens fit, lens surface and endothelium. Finally, conical beam with high magnification to observe flare and cells in anterior chamber.

Illumination settings

- 30 to 45 angle between illumination system and the microscope. Variation in angle is made provided they focus on the same point.
- Slit beam narrow to wide
- Vary height of light for conical beam
- Medium to high illumination

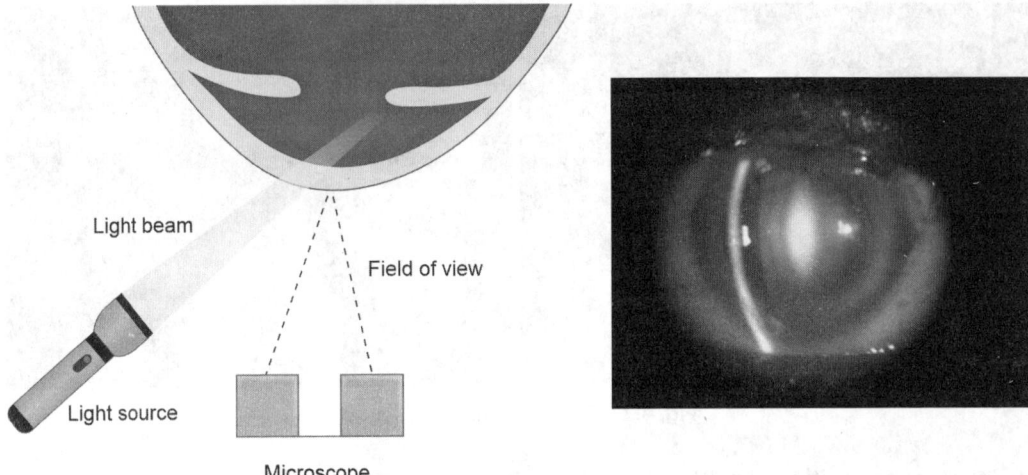

Fig. 4.28: Direct illumination.

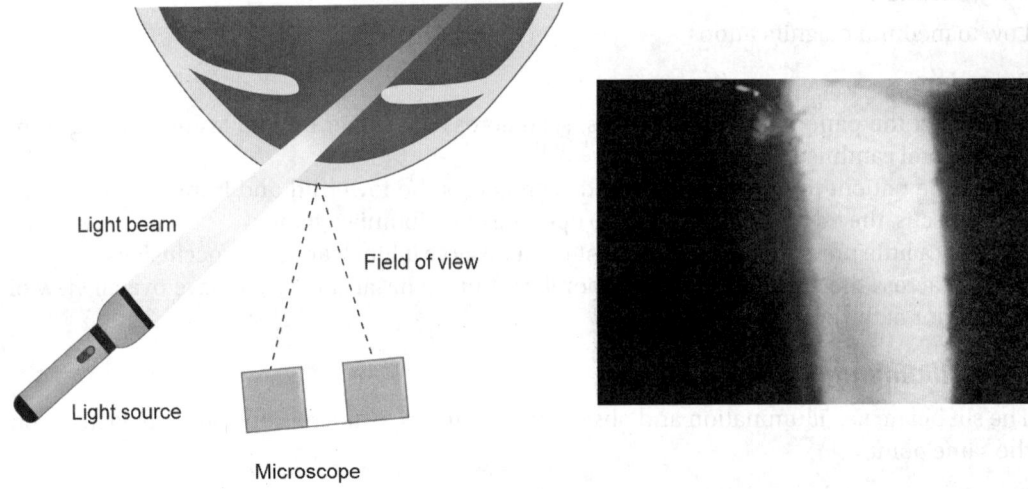

Fig. 4.29: Peripheral corneal erosion observed with indirect illumination.

Magnification

Medium to high magnification.

Procedure

- Instruct the patient to look straight ahead and angle the illumination arm and scan across the central portion of the cornea.
- When you reach the apex of the cornea, swing the illumination arm to other side, set it at the proper angle and continue scanning.
- Elevate the upper lid to scan across superior one third cornea. Pull down the lower lid with your index finger, and scan across the lower portion of cornea.

Indirect Illumination (Fig. 4.29)

Focus the light beam on a position just beside the area to be examined.

Significance

With indirect illumination the light does not fall directly on the pathology.

Application

Useful for observing specific conditions, including:
- Corneal microcysts
- Epithelial vesicles
- Epithelial erosions
- Iris sphincter details
- Ideal for examining objects near corneal areas with reduced transparency, such as infiltrates, scars, deposits, or defects

Illumination settings

- Can be applied with low, medium, and high illumination intensity.
- Moderate slit beam width, adjustable as needed.
- The slit beam can be offset by rotating the prism or mirror at the head of the illumination system.
- Maintain a 30 to 45-degree angle between the illumination arm and the microscope.

Magnification

Low to high magnification.

Procedure

- With this method, light enters the eye through a narrow to medium slit (2 to 4 mm) to one side of the area to be examined. Introduce light through a narrow to medium slit (2 to 4 mm) positioned just beside the area of interest. Observation is thus against a comparatively dark background. The observed corneal area is situated between the incident light section through the cornea and the illuminated area of the iris. Observation occurs against a comparatively dark background, enhancing visibility and contrast.
- Helpful for detecting corneal microcysts, vesicles, and erosions.
- Facilitates examination of corneal areas with reduced transparency.
- Enables detailed observation of the iris sphincter for functional and structural assessments.

Retro-illumination (Fig. 4.30)

Object of interest is illuminated by the light reflected from the structure behind that. Light is focused on the iris, or crystalline lens or fundus while the microscope is focused on the cornea or iris or lens.

Significance

In certain cases, illumination by optical section does not yield sufficient information or is impossible when larger, extensive zones or spaces of the ocular media are opaque.

Then the scattered light that is not very bright normally is absorbed. A similar situation arises when areas behind the crystalline lens are to be observed.

In this case, the observation beam must pass a number of interfaces that may reflect and attenuate the light. In such cases, retro-illumination often proves to be useful.

Application

Observe cornea for neovascularization, edema, microcysts, vacuoles, infiltrates, crystalline lens opacities, contact lens front and back surface deposits.

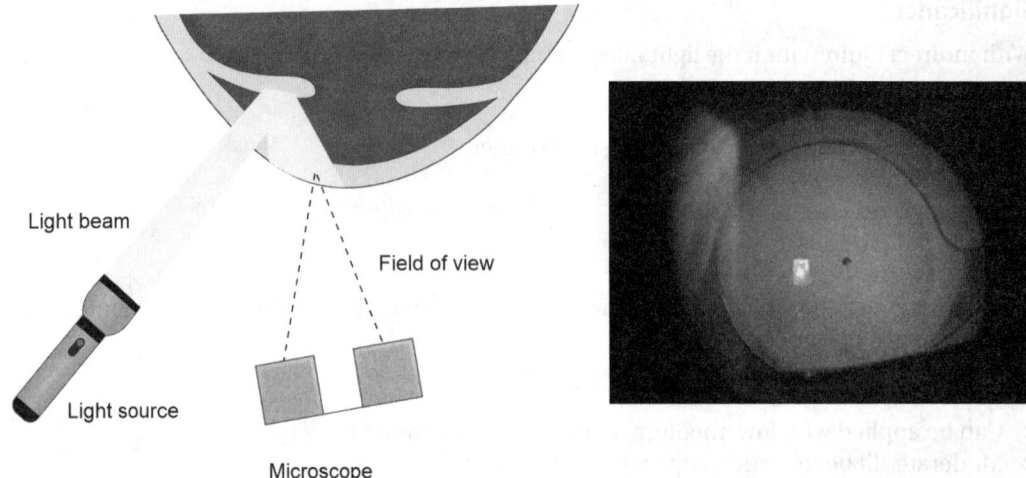

Fig. 4.30: Retro-illumination.

Illumination settings
- Wide beam of 2 to 3 mm or parallelepiped, also narrow slit beam when the retro illumination is from retina.
- Vary angle between illumination arm and microscope, also smallest angle when retro-illumination is from retina.
- Slit beam is offset by rotation of the prism at the head of the illumination system.

Magnification
Medium to high magnification.

Procedure
Basically, there are two types of retro-illumination:
1. Direct retro illumination
2. Indirect retro illumination

Direct retro-illumination is caused by direct reflection at the surfaces, such as the iris, lens or fundus. Indirect retro-illumination is caused by the diffuse reflection in the medium, i.e., all scattering light in the anterior and posterior segments.

Retro-illumination from the iris
Retro-illumination from the iris is very strong and hence the slit is kept narrow. Retro-illumination from the iris can be used to observe corneal opacities, foreign bodies in the cornea, vascularization, microcysts, vacuoles, edema. Examination is done in the yellow field.

Retro-illumination from the crystalline lens
The light may be put either on the front surface of the lens or onto the back surface and the examination is done in the greyish white field of light. The light from the front surface of lens can be used to observe defects in the pigment leaf of the iris, corneal defects and scars. The light from the back surface of the lens can be used to observe structures in the crystalline lens.

Retro-illumination from retina
Illumination system and observation system are set at 0 degree and examination is done in the red field. A reddish corneal reflection appears that is not very bright. Observation of superficial

corneal defects, scars, cataract can be observed. With this type of retro-illumination, pupil has to be dilated as otherwise the relatively small field of view through the normal pupil size makes observation almost impossible.

Specular Illumination

Specular illumination **(Fig. 4.31)** is a specialized technique that enables the observation of delicate structures within the eye, including the cornea's endothelial cells and both surfaces of the crystalline lens. This method involves positioning the illumination system and biomicroscope at equal angles of incidence and reflection.

Significance

This technique is the sole method for visualizing the endothelial cells of the cornea and the epithelial cells on the back surface of the lens. The observed cells are visible to only one eye, appearing in the ocular opposite to the direction of the illumination light source.

Application

Valuable for viewing endothelium cells, tear film debris, tear film lipid layer.

Illumination settings

- Slit beam to medium width parallelepiped
- Start with 45 to 60 degree angle between microscope and illumination system
- High illumination

Magnification

High magnification.

Procedure

- Position the biomicroscope directly in front of the patient's eye, with the illumination light source at a 45 to 60-degree angle.
- Just off the limbus, focus on creating a sharply defined parallelepiped of the cornea.
- Slowly advance the parallelepiped across the cornea until a dazzling reflection of the filament is observed within the biomicroscope.

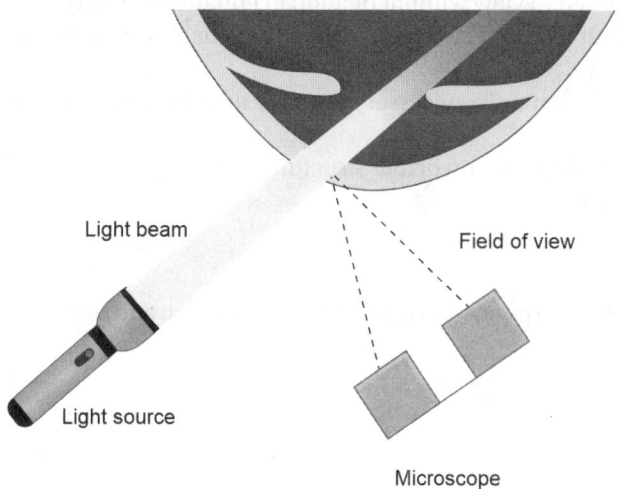
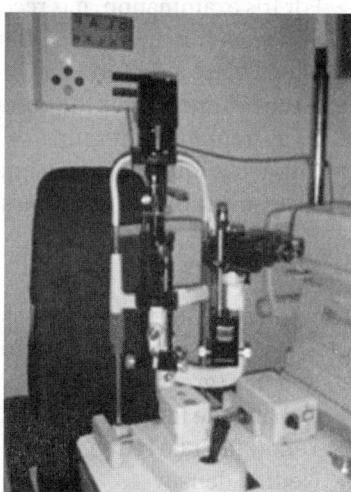

Fig. 4.31: Specular illumination.

- Keep the reflected light within the biomicroscope's field of view and move the focus back toward the endothelial cells.
- Reach a point where two images of the filament are visible—one bright and the other ghostlike or copper-yellow in color.
- Critically focus the biomicroscope on the latter until a mosaic of hexagonal cells becomes apparent.

Tangential Illumination

Tangential illumination is a specialized technique employed for the examination of the iris, offering a unique perspective by utilizing extremely oblique illumination. In this method, the observation system is positioned directly in front of the eye under examination.

Significance

The primary significance of tangential illumination lies in its ability to reveal surface texture. Unlike direct illumination, which tends to produce a flat view, tangential light projected from an oblique angle creates shadows that accentuate surface irregularities. This effect is analogous to the way shadows add depth to drawings.

Application

This technique is particularly valuable for the detailed observation of iris freckles, tumors, and the overall integrity of the cornea and iris.

Illumination settings

- Large angle between the illumination system and the observation system, approximately 70 to 80 degrees.
- Microscope should be pointed straight ahead.

Magnification

Choose magnification levels of 10X, 16X, or 25X for optimal results.

Procedure

- For iris examination, it is recommended to view without dilation to enhance visibility.
- For details on the cornea or lens, dilation is preferred, as it creates a dark background against which these structures can be viewed.
- If the headrest limits the oblique angle, it may be necessary to gently turn the patient's head away from the light source.
- This technique provides a nuanced perspective on ocular structures, allowing for a detailed assessment of the iris and associated features.

Use of Filters

An additional filter lens system is usually incorporated to control the illumination and maximize the view. The common filters are:
- Red free (green)
- Cobalt blue filter (Wratten #47 A)
- Yellow filter (Wratten #12)
- Neutral density

They all enhance the visibility of certain conditions.

Red Free Filter

Red free filter is used to differentiate vascular from pigmented lesions. Blood vessels and small hemorrhages will take on a dark appearance with the use of the red free filter, whereas pigmented lesions will remain dark. This enhances the contrast while looking for corneal and iris vascularization as red appears black.

Cobalt Blue Filter

The cobalt blue filter serves as a valuable tool in ocular examinations, specifically for assessing ocular surface integrity and optimizing contact lens fitting. Its ability to excite sodium fluorescein, a fluorescent dye, enables the visualization of subtle abnormalities and assists in diagnosing conditions like keratoconus. Illumination of sodium fluorescein with the cobalt blue filter (460 nm to 490 nm) induces a greenish light emission with a peak at 520 nm. This fluorescence highlights any areas where fluorescein is absorbed, revealing them as fluorescent green against a general blue background. This is useful technique to examine:
- Ocular surface integrity
- Contact lens fitting
- Diagnosis of keratoconus
- Enhanced contrast for iron pigment

Yellow Filter

The yellow filter serves as a supplementary barrier filter, strategically positioned in front of the viewing system rather than being integrated into the illumination system. This positioning is crucial for its specific function in enhancing contrast during ocular examinations. When used in conjunction with the cobalt blue filter, the yellow filter plays a key role in optimizing contrast for fluorescein staining. While the cobalt blue filter excites fluorescein, causing it to emit green fluorescence, the yellow filter selectively transmits this green fluorescent light. Simultaneously, it effectively blocks the blue light that may be reflected from the corneal surface. The yellow filter's ability to permit the transmission of green fluorescent light while attenuating the blue light results in improved visualization of fluorescein staining. This selective transmission enhances the contrast between the stained areas, represented by green fluorescence, and the surrounding structures. It is essential to note that the yellow filter, by design, introduces light loss due to its selective transmission properties. Consequently, a compensatory adjustment in illumination intensity is required to maintain adequate brightness during the examination. A high illumination level becomes necessary to counteract the light loss attributed to the filter. The yellow filter is particularly valuable when examining ocular surfaces for subtle abnormalities or irregularities highlighted by fluorescein staining. It provides enhanced clarity and definition in the visualization of stained areas. Conditions where precise discrimination of fluorescein patterns is crucial, such as in assessing corneal integrity and contact lens fitting benefit significantly from the combined use of cobalt blue and yellow filters.

Neutral Density

Neutral density (ND) filters integrated into slit lamps serve a dual purpose—managing light intensity for optimal imaging and enhancing patient comfort by absorbing excess heat. These filters are designed to selectively attenuate light across the visible spectrum without altering its color characteristics. ND filters are particularly useful during slit lamp photography, where precise control over light intensity is essential for capturing high-quality images without causing glare or discomfort to the patient. For examinations that require extended periods of time, such as complex anterior segment assessments or contact lens fittings, the inclusion of ND filters contributes to a more tolerable experience for the patient.

Van Herrick Technique

Van Herrick technique **(Fig. 4.32)** is used to evaluate anterior chamber angle without gonioscopy. Set the illumination arm at 60 degree to the temporal or nasal side of the patient's line of fixation. Alternatively, illumination may be set at 30 degree to one side and microscope 30 degree to the other side, yielding a 60 degree angle **(Fig. 4.33)**.

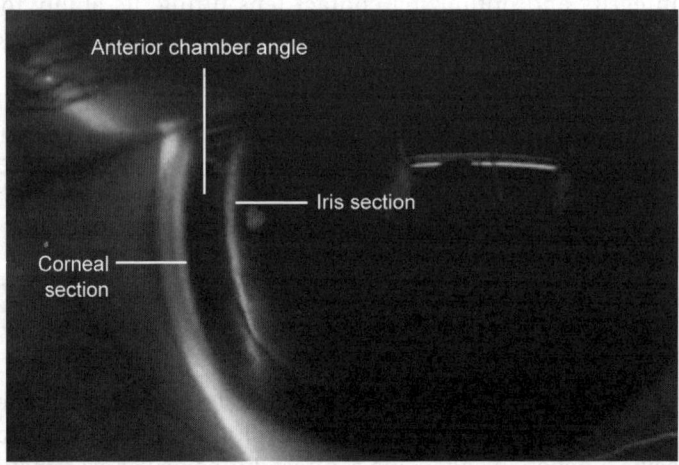

Fig. 4.32: Assessment of anterior chamber angle using Van Herrick technique.

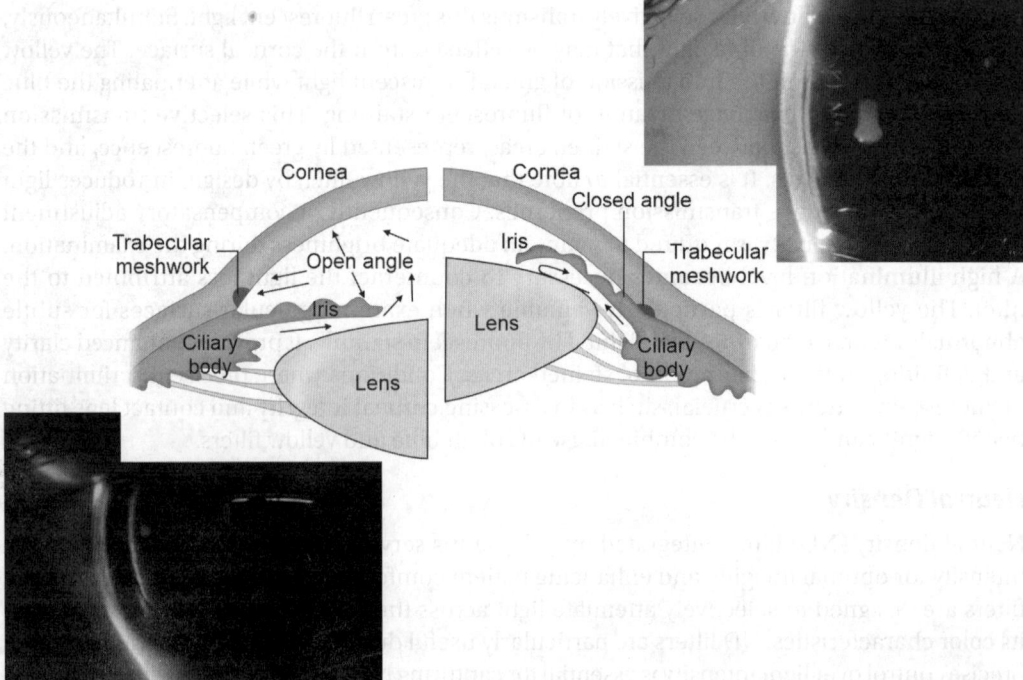

Fig. 4.33: Representation of angle of anterior chamber as observed using Van Herrick technique.

Magnification should remain on medium setting. Narrow the beam to optic section and instruct the patient to look straight ahead and now focus the light sharply on the cornea at the very edge of the temporal limbus.

Depth of anterior chamber is evaluated to the thickness of cornea. Compare the width of the shadow formed on the iris (representing the depth of the anterior chamber) to the width of the optic section (representing the thickness of the cornea). The shadow is actually a dark interval between the light on the cornea and the light on the iris represents the optically empty aqueous in the anterior chamber.

- Grade 4—open anterior chamber angle 1:1 ratio
- Grade 3—open anterior chamber angle 1:2 ratio
- Grade 2—narrow anterior chamber angle 1:4 ratio
- Grade 1—risky narrow anterior chamber angle less than 1:4 ratio
- Grade 0—closed anterior chamber, cornea "sits" on iris

Routine clinical procedure for slit lamp examination

In a routine clinical practice, a complete slip lamp examination does not take more than 2 to 3 minutes. But in order to complete the comprehensive slit examination quickly, certain sequential steps are necessary and a correct set-up of the instrument is essential. The illumination and observation systems must be coupled and in focus for the observer, and the patient must be seated comfortably, with his chin in the rest, head firmly against the headrest and eye level at the center of the vertical travel of the instrument.

The sequential steps needed to achieve this are:
- Instrument focusing
- Patient position
- Focusing check
- PD adjustment
- Operator's posture
- Viewing angle
- Patient examination

- Using the focusing rod provided with the slit lamp ensures a narrow slit beam is clearly in focus through each eyepiece individually, and then binocularly.
- Explain to the patient the nature of the examination and ensure they are seated comfortably with eye level at the middle of the instrument's vertical travel. If the eye level is not in the middle of the instrument's vertical travel, the examiner will have difficulty looking at the inferior and superior parts of the eye. Most slit-lamps have a notch on the headrest which should be lined up with the outer canthus of the eye to ensure the head position is optimal. Adjust the height of the instrument table to be comfortable to both for patient as well as practitioner.
- With the eyelids closed the examiner should focus the light on the lids and check its focus by rotating the illumination system from side to side. As it rotates, the light should remain stationary on the lid. If it is showing relative movement, the instrument is not in focus.
- Set the slit lamp to your PD by adjusting the separations of oculars. The correct setting of PD will ensure that you get correct binocular view when looking through the oculars.
- Use one of your hands to operate the joystick and the elevation knob and the other hand to control the slit beam and to vary the angle between the lamp and the microscope, and to manipulate the patient eyelids.
- Set the illumination arm at a suitable angle. Illumination arm and viewing angles are regularly adjusted during the procedure. Larger angle allows identifying different layers more easily.

- Reduce the room illumination and start the examination now. Instruct the patient to close his eyes. Turn on the instrument.
- Using the patient's eyelashes for fixation, examine the various structures of the eye in an anterior-to-posterior sequence.
- In the routine examination, the right eye is usually examined first and then the left eye.

Lids and lashes examination

Perform a meticulous lids and lashes examination using diffuse illumination, setting the light arm at a 30-degree angle. Keep magnification low and instruct the patient to close their eyes, scanning from the temporal canthus across upper lids and lashes. Sweep the adnexa with a broad beam to identify signs of marginal blepharitis or styes. With eyes open, examine the lid margin for tear duct and meibomian gland patency, assessing the tear meniscus for any anomalies. This approach ensures a comprehensive evaluation of adnexal structures, aiding in the detection of ocular surface issues and contributing to overall eye health assessment.

Conjunctiva examination

For a comprehensive conjunctival examination, employ a narrow slit beam widened to a parallelepiped, positioning the illumination arm at approximately 30 degrees from the straight-ahead position. Keep magnification low and instruct the patient to open their eyes, looking up initially. Evert the lower lid by placing the index finger near the lower margin, scanning the inferior palpebral and bulbar conjunctiva for irregularities, elevations, or discolorations, while evaluating the inferior punctum. As the patient looks down, use the thumb to lift the upper lid, examining the superior bulbar conjunctiva. Instruct the patient to look left and right for a thorough assessment of the nasal and temporal conjunctiva. Conclude by everting the upper lid, systematically scanning from temporal to nasal, ensuring a comprehensive evaluation of hyperemia, follicles, papillae, and the potential presence of pingueculum or pterygium.

Cornea and tear film examination

After completing the conjunctival examination, transition to the cornea assessment using a parallelepiped or wide beam with a 2 to 3 mm aperture. Set the illumination arm at a 30 to 45-degree angle, utilizing medium magnification. Scan the entire cornea, noting opacities or irregularities from the limbus to the apex. Employ a red-free filter for enhanced vascularization detection. Ensure a comprehensive view by adjusting the patient's gaze and elevating lids as needed. Subsequently, narrow the beam for cross-sectional examination with high illumination and magnification to evaluate opacifications, microcysts, stromal striae, and anterior chamber angle depth. Conclude with a crucial fluorescein staining examination, using sodium fluorescein to reveal even minute corneal abrasions. Enhance visibility with a yellow barrier filter, optimizing diagnostic precision in assessing corneal and conjunctival integrity, particularly valuable in contact lens practice.

Angle of anterior chamber examination

For optimal examination of the anterior chamber angle, position the illumination arm at a 60-degree angle to either the temporal or nasal side of the patient's line of fixation. Alternatively, set the illumination arm at 30 degrees to one side and the microscope at 30 degrees to the other side, achieving a 60-degree angle between the lamp and microscope. Maintain medium magnification. Narrow the beam to optic section, instructing the patient to look straight ahead. Focus the light sharply on the cornea at the temporal limbus edge. Compare the width of the shadow on the iris, indicating anterior chamber depth, to the width of the optic section, representing corneal thickness. The shadow, a dark interval between corneal and iris light, signifies the optically empty aqueous in the anterior chamber. If the angle width is less than ¼:1, consider performing gonioscopy for a more detailed assessment.

Iris examination

To examine the iris, widen the slit width to approximately 3 mm, configuring it as a wide parallelepiped. Set the illumination arm at 30 to 45 degrees from the straight-ahead position, maintaining a medium magnification setting. Instruct the patient to gaze straight ahead and scan the iris surface for irregularities. Observe the papillary reflex, noting that the pupil should constrict as the slit lamp beam reaches the papillary margin. This approach ensures a focused and efficient assessment of the iris, providing valuable insights into its structure and responsiveness.

Crystalline lens examination

To assess the crystalline lens, angle the illumination arm at 10 to 20 degrees from the straight-ahead position, maintaining medium magnification. Narrow the slit beam to a thin parallelepiped. Gradually approach the patient until the light penetrates the pupil, sharply focusing on the anterior lens surface. Systematically scan the front surface before moving the biomicroscope closer to inspect deeper layers. Focus on the posterior lens surface, checking for irregularities or discolorations. Swing the illumination arm to the opposite side, ensuring a thorough examination from anterior to posterior. If opacities are identified, narrow the slit beam to optic section for precise determination of their depth within the lens. This method ensures a detailed and focused evaluation of the crystalline lens.

Contact lens surface quality assessment

To assess a contact lens using a slit lamp, clean and rinse it, then position with tweezers, holding the surface towards the biomicroscope lens. Employ low magnification with a wide parallelepiped and focus by adjusting lens or instrument. Check for films, spots, or damage. If clean, record as such. For deposits or damage, describe findings. Protein films may be transparent or opaque, lipid deposits appear greasy and shiny, jelly bumps are raised spots, and calcium deposits form a whitish film or discrete deposits, and fungal growths show filamentary patterns in various colors. Cracking and crazing manifest as lattice-type cracks **(Fig. 4.34)**.

Contact lens surface wettability assessment

To assess contact lens surface wettability **(Fig. 4.35)**, place the lens on the patient's eye and allow 15–20 minutes for stabilization. Set the slit lamp for a specular reflection on the lens surface using medium parallelepiped and low to moderate light intensity. Instruct the patient to blink, observing tear break-up time as an indicator of lens drying time. Rapid tear disruption points to poor wettability, often caused by deposits, polish residues, or surface damage. This method provides a quick and effective evaluation of the lens' interaction with tears and its overall surface condition.

Additional Use of Slit Lamp

The applications of slit lamp in the clinical practice can be extended by additional attachments for comprehensive eye examinations and various ophthalmic procedures. The common attachments are:

- ❖ **Applanation tonometry:** Applanation tonometry can be attached to a slit lamp to measure intraocular pressure.
- ❖ **Pachymetry:** A pachometer can be used with a slit lamp to measure corneal thickness.

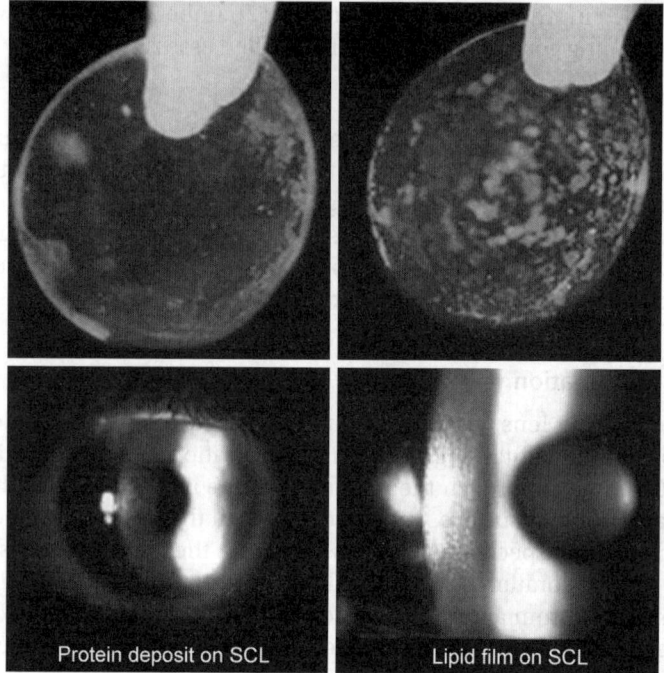

Fig. 4.34: Protein and lipid deposits on soft contact lenses.

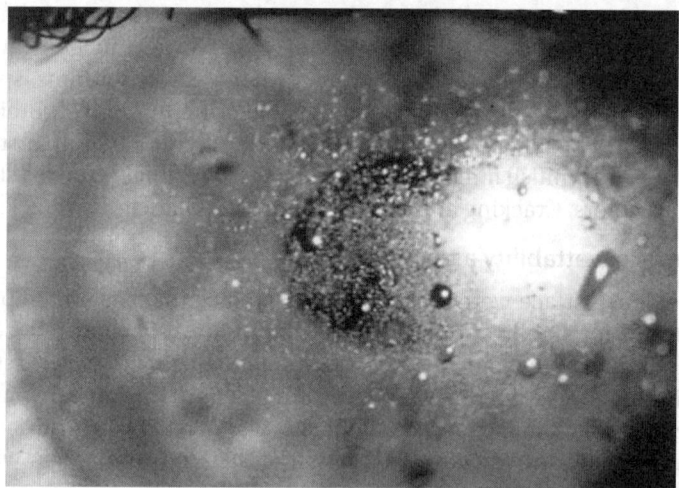

Fig. 4.35: Poor surface wettability of SCL.

- **Gonioscopy:** A gonioscope attachment allows the assessment of the anterior chamber angle.
- **Volk lens or Hruby lens:** These lenses are used for binocular indirect ophthalmoscopy.
- **LASER treatment:** Some slit lamps can be equipped with a laser delivery system for specific treatments.
- **Aesthiometry:** Aesthiometry can be used to measure corneal sensitivity.
- **Photography:** Camera attachments can be used for photographing the eye during examinations.

GONIOSCOPE

INTRODUCTION

A gonioscope is a specialized ophthalmic instrument utilized in eye care clinics to meticulously examine the angle of the anterior chamber of the eye. Comprising a lens system and mirrored prism, the gonioscope enables the examiner to visualize the angle structures within the eye. By delicately placing the gonioscope on the cornea, the examiner gains a direct view of the angle formed between the cornea and the iris. This angle plays a crucial role in evaluating and diagnosing various eye conditions, particularly those associated with the drainage of aqueous humor—the vital fluid that nourishes the eye. The gonioscope's precise examination of these structures is instrumental in diagnosing conditions like glaucoma and guiding appropriate treatment strategies.

Parts of Gonioscope

The gonioscope, a specialized instrument in ophthalmic examination, consists of several key components:
- Gonioscope lens
- Mirrored prism
- Light source
- Viewing window

Gonioscope Lens

The lens system of the gonioscope is designed to provide a clear and magnified view of the anterior chamber angle structures when placed on the patient's eye.

Mirrored Prism

The mirrored prism is a crucial component that reflects light and redirects the image, allowing the examiner to visualize the angle formed between the cornea and the iris.

Light Source

An integral part of the gonioscope, the light source ensures proper illumination during the examination. This illumination is essential for obtaining a detailed and well-lit view of the angle structures.

Viewing Window

The viewing window is the part of the gonioscope through which the examiner observes the reflected image and the angle structures of the eye. It provides a clear line of sight for a comprehensive examination.

These components work in tandem to facilitate a thorough evaluation of the anterior chamber angle, aiding in the diagnosis and management of various eye conditions, particularly those related to the drainage of aqueous humor. The gonioscope's precise design and functionality contribute to its effectiveness in ophthalmic examinations, ensuring accurate assessments of critical eye structures.

Types of Gonioscope

There are different types of gonioscopes, each designed for specific purposes. The choice of gonioscope depends on the specific requirements of the examination, the patient's anatomy, and the preferences of the ophthalmologist. Each type of gonioscope has its advantages and is suited for different clinical scenarios.

Goldmann-type Gonioscope

This is one of the most widely used types. It consists of a glass or plastic prism that is applied to the patient's eye after applying a viscous coupling gel. The Goldmann-type gonioscope allows for a clear view of the angle structures.

Zeiss-type Gonioscope

Similar to the Goldmann-type, the Zeiss-type gonioscope is designed for examining the anterior chamber angle. It employs a prism to enable visualization of the trabecular meshwork and other angle structures.

Sussman Gonio Lens

The Sussman gonio lens is a mirrored lens that provides a wide and panoramic view of the angle structures. It is particularly useful for assessing peripheral structures and variations in the angle. The type is especially designed for infants and children. It has a small size lens and a short handle for easier maneuverability in children patient.

Koeppe Gonio Lens

The Koeppe gonio lens is a small handheld lens with mirrors, allowing for a direct view of the angle structures. It is often used in combination with a slit lamp for detailed examination.

Swan-Jacobs Gonio Lens

This type of gonioscope is designed for dynamic gonioscopy, which involves observing changes in the angle structures during different lighting conditions or with alterations in eye position.

Four Mirror Gonio Lens

As the name suggests, this gonio lens has four mirrors, allowing for a comprehensive view of all quadrants of the angle. It is particularly useful for assessing the entire circumference of the angle.

Hruby Lens

Although primarily used for fundus examination, the Hruby lens can also be used for indirect gonioscopy. It provides a wider field of view compared to traditional gonioscopes.

PACHYMETER

INTRODUCTION

A pachymeter is a medical device used to measure the thickness of the cornea. Corneal thickness is an important parameter in various ophthalmic assessments, particularly in the context of glaucoma management and refractive surgery. The accurate measurement of the thickness of the cornea is crucial in assessing intraocular pressure and planning surgical interventions. Corneal thickness is a factor in the accurate measurement of IOP. Thicker or thinner corneas can influence IOP readings. In refractive surgery, such as LASIK (Laser-Assisted In Situ Keratomileusis), pachymetry is crucial for determining the amount of corneal tissue that can be safely removed to achieve the desired refractive correction. Pachymetry is also used to screen for conditions like keratoconus, a progressive thinning and distortion of the cornea. Changes in corneal thickness can be indicative of early stages of keratoconus.

Measurement Technique

Pachymetry is typically performed using ultrasound or optical methods.

Ultrasound Pachymetry

In ultrasound pachymetry, a probe is placed on the corneal surface, and the time delay of ultrasound waves is measured. This method is commonly used and provides accurate and reliable measurements.

Optical Coherence Tomography

Optical pachymetry utilizes optical coherence tomography (OCT) to obtain corneal thickness measurements. OCT uses light waves to create detailed cross-sectional images of the cornea, allowing for precise thickness measurements.

Corneal Thickness Mapping

Pachymeters can generate corneal thickness maps, providing a visual representation of thickness variations across the cornea. This information is valuable in detecting conditions such as corneal ectasia.

Non-invasive Techniques

Some pachymeters use non-contact or air-puff methods to measure corneal thickness. While these methods are less invasive, they may be less accurate compared to direct contact methods.

ISHIHARA CHART

INTRODUCTION

The Ishihara color test is a diagnostic tool used to assess color vision deficiencies, particularly red-green color blindness. Named after its creator, Dr Shinobu Ishihara, the Ishihara Chart consists of plates containing circles of dots with varying colors and sizes.

Purpose

The Ishihara Chart is widely used in various settings, including eye clinics, occupational health screenings, and the military, to identify individuals with color vision deficiencies. The primary purpose of the Ishihara Chart is to identify and diagnose red-green color deficiencies, which are the most common types of color blindness.

Design

Each plate of the Ishihara Chart is designed to present numbers or patterns embedded within a background of dots. These numbers or patterns are distinguishable to individuals with normal color vision but may be challenging for those with color vision deficiencies.

Color Vision Deficiencies

The most common color vision deficiencies involve difficulty distinguishing between red and green hues. The Ishihara Chart helps identify the type and severity of these deficiencies.

Testing Procedure

During the Ishihara Color Test, an individual is asked to identify numbers or patterns on the plates. The responses provide information about their color vision abilities.

Hidden Figures

For individuals with red-green color deficiencies, the numbers or patterns on the plates may appear indistinct or hidden within the background dots, making them challenging to discern.

Types of Plates

The Ishihara Chart consists of various plates, each designed to reveal specific types of color vision deficiencies. Some plates are more challenging than others, allowing for a detailed assessment of color perception.

Protanopia and Deuteranopia

Protanopia is a form of red color blindness, while deuteranopia is a form of green color blindness. The Ishihara Chart helps differentiate between these types and assess their severity.

Tritanopia

While the Ishihara Chart primarily focuses on red-green deficiencies, it may also include plates to assess tritanopia, a rare blue-yellow color vision deficiency.

Limitations

The Ishihara Chart has limitations, and individuals with milder color vision deficiencies may still pass the test. Additional testing methods may be required for a comprehensive assessment.

Standardization

The Ishihara Chart is available in standardized versions with specific sequences of plates. Standardization ensures consistency in testing procedures and results.

Ishihara Plates Book

The Ishihara Chart is often presented as a book containing multiple plates. The book format allows for systematic testing and evaluation.

Alternative Color Vision Tests

In addition to the Ishihara Chart, other color vision tests, such as the Farnsworth-Munsell 100 Hue Test, may be used for more detailed assessments.

The Ishihara Chart remains a widely recognized and practical tool for quickly assessing red-green color deficiencies, aiding in the diagnosis and understanding of color vision impairments.

PERIMETER

INTRODUCTION

A perimeter is a visual field testing device. Visual field testing assesses the full horizontal and vertical range that an individual can see while keeping their eyes fixed on a central point.

Purpose

Visual field testing with a perimeter is performed to evaluate the complete extent of a person's vision, detecting any abnormalities or defects in their visual field.

Conditions Assessed

Visual field testing is crucial for diagnosing and monitoring conditions such as glaucoma, retinal disorders, neurological disorders (e.g., optic nerve damage, tumors), and other visual pathway abnormalities.

Glaucoma Monitoring

In glaucoma, visual field testing helps assess peripheral vision loss, which is a common early sign of the condition. Monitoring changes in the visual field is essential for managing and adjusting glaucoma treatment.

Types of Perimeters

There are different types of perimeters, including manual perimeters and automated perimeters. Automated perimeter, often computerized, is more commonly used in modern eye care.

Automated Perimetry

Automated perimetry involves the use of a computerized device to present stimuli at various locations within the visual field. The patient responds to the stimuli, and the results are recorded and analyzed by the computer.

Testing Procedure

During visual field testing, the patient focuses on a central target, and lights or other stimuli are presented in different areas of their visual field. The patient indicates when they perceive the stimuli.

Types of Visual Field Tests

Common visual field tests include the Humphrey visual field test, Octopus perimetry, and Goldmann visual field test.

Humphrey Visual Field Test

Humphrey visual field test is one of the most widely used automated perimetry tests. It assesses the central and peripheral visual field and is commonly employed in glaucoma management.

Octopus Perimetry

Octopus perimetry is another automated visual field test that evaluates the entire visual field. It is versatile and can be used in various clinical situations.

Goldmann Visual Field Test

Goldmann visual field test is a manual test that uses a kinetic stimulus. It is often used for specific clinical purposes, and the results are recorded manually.

Mapping Visual Field Defects

Visual field testing provides a map of any defects or abnormalities in the visual field, aiding in diagnosis and treatment planning.

EXOPHTHALMOMETER

INTRODUCTION

An exophthalmometer **(Fig. 4.36)** is used to measure the degree of proptosis or exophthalmos, which is the protrusion of the eyeball from the orbit. This measurement is particularly relevant in the evaluation of conditions such as thyroid eye disease (Graves' disease) and other orbital disorders.

Purpose

The primary purpose of an exophthalmometer is to measure and quantify the degree of forward displacement or protrusion of the eyeball from its normal position within the eye socket (orbit).

Proptosis Measurement

Proptosis is measured in millimeters and is the distance between the anterior corneal surface (front of the eye) and a reference point on the orbital rim. This reference point is typically the lateral orbital rim.

Conditions Assessed

Exophthalmometry is commonly performed in cases of thyroid eye disease (Graves' disease), a condition where inflammation and swelling of the eye muscles can lead to proptosis. It is also used to assess other orbital conditions.

Exophthalmometry Techniques

Various techniques and instruments are used for exophthalmometry, with one common approach involving the use of an exophthalmometer instrument.

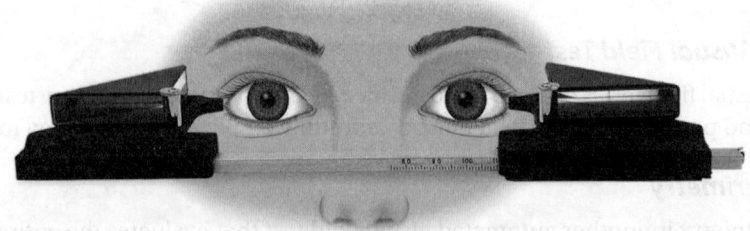

Fig. 4.36: Exophthalmometer.

Hertel Exophthalmometer

The Hertel exophthalmometer is a widely used instrument for measuring proptosis. It typically consists of two prongs or arms that are placed against the lateral orbital rims of both eyes simultaneously.

Measurement Procedure

The patient is positioned with the head in a standardized position, and the exophthalmometer is gently placed against the lateral orbital rims. The distance between the prongs and the corneal surface is measured.

Bilateral Measurement

Exophthalmometry is usually performed bilaterally, measuring both eyes simultaneously. The difference in proptosis between the two eyes can provide additional diagnostic information.

Baseline Measurement

A baseline exophthalmometry measurement is often recorded for comparison during follow-up visits. Changes in proptosis over time can be indicative of disease progression or response to treatment.

Limitations

Exophthalmometry measurements may have limitations, and factors such as patient cooperation, head positioning, and examiner technique can influence the accuracy of the results.

Management Implications

Exophthalmometry results can guide treatment decisions, such as the need for medical management, surgical intervention, or monitoring in cases of thyroid eye disease or other orbital disorders.

Comparison with Normative Values

The measured proptosis values are often compared with normative values for the population to determine the extent of the deviation from the normal range.

A AND B SCAN

A-scan and B-scan are types of ultrasound imaging techniques used in ophthalmology for evaluating the structures within the eye.

A-SCAN (AMPLITUDE SCAN)

Purpose

A-scan ultrasound is used to measure the axial length of the eye and is particularly valuable in the preoperative assessment of intraocular lens power for cataract surgery.

Measurement

It measures the time it takes for sound waves to travel from the cornea to the retina and back. The axial length obtained helps determine the appropriate intraocular lens power.

Components

A typical A-scan consists of a single-dimensional display, representing the amplitude or intensity of echoes along the axis of the eye.

Procedure

During the A-scan procedure, a probe is placed on the cornea, and high-frequency sound waves are emitted. The reflections from different intraocular structures are analyzed to determine the axial length.

Applications

A-scan ultrasound is commonly used in cataract surgery planning, especially for calculating the power of intraocular lenses to be implanted.

B-SCAN (BRIGHTNESS SCAN)

B-scan ultrasound provides a two-dimensional, cross-sectional view of the eye's internal structures. It is useful for evaluating the posterior segment of the eye, including the retina and vitreous.

Imaging Technique

B-scan generates a real-time, dynamic image by using sound waves to produce a series of cross-sectional scans. The brightness of the image corresponds to the amplitude of the echoes received.

Components

The B-scan displays a bright line for each echo received, creating a visual representation of the internal structures in the eye.

Procedure

Similar to A-scan, B-scan involves placing a probe on the eye's surface. The ultrasound waves penetrate the eye, and the echoes are translated into a two-dimensional image on the screen.

Applications

B-scan is used for assessing various ocular conditions such as retinal detachments, vitreous opacities, tumors, and other abnormalities in the posterior segment of the eye.

Types

There are different types of B-scan imaging, including longitudinal scans (sagittal or coronal views) and transverse scans (axial views). The choice of scan depends on the structures being evaluated.

Diagnostic Aid

B-scan is a valuable diagnostic tool when direct visualization of the posterior segment is challenging, as in the case of opaque media (e.g., dense cataracts or vitreous hemorrhage).

Patient Comfort

B-scan is a non-invasive procedure that does not involve exposure to ionizing radiation, making it comfortable and safe for patients.

In summary, A-scan is primarily used for measuring axial length in cataract surgery planning, while B-scan provides cross-sectional imaging of the posterior segment for the evaluation of various ocular conditions.

ERG, EOG AND VER

In ophthalmology, ERG, EOG and VER are abbreviations for specific electrodiagnostic tests that help evaluate the function of different parts of the visual system.

ERG (ELECTRORETINOGRAM)

ERG is a test that measures the electrical activity of the retina in response to light stimulation. It assesses the function of the photoreceptor cells (rods and cones) and the inner retinal layers.

Procedure

During an ERG, the patient's eyes are exposed to flashes of light, and electrodes placed on the cornea and skin record the electrical responses generated by the retina.

Applications

ERG is used to diagnose and monitor various retinal disorders, including inherited retinal diseases, retinal degenerations, and certain toxic effects on the retina.

EOG (ELECTROOCULOGRAM)

EOG measures the electrical potential of the eye's surface related to changes in the position of the eyeball. It evaluates the function of the retinal pigment epithelium (RPE).

Procedure

Electrodes are placed around the eyes to measure the voltage changes that occur when the eyes move between light and dark conditions. The movement of the eyes generates a characteristic waveform.

Applications

EOG is particularly useful in assessing disorders such as best vitelliform macular dystrophy and other conditions affecting the RPE.

VER (VISUAL EVOKED RESPONSE OR VISUAL EVOKED POTENTIAL)

VER measures the electrical activity of the visual cortex in response to visual stimuli. It assesses the transmission of visual signals along the optic nerve and the visual pathways.

Procedure

Visual stimuli, such as pattern-reversal or light flashes, are presented to the patient while electrodes placed on the scalp record the electrical responses generated in the brain.

Applications

VER is used in the diagnosis of optic nerve disorders, demyelinating diseases (e.g., multiple sclerosis), and conditions affecting the visual pathways. It is also employed in monitoring visual function during surgery involving the optic nerve.

These electrodiagnostic tests provide valuable information about the integrity and function of different components of the visual system. They are important tools in the diagnosis, monitoring, and management of various ophthalmic conditions, especially those involving the retina, retinal pigment epithelium, optic nerve, and visual pathways.

SYNOPTOPHORE

INTRODUCTION

The synoptophore is an orthoptic instrument designed for the assessment and treatment of binocular vision disorders. It has several uses and functions, making it a valuable tool in the field of orthoptics. Synoptophore consists of several parts:
- Chinrest
- Forehead rest
- Two tubes
- Controls
- Mirrors
- Scales
- Illumination system
- Keys

The synoptophore is equipped with two tubes, each housing a slide carrier at the outer end. These carriers hold picture slides, allowing for separate stimulation of each eye through angled eyepieces. Positioned horizontally, the tubes are attached to a movable column, enabling horizontal adjustments. The total tube length equals the focal length of the lens, and slides are placed at the focal distance of a +6.50D or +7.00D lens, ensuring parallel emergent rays and eliminating the need for patient accommodation.

The tubes' distance is adjustable to match the patient's inter-pupillary distance, and they can be locked together for simultaneous horizontal movement. Some modern synoptophores also allow vertical adjustments. Scales on the instrument facilitate the measurement of displacement in both arc degrees and prism diopters. The illumination system can be individually controlled for each target, with manual flashing keys for individual targets. Certain models offer controlled flashing, afterimage production, and features like Haidinger's brushes, which assess macular function and projection. This comprehensive design provides versatility in diagnosing and treating binocular vision disorders.

Uses of Synoptophore

The synoptophore can be used for diagnostic and therapeutic purpose. The diagnostic applications of the synoptophore encompass the following:

- **Measurement of angle of deviation:** The synoptophore is utilized for precise measurement of the angle of deviation, providing accurate information about the misalignment of the eyes.
- **Measurement of angle kappa:** It facilitates the measurement of angle kappa, which is the angular difference between the visual axis and the pupillary axis.
- **Measurement of primary and secondary deviation:** The instrument aids in measuring both primary deviation (the initial misalignment) and secondary deviation (the additional deviation when the fixing eye is covered).
- **Measurement of deviation in cardinal directions of gaze:** The synoptophore assists in measuring deviations in the cardinal directions of gaze, allowing for a comprehensive evaluation of eye movements.
- **Estimation of retinal correspondence:** It is employed to estimate retinal correspondence, distinguishing between normal and abnormal correspondence. It helps identify the presence and type of suppression and evaluates the existence of fusion.
- **Measurement of fusional amplitudes:** The instrument is utilized for measuring fusional amplitudes, providing insights into the range of binocular fusion abilities.
- **Presence of stereopsis:** The synoptophore assesses the presence of stereopsis, which is the ability to perceive depth and three-dimensional vision.
- **Assessment of grades of binocular vision:** It aids in grading binocular vision, allowing for a classification of the patient's ability to use both eyes together effectively.

The therapeutic applications of the synoptophore include the following:

- **Treatment of suppression:** The synoptophore is employed in the therapeutic management of suppression, a condition where the brain ignores the visual input from one eye.
- **Treatment of abnormal retinal correspondence:** It is utilized to address abnormal retinal correspondence, helping to establish a more appropriate alignment of corresponding retinal points.
- **Eccentric fixation (with Haidinger brushes):** When equipped with Haidinger brushes, the synoptophore can aid in the treatment of eccentric fixation, a condition where the patient develops a preferred, non-central point of fixation.
- **Accommodative esotropia (dissociation training):** The instrument is used in the therapeutic intervention for accommodative esotropia, involving dissociation training to improve eye coordination and alignment during focusing tasks.
- **Heterophoria and intermittent heterophorias:** Synoptophore therapy is applied in the treatment of heterophoria (latent misalignment) and intermittent heterophorias, working to enhance binocular vision and coordination during various visual tasks.

OTHER ORTHOPTIC INSTRUMENTS

AMBLYOSCOPES

Amblyoscopes are devices used to train the amblyopic (lazy) eye. They often incorporate mechanisms to occlude or blur one eye, encouraging the use and development of the weaker eye.

HAPLOSCOPES

Haploscopes are instruments designed for the evaluation of binocular vision and stereopsis. They use prisms and lenses to create conditions that challenge the eyes to work together.

BAGOLINI STRIATED GLASSES

These glasses are used to assess and train fusional abilities. They contain vertical and horizontal lines that can be rotated to stimulate different visual responses.

MADDOX ROD

The Maddox Rod is a cylindrical lens that creates a line of light when superimposed on an image. It is used for assessing and measuring eye deviations and phorias.

WORTH 4-DOT TEST

This test uses red and green filters to assess binocular vision and identify suppression or misalignment of the eyes.

These instruments are essential in the field of orthoptics, enabling eye care professionals to diagnose and manage various binocular vision disorders. They play a crucial role in the evaluation, treatment, and rehabilitation of conditions that affect how both eyes work together to provide clear and comfortable vision.

KERATOMETER

Keratometry is an instrument used to measure the front surface curvature of the cornea. The readings provide information as to the corneal astigmatism which may be used as baseline cylinder correction needed for the patient. The other uses of keratometer are:
- Keratometer is of great importance for fitting contact lenses.
- Keratometer can be used for calculating the power of intraocular lens to be implanted.
- Keratometer is useful to monitor pre and post-surgical astigmatism.
- Keratometer is helpful equipment for qualitative assessment of corneal integrity.

GENERAL PRINCIPLE OF KERATOMETER

Keratometer is based on the principle of convex mirror optics. It is based on the fact that the anterior surface of the cornea acts as a convex mirror. The size of image formed by cornea varies with its curvature. The greater the curvature of the cornea, smaller is the image size. Therefore, from the size of the image formed by the anterior surface of cornea, i.e, first purkinje image, the radius of the curvature of cornea can be calculated. However, it is difficult to measure the reflected image directly, because it is constantly moving as a result of microscopic eye movements. To overcome this problem, the principle of doubling is applied by using suitable prism midway in the observation system that forms a second image of the target and the effect of eye movement is nullified as both images move with the eye.

Keratometer measures the radius of curvature of very small portion of central cornea. The reflected image formed is very small in size and lies in anterior chamber of the eye, it is inaccessible for direct measurement. That is why a telescope is used to magnify the reflected image and forms the second image of the mire which is accessible for measurements.

Types of Keratometer

There are two types of keratometer available:
1. Two-position keratometer
2. One-position keratometer

Two-position Keratometer

The two-position keratometer **(Fig. 4.37)** requires rotation about the axis to measure each of the principal meridians. Javal-Schiotz keratometer is two position keratometer. Javal-Schiotz keratometer is based on the principle of variable object size and constant image size. The mires have variable separations and are mechanically arranged so as to allow the radius of curvature of the surface to be read from their separation.

One-position Keratometer

One-position keratometer **(Fig. 4.38)** does not require rotation about the axis. Simultaneous doubling of perpendicular pairs of mires is produced by doubling devices in each of the corresponding meridians. Bausch and Lomb keratometer is one position keratometer. The object in the B and L keratometer is the circular mire with two plus and two minus signs. A lamp illuminates the mire by means of a diagonally placed mirror. Light from the mire strikes the patient's cornea and produces a diminished image behind it. This image becomes the object for the remainder of optical system.

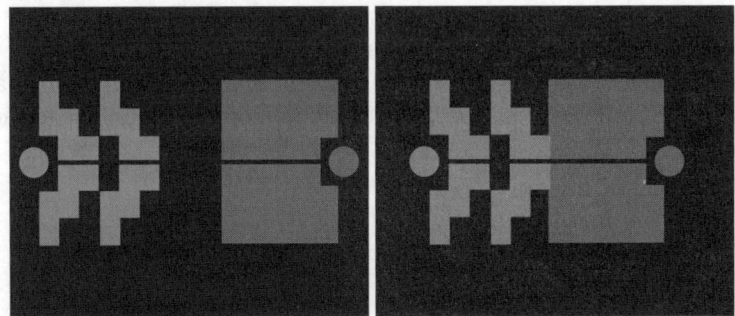

Fig. 4.37: Two-position keratometer.

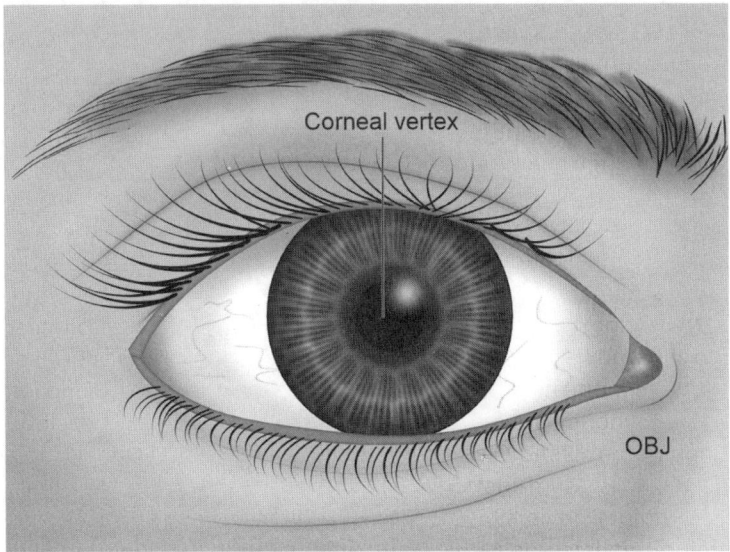

Fig. 4.38: One-position keratometer.

Estimation of Total Corneal Power

Keratometer gives only anterior corneal radius—it cannot measure posterior radius. The total corneal power reading is only an estimate. And this estimate is reasonable because the anterior cornea carries so much of the total corneal power. To do this keratometer uses a fudge factor in the index of refraction to account for the posterior corneal power and also to allow 45.00D to equal 7.50 mm radius of curvature.

Therefore, instead of calibrating the instruments for the true refractive index of the cornea (1.376) which would give a reading of the front surface power, a lower refractive index is assumed. Most instruments use 1.3375.

Axis of the corneal astigmatism can be measured by rotating the keratometer tube until the left mire and the focusing mire plus signs are not staggered but rather perfectly in line. For moderate to high corneal astigmatism, this is simple. To verify alignment for low astigmatism, the focusing mire can be thrown slightly out of focus, and the left mire plus sign should line up exactly between the doubled plusses.

An estimation of corneal astigmatism can be done by measuring the curvatures of the cornea at two principle meridian and recording the values as under:
- Flat K values: 44.00D @ 180 or 7.80 mm @ 180
- Steep K values: 45.00D @ 90 or 7.70 mm @ 90
- Estimated corneal astigmatism: -1.00D @ 180 degree

However, the amount of astigmatism derived by keratometer may differ from that of spectacle refraction. It may be more than the spectacle refraction, or less than the spectacle refraction or may be same.

CHAPTER 5

Community Ophthalmology

Ajay Kumar Bhootra, Sumitra Agarwal

INTRODUCTION

Community ophthalmology stands as a pivotal branch of medicine dedicated to delivering eye care services directly to the community, signaling a shift from traditional hospital-centric approaches. This specialized field prioritizes the prevention and management of eye diseases while fostering overall eye health within localities **(Flowchart 5.1)**. Recognized by various names such as public health ophthalmology or preventive ophthalmology, it has garnered significant attention within the broader ophthalmological community.

Flowchart 5.1: Components of community ophthalmology.

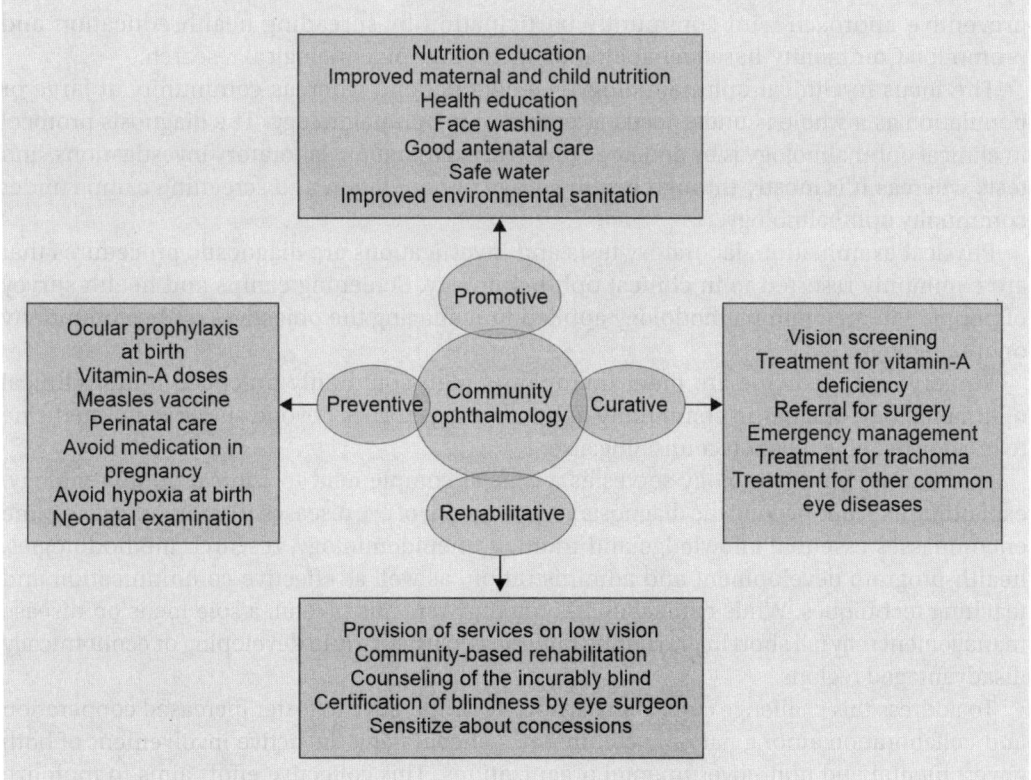

Source: Philippine Journal of Ophthalmology, Vol. 34, January-June 2009.

At its essence, community ophthalmology adopts a comprehensive approach encompassing preventive, curative, promotive, and rehabilitative activities. This holistic methodology integrates basic, clinical, and public health sciences, reflecting a departure from solely individualized care to a more community-centric paradigm. The core tenet of this approach is the realignment from exclusive hospital or clinic-based practices to inclusive community-based eye care services.

Unlike the confined setting of clinical ophthalmology, community ophthalmology extends its reach beyond the hospital walls, aiming to initiate eye care at the grassroots level. It envisions a health-management strategy geared towards preventing eye diseases, reducing eye morbidity rates, and fostering eye health through active community participation. The delivery of comprehensive eye care services is designed to commence where people reside and work, thereby addressing the unique needs of each community.

In essence, community ophthalmology transcends the confines of traditional medical settings, evolving into a dynamic and proactive health-management approach. The emphasis lies not only on treating individuals but on instigating preventive and promotional measures at the community level. As a result, public eye health emerges as one of the most challenging and crucial aspects of contemporary eye care. Through community engagement and a ground-up approach, community ophthalmology aims to redefine and elevate the standards of eye care, ensuring a healthier vision for entire communities.

Community ophthalmology differs from clinical ophthalmology in more than one ways. The primary goal of clinical ophthalmology is treatment and care. The goal in community ophthalmology goes beyond treatment and care and it also includes implementation of preventive approach with community participation by spreading health education and promotion Community-based rehabilitation including epidemiological research.

The focus in clinical ophthalmology is single patient, whereas community at large or population as a whole is under focus in community ophthalmology. The diagnosis protocol in clinical ophthalmology is by and large physical examination, laboratory investigations, and tests whereas it is mostly through health survey of population and screening camps under community ophthalmology.

Physical examination, laboratory tests and investigations are diagnostic procedures that are commonly resorted to in clinical ophthalmology. Screening camps and health survey of population are main methodology applied in managing the objectives of the community ophthalmology.

Surgery and medicine are main therapeutic plan commonly practiced under clinical ophthalmology whereas in community ophthalmology it goes beyond surgery and medicine to include health education counseling also.

Community ophthalmology serves as a crucial complement to clinical ophthalmology, expanding its scope beyond the diagnosis and treatment of eye diseases. This broader discipline encompasses essential knowledge and training in epidemiology, research methodologies, health-program development and administration, as well as effective communication and teaching techniques. While clinical ophthalmology remains pivotal, a sole focus on disease management may fall short in preventing blindness, particularly in developing or economically disadvantaged regions.

To address this challenge comprehensively, it is imperative to foster increased cooperation and collaboration among national committees, encouraging the active involvement of both governmental and non-governmental organizations. This collective effort aims to mobilize essential resources and cultivate political will to establish robust and effective blindness-prevention programs integrated into the broader national healthcare framework.

NATIONAL PROGRAMME FOR CONTROL OF BLINDNESS

The National Programme for Control of Blindness (NPCB) was initiated by India in 1976 as a 100% centrally sponsored program. The primary objectives of the program are as follows:

OBJECTIVES OF NATIONAL PROGRAMME FOR CONTROL OF BLINDNESS

Reduce Blindness Backlog

Identify and treat individuals suffering from blindness to alleviate the existing backlog of cases.

Develop Comprehensive Eye Care Facilities

Establish comprehensive eye care facilities in every district to ensure widespread access to eye care services.

Build Human Resources for Eye Care Services

Develop and enhance the pool of skilled human resources dedicated to providing eye care services.

Improve Quality of Service Delivery

Enhance the quality of service delivery for individuals affected by blindness, focusing on providing effective and efficient care.

Engage Voluntary Organizations/Private Practitioners

Encourage and involve voluntary organizations and private practitioners in the delivery of eye care services.

Raise Community Awareness

Increase awareness within the community about the importance of eye care, prevention of blindness, and the availability of services.

Provide Optimal Treatment for Curable Blindness

Ensure the availability and accessibility of the best possible treatment for curable blindness at the district and regional levels.

Establish Referral Mechanism and Coordination

Set up a robust mechanism for coordinating referrals, feedback, and collaboration between organizations dedicated to the prevention, treatment, and rehabilitation of blindness.

A significant prevalence of blindness within a population often indicates a combination of factors related to socioeconomic development and the efficiency of the country's eye care services. This is particularly concerning given that approximately 80-90% of cases of blindness are either curable or preventable. Notably, several key observations highlight the challenges and disparities in visual outcomes, especially after cataract surgery. The National Programme for Control of Blindness, therefore underwent pivotal moments in its evolution, marking notable milestones in its mission:

- A pivotal moment for NPCB occurred with its inclusion in the Prime Minister's-20 Point Programme in 1982. This recognition elevated the program's status, signifying its importance in the broader national health agenda.
- In 1983, the National Health Policy of India reiterated that blindness was an important public health problem and set a target to reduce the blindness prevalence rate from 1.4 to 0.3%.
- Another significant advancement for NPCB came with the initiation of the Cataract Blindness Control Project, supported by the World Bank from 1994 to 2001. This project targeted the reduction of cataract backlogs in seven states identified with the highest prevalence of cataract blindness based on a WHO—NPCB survey conducted from 1986 to 1989. These states, in descending order, were Uttar Pradesh, Tamil Nadu, Madhya Pradesh, Maharashtra, Andhra Pradesh, Rajasthan, and Orissa.
- The adoption of Vision 2020: Right to Sight in 2001 marked a prestigious milestone for NPCB. Aligned with the global initiative, this adoption reflected a commitment to eliminating avoidable blindness and enhancing vision care services. Vision 2020 emphasized collaborative efforts, technological advancements, and a comprehensive approach to eye care.

These transformative moments not only showcased the growing recognition of NPCB's importance but also demonstrated a commitment to strategic initiatives, international collaboration, and a holistic vision for eye care in India. The program's evolution from being part of a national agenda to targeted projects and global frameworks underscores its adaptability and commitment to addressing the multifaceted challenges of blindness prevention and control.

As of the present, the National Programme for Control of Blindness has evolved to encompass a broader spectrum of eye care initiatives. The program is currently funded to manage various eye health issues through successful public private partnership (PPP). Key focus areas include:
- NPCB is actively involved in the management of diabetic retinopathy, recognizing the increasing prevalence of diabetes-related eye complications.
- The program addresses the prevention and management of Glaucoma, a condition that can lead to irreversible vision loss if not detected and treated early.
- NPCB includes efforts to manage and prevent ocular trauma, recognizing the impact of injuries on vision and the need for timely intervention.
- Childhood blindness is a targeted focus, emphasizing the importance of early detection and intervention to prevent visual impairment in children.
- The program supports efforts related to keratoplasty, highlighting the importance of corneal transplantation for restoring vision in certain cases.
- Squint management is addressed, recognizing the significance of corrective measures for this condition that affects eye alignment.
- NPCB is involved in addressing low vision issues, emphasizing solutions and support for individuals with visual impairments.
- Special attention is given to retinopathy of prematurity, a condition affecting premature infants, with a focus on early diagnosis and intervention.

In addition to these specific focus areas, NPCB continues to implement ongoing schemes through effective PPP arrangements. The program also organizes the annual Eye Donation Fortnight from 25th August to 8th September, aiming to promote eye donation and eye banking. Several states, including Gujarat, Tamil Nadu, Maharashtra, Delhi, Chandigarh, Andhra Pradesh, Kerala, and Karnataka, are actively engaged in advancing these initiatives and are recognized as leaders in eye care activities.

This multi-faceted approach reflects NPCB's commitment to addressing a diverse range of eye health challenges and promoting collaboration between public and private sectors to enhance the overall eye care landscape in the country.

PLAN OF ACTION

The basic action plan of NPCB, since its inception in 1976, includes three activities as shown in **Flowchart 5.2**.

Extension of Eye Care Services

The initiatives aim to extend eye care services comprehensively, ensuring that even in challenging geographical and socioeconomic conditions; individuals have access to quality eye care. The focus is to reach the community through different channels. The three channels have been implemented, they are:
1. **Eye camps and mobile eye units:** Implementation of eye camps and mobile eye units to reach remote and underserved areas.
2. **Multipurpose district mobile ophthalmic units (MDMOU):** The initiative involves the development of MDMOU with the primary goal of expanding eye-care coverage. The objective is to bring comprehensive eye care to remote and underserved areas, addressing the unique challenges faced by these communities. Four-hundred multipurpose district mobile ophthalmic units have been approved for district hospitals in a phased manner. Preference will be given to remote/hilly areas including NE states and underprivileged regions to expand eye-care services.
3. **Tele-ophthalmology network units:** Tele-ophthalmology network units with linkage to ophthalmic consultation units in the medical colleges and RIOs are to be set up. The linkage and exchange of data is provided by internet.

Establishment of Permanent Infrastructure

The primary eye care at peripheral level has been strengthen by providing necessary equipment, posting a paramedical ophthalmic assistant, and organizing refresher courses for doctors and other staff of peripheral health centers on prevention of blindness.

Secondary eye care, at intermediate level, tertiary eye care, at central level, and center of excellence, at apex level for high quality tertiary eye care, and to provide guidance and leadership for technical matters.

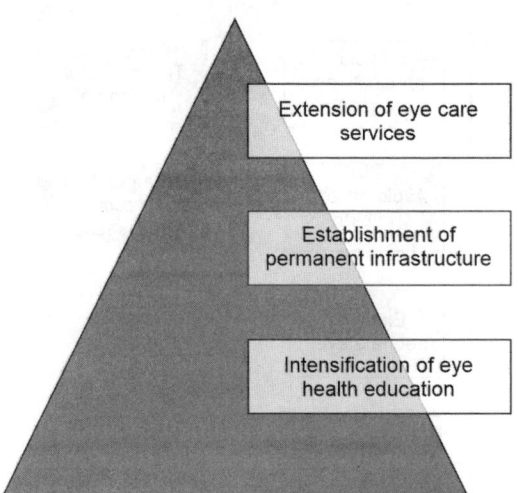

Flowchart 5.2: Plan of action and activities of NPCB.

Community ophthalmic practice at primary care level is summarized in **Flowchart 5.3**. By implementing these measures, the eye care system ensures comprehensive services at different levels, emphasizing prevention, accessibility, and quality care.

Intensification of Eye Health Education

Intensification of eye health education under 'Vision 2020: Right to Sight'—National Programme for Control of Blindness.

Adoption and Planning

- ❖ The Government of India adopted 'Vision 2020: Right to Sight' under the 'National Programme for Control of Blindness' during a meeting in Goa on October 10–13, 2001.

Flowchart 5.3: Community ophthalmology practice at primary level.

Promotive	Preventive	Curative	Rehabilitative
Nutrition education	Ocular prophylaxis at birth	Vision screening	Low vision services
Improved maternal and child nutrition	Vitamin A doses	Treatment for Vita A deficiency	Community-based rehabilitation
Health education	Measles vaccine	Referral for surgery	Counseling of incurable blind
Face washing	Prenatal care	Emergency management	Certification of blind by blind surgeon
Good antenatal care	Avoid medication in pregnancy	Treatment for trachoma	Sensitize about concessions
Safe water	Avoid hypoxia at birth	Treatment for other common eye diseases	
Improved environmental sanitation	Examine neonate eyes		
	Nutrition supplement		

❖ A dedicated working group was constituted to plan the action and activities for the effective implementation of the vision care initiative.

Implementation as per 'Vision 2020: Right to Sight India'

The vision care initiative, known as 'Vision 2020: Right to Sight India,' is now being implemented in alignment with the principles outlined in the original Vision 2020 program.

Educational Activities

❖ Eye health education activities are an integral part of 'Vision 2020: Right to Sight India.'
❖ Educational initiatives encompass awareness campaigns, school outreach programs, community workshops, and other targeted efforts to educate diverse populations about eye health.

School and Community Engagement

❖ Collaboration with schools to integrate eye health education into the curriculum, including regular eye screenings for students.
❖ Community engagement strategies involve interactive workshops, mobile health units, and digital platforms to disseminate eye health information widely.

Partnerships and Working Groups

❖ Forge partnerships with NGOs, media outlets, and local leaders to strengthen the impact of eye health education.
❖ Collaborate with working groups to plan and execute educational initiatives that align with the goals of 'Vision 2020: Right to Sight.'

Incorporation of Feedback Mechanism

❖ Establish and maintain a robust feedback mechanism to gather insights from the community.
❖ Utilize feedback to adapt and refine eye health education programs based on the specific needs and concerns of the target audience.

Alignment with NPCB

❖ 'Vision 2020: Right to Sight India' operates under the umbrella of the 'National Programme for Control of Blindness'.
❖ The initiative leverages the existing infrastructure and resources of NPCB to maximize the impact of eye health education and control blindness at the national level.

By refining and implementing these strategies under 'Vision 2020: Right to Sight India,' the Government of India aims to intensify eye health education, making significant strides in preventing blindness and promoting comprehensive eye care across the nation.

ACTIVITIES

The activities of "National Programme for Control of Blindness and Vision Impairment being implemented through Vision 2020: The Right to Sight launched in October 2001, 13 with strategies as shown in **Flowchart 5.4**.

Flowchart 5.4: Strategies under Vision 2020: The Right to Sight program.

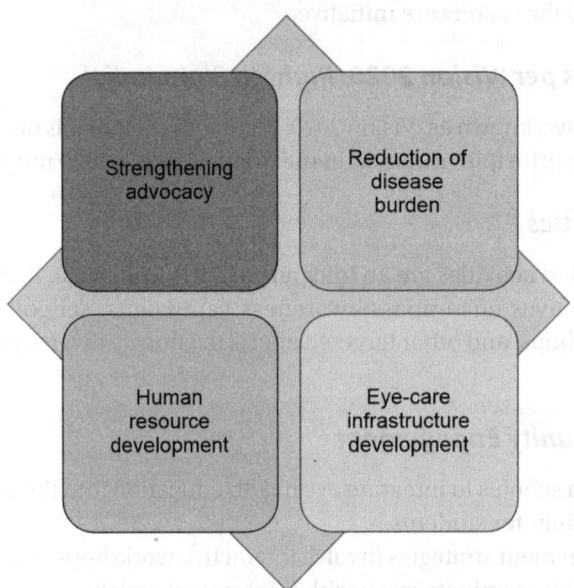

Strengthening Advocacy

To enhance the effectiveness of advocacy and raise public awareness on eye care and blindness prevention, a comprehensive strategy is proposed at the national, state, and district levels. The following activities aim to maximize impact:

Media Outreach

- Implement frequent press releases and articles in leading newspapers to disseminate information on eye care and blindness prevention.
- Increase the frequency of broadcast and telecast of messages related to eye care through various media channels.
- Incorporate eye care topics into school curricula to ensure early education on the importance of vision health.

Professional Organization Collaboration

- Foster collaboration with professional organizations such as the All India Ophthalmological Society (AIOS), Eye Bank Association of India (EBAI), and the Indian Medical Association (IMA) in the National Programme for Control of Blindness.
- Facilitate joint initiatives and campaigns to leverage the expertise and resources of these organizations.

Information Dissemination

- Publish quarterly newsletters and articles in scientific journals to update the public and professionals on advancements in eye care.
- Develop prototype print materials to be distributed widely, emphasizing the importance of regular eye check-ups and preventive measures.

District-Level Initiatives
- Strengthen the functioning of District Blindness Control Societies (DBCS) through capacity building, training, and resource allocation.
- Enhance collaboration with NGOs, local community societies, and community leaders to ensure grassroots involvement and a tailored approach to local needs.

Hospital Retrieval Programs
- Reinforce hospital retrieval programs for eye donation by implementing effective grief counseling.
- Involve volunteers, forensic departments, and the police in the process to streamline and improve the eye donation system.

Customized Public Awareness
- Tailor public awareness activities to local needs through effective media campaigns, considering cultural nuances and regional preferences.
- Engage with community influencers and leaders to amplify the reach and impact of awareness initiatives.

Reduction of Disease Burden
Target diseases identified for intervention include:
- Cataract
- Childhood blindness
- Refractive errors and low vision
- Glaucoma
- Diabetic retinopathy
- Corneal blindness

Cataract
Cataract remains the predominant cause of blindness, constituting 62.2% of blindness in the Indian population aged 50 and above, as per the latest National Survey (2015-2019). The primary objective is to enhance both the quantity and quality of cataract surgery. Efforts should be directed towards:

Increased quantity of cataract surgery
- Implement awareness campaigns to educate the public on early detection and the availability of cataract surgeries.
- Strengthen collaboration with healthcare providers and organizations to scale up cataract surgery outreach programs.
- Focus on reducing waiting times for cataract surgery through streamlined processes and increased surgical capacity.

Improved quality of cataract surgery
- Enhance training programs for ophthalmic professionals to ensure a higher standard of surgical procedures.
- Promote the use of advanced surgical techniques and technology for better outcomes.
- Implement regular monitoring and evaluation mechanisms to maintain and improve the quality of cataract surgeries.

By refining both the quantity and quality of cataract surgery, it is possible to significantly reduce the burden of cataract-related blindness in the population. This involves a comprehensive approach that combines awareness, accessibility, and continuous improvement in surgical practices.

Childhood Blindness

Childhood blindness poses a significant public health challenge in developing countries, given its social and economic impact. While the prevalence of childhood blindness is relatively low compared to blindness in the elderly, its significance lies in the substantial number of disability years for each blind child.

In India, the projected prevalence of childhood blindness is 0.8/1000 children, estimated through a correlation with under-five mortality rates. Common causes include vitamin A deficiency, measles, conjunctivitis, ophthalmia neonatorum, injuries, congenital cataract, retinopathy of prematurity (ROP), childhood glaucoma, and refractive errors which are the most common cause of visual impairment in children.

The primary aim is to eliminate avoidable causes of childhood blindness. To achieve this, a recommended schedule for ophthalmic examinations in children is as follows:

At the time of primary immunization

Integrate eye screenings with primary immunization programs to identify and address early childhood eye disorders.

At school entry

Conduct comprehensive eye examinations as children enter school to detect and address visual impairments, refractive errors, squints, amblyopia, and corneal diseases.

Establish a routine of periodic check-ups

- Every 3 years for children with normal vision.
- Annually for those with visual defects or identified eye disorders.

By following this schedule, the goal is to proactively detect and manage eye disorders in children, ensuring timely intervention and preventing avoidable causes of childhood blindness. This strategy emphasizes integration with existing healthcare programs and regular check-ups to address visual issues in a timely manner.

Refractive Errors and Low Vision

As per the 'Rapid Assessment of Avoidable Blindness (RAAB)' conducted in 2015–2019, refractive errors accounted for 13.4% of vision impairment in individuals aged over 50 and 29.6% in those aged 0 to 49.

To address refractive errors and low vision in India, the following targets have been established:

Widespread refraction services

Ensure the availability of refraction services in all primary health centers, facilitating easy access to eye examinations for individuals of all age groups.

Affordable spectacles for children

Guarantee the provision of low-cost, high-quality spectacles, particularly targeting children, to address and correct refractive errors at an early stage.

Establishment of low vision service centers

Set up low vision service centers at 150 tertiary-level eye-care institutions to cater to individuals with significant visual impairment, offering specialized services and aids.

By achieving these targets, the goal is to enhance accessibility to vision correction services, particularly for refractive errors, and provide support for individuals with low vision. This strategy aims to reduce the prevalence of avoidable visual impairment and promote overall eye health across different age groups in the population.

Glaucoma

According to the 'National Blindness and Visual Impairment Survey' (2015–2019), glaucoma accounts for 5.5% of blindness in the population aged 50 and above. Preventing blindness resulting from glaucoma is challenging, primarily due to difficulties in early detection.

To address this issue, the recommended strategy for glaucoma screening involves opportunistic interventions rather than population-based screening in developing countries. The refined approach includes:

Opportunistic screening at eye care institutions

Conduct screenings at eye care institutions for individuals aged 35 and above, those with diabetes mellitus, and those with a family history of glaucoma. This targeted approach ensures that high-risk individuals receive timely attention.

Community-based referral by multipurpose workers

Utilize multipurpose workers to refer individuals with symptoms such as diminution of vision, colored haloes, rapid changes in glasses prescription, ocular pain, and a family history of glaucoma to eye care services within the community.

Opportunistic screening at eye camps

Integrate glaucoma screening into eye camps, targeting individuals aged 35 and above. This ensures broader coverage and accessibility for those who may not routinely access eye care institutions.

By emphasizing opportunistic screening in high-risk groups and integrating it into existing healthcare structures, the strategy aims to enhance the early detection of glaucoma and improve the management of individuals at risk of glaucomatous blindness.

Diabetic Retinopathy

Diabetic retinopathy (DR) is gaining significance, contributing to 1.2% of blindness cases in the population aged 50 and above (National Blindness and Visual Impairment Survey 2015–2019).

To prevent visual loss resulting from diabetic retinopathy, timely intervention through periodic follow-up is crucial. The refined recommendations include:

Awareness generation by health workers

Health workers should actively engage in creating awareness about diabetic retinopathy, emphasizing the importance of regular eye check-ups among diabetic individuals.

Examination and referral by ophthalmic assistants

All known diabetic patients should undergo regular eye examinations conducted by ophthalmic assistants, who will then refer them to eye surgeons for further evaluation.

Confirmation by fundus fluorescein angiography and tertiary level treatment

Confirm the diagnosis using fundus fluorescein angiography (FFA) and provide treatment for diabetic retinopathy at the tertiary level, including laser treatment when necessary.

Medical management at secondary level

Implement a strategy to reduce the medical management of diabetic retinopathy at the secondary level, focusing on early detection and referral to tertiary care for advanced cases.

By integrating these recommendations into the healthcare system, the aim is to enhance awareness, improve the accessibility of eye examinations for diabetics, and ensure timely and appropriate intervention for diabetic retinopathy at the tertiary level. This approach can significantly contribute to preventing visual impairment caused by diabetic retinopathy.

Corneal Blindness

Corneal blindness poses a significant challenge, with 7.4% of cases in those aged >50 and 37.5% in those aged 0–49, according to the National Blindness and Visual Impairment Survey 2015–2019. Approximately 1,20,000 corneal blinds exist, with 25,000 to 30,000 new cases annually.

To address this, collaborative efforts from the public, government, education department, school teachers, general medical practitioners, and ophthalmologists are crucial.

General strategies

- Identify infants at risk through RCH programs.
- Conduct door-to-door surveys for pre-school children.
- Utilize school health services to identify at-risk school children.
- Identify senior citizens with post-cataract surgery bullous keratopathy.
- Ensure the supply of essential drugs for primary care.

Disease-specific strategies

- Health education and improved personal hygiene to reduce conjunctivitis and prevent corneal blindness.
- Educate people on avoiding ocular trauma from various sources.
- Address trachoma, which contributes to 0.8% of corneal blindness in India.
- Prevent xerophthalmia to reduce corneal blindness cases.
- Implement a total ban on quack ophthalmic practices and harmful eye medicines.
- Provide protective measures for industrial workers and agriculturists, including the use of goggles and eye shades.

Eye donation and keratoplasty

- Increase awareness through intensive publicity.
- Cooperate with government and non-government agencies.
- Organize eye donation fortnights annually (25th August to 8th September).
- Establish more eye banks and train ophthalmic surgeons for corneal grafting.
- Emphasize the hospital retrieval system for better donor material.
- Include a line on eye donations in death certificates.

Efforts are needed to bridge the gap between the annual need for 2 lakh corneas and the current collection of 60,000 eyes, highlighting the urgency for increased voluntary eye donations and improved infrastructure for transplantation.

Human Resource Development

For the 'Vision 2020' initiative in India, addressing the human resource needs to combat blindness by 2020 requires the development of mid-level ophthalmic personnel (MLOP) in addition to ophthalmic surgeons. The term MLOP encompasses various paramedics working full-time in eye care, categorized into two streams:

Hospital-based MLOP

This category includes ophthalmic nurses, ophthalmic technicians, optometrists, orthoptists, and similar professionals primarily working within hospital settings. Their roles involve assisting ophthalmologists, conducting diagnostic tests, and providing support in various ophthalmic procedures.

Community-based MLOP

This group involves individuals engaged in outreach and field functions, playing a crucial role in bringing eye care services to communities. It encompasses primary eye-care workers and ophthalmic assistants who operate beyond traditional hospital settings, focusing on community-level eye care.

The refinement emphasizes the diversified roles within MLOP, recognizing the specific skills and responsibilities associated with hospital-based and community-based personnel. By strategically developing and deploying MLOP, the Vision 2020 initiative aims to enhance the accessibility and effectiveness of eye care services, thereby contributing to the broader goal of reducing and preventing blindness in India.

Eye Care Infrastructure Development

Based on WHO recommendations, the development of eye-care infrastructure is envisioned through a hierarchical pyramid, addressing various levels of care:

Primary Level: Vision Centers

Establish 20,000 vision centers, each staffed with one ophthalmic assistant or equivalent (Community-based MLOP). These centers aim to cover a population of 50,000, ensuring primary eye care and early intervention.

Secondary Level: Service Centers

Develop 2,000 service centers at the secondary level, each equipped with two ophthalmologists, 8 paramedics (Hospital-based MLOP), and one eye-care manager. These centers are designed to serve a population of 5,00,000, providing more comprehensive eye care services.

Tertiary Level: Training Centers

Establish 200 training centers for ophthalmologists at the tertiary level. Each training center will cater to a population of 5 million, ensuring the continuous development of skilled professionals.

Center of Excellence (COE)

Develop 20 centers of excellence (COE) with well-developed sub-specialties of ophthalmology. Each advanced tertiary-level COE will cater to a larger population of 50 million, serving as hubs for specialized and advanced eye care services.

This refined infrastructure pyramid outlines the strategic distribution of eye-care facilities at different levels, ensuring a comprehensive approach to address eye health needs at the primary, secondary, and tertiary levels. The plan not only focuses on service delivery but also emphasizes the crucial aspects of training and specialization in ophthalmology.

BLINDNESS: CAUSES AND ITS PREVENTION

Blindness is a broad term encompassing various degrees of vision loss, including individuals with low vision who retain some visual capacity but require visual aids or adaptive tools for specific tasks.

Visual impairment is a comprehensive term that spans a spectrum of vision loss, ranging from mild to severe. This umbrella term encompasses various conditions, including partial vision, low vision, and other visual challenges impacting daily tasks. Levels of visual impairment, such as low vision or moderate visual impairment are used to categorize the severity of vision loss. Moderate visual impairment refers to individuals experiencing more substantial vision loss than those with low vision but still retaining some functional vision. Severe visual impairment denotes a higher degree of vision loss, necessitating a greater reliance on non-visual methods for daily activities.

Blindness generally denotes a complete or near-complete absence of vision, leaving individuals with minimal to no ability to see. Those who are blind often depend on alternative senses and tools, such as Braille, guide dogs, or canes, to navigate their surroundings. The legal definition of blindness varies among countries but frequently hinges on specific criteria, such as a defined threshold for visual acuity or field of vision.

In 1970, the term "Total Blindness" was utilized in India, specifically referring to individuals with no perception of light. A multicentric survey on blindness conducted in seven centers by the Indian Council of Medical Research between 1971 and 1974 reported on the prevalence of various categories, including "Total Blindness" (visual acuity less than 20/400 in the better eye with spectacle correction), "Economic Blindness" (visual acuity less than 20/200 in the better eye with spectacle correction), and "One Eye Blindness" (visual acuity less than 20/400 in one eye and better than 20/200 in the other eye with spectacle correction).

A Central Coordination Committee provided the definition of blindness as (a) vision of 20/200 or less with the best possible spectacle correction, (b) diminution of the field of vision to 20° or less in the better eye, or (c) one eye having vision of 20/200 or less with the best possible spectacle correction and the other eye having a visual field of 20° or less.

The current definition of blindness, as adopted under the NPCB, is characterized by presenting distance visual acuity (VA) less than 20/200 in the better eye. Additionally, a limitation of the field of vision to under 20° from the central point of fixation in the better eye is also considered indicative of blindness.

CAUSES OF BLINDNESS

There can be many different causes of blindness. The leading causes of blindness worldwide are depicted in **Flowchart 5.5**.

Refractive Error

Refractive error is a common cause of visual impairment, but it is not typically a direct cause of blindness. Refractive error refers to the inability of the eye to properly focus light on the

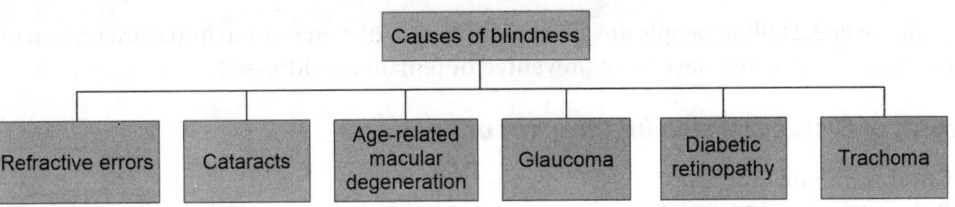

Flowchart 5.5: Causes of blindness.

retina, resulting in blurred vision. While refractive errors themselves do not cause blindness, uncorrected refractive errors can certainly lead to significant visual impairment and reduce the overall quality of life. Regular eye check-ups are essential to identify and address any vision issues promptly.

Cataracts

Cataract is a condition that causes yellowing and hardening of the lens in the eye, is the leading cause of blindness worldwide in developing and developed countries. Cataracts are generally treatable with surgery to replace the cloudy lens with an artificial one.

Age-related Macular Degeneration

ARMD, a condition that damages a part of the retina known as the macula, is the leading cause of blindness in Caucasians and those aged 65 and older. Certain lifestyle changes and early detection through regular eye exams can help manage ARMD.

Glaucoma

Glaucoma is a condition that damages the optic nerve, is the leading cause of blindness in African Americans. Regular eye check-ups and timely treatment, often with eye drops or surgery, can help prevent progression.

Diabetic Retinopathy

Diabetic retinopathy is a condition due to systemic diabetes, is the leading cause of new blindness in adults between 25 and 64 years of age. Managing diabetes through lifestyle changes, medication, and regular eye exams is crucial in preventing diabetic retinopathy.

Trachoma

Trachoma is also on the list of leading causes. However, the incidence is decreasing due to public health action.

Global disparities in the causes of vision impairment stem from variations in the availability, affordability, and accessibility of eye care services, coupled with differences in population education levels. In low- and middle-income countries, unoperated cataracts constitute a substantial proportion of vision impairment cases. Conversely, high-income countries exhibit a higher prevalence of conditions like glaucoma and age-related macular degeneration. For children in low-income countries, congenital cataracts are a major cause of vision impairment, while middle-income countries see a higher likelihood of retinopathy of prematurity. Notably, uncorrected refractive error persists as a leading cause of vision impairment across all countries for both children and adults, emphasizing the universal challenge of ensuring accessible and affordable vision care services worldwide.

Prevalence

Globally, over 2.2 billion people are affected by near or distance vision impairment, and nearly half of these cases could have been prevented or remain unaddressed.

Causes of Distance Vision Impairment or Blindness

- **Cataract:** 94 million cases
- **Refractive error:** 88.4 million cases
- **Age-related macular degeneration:** 8 million cases
- **Glaucoma:** 7.7 million cases
- **Diabetic retinopathy:** 3.9 million cases

Cause of Near Vision Impairment

- **Presbyopia:** 826 million cases.
- **Regional disparities:** Distance vision impairment is prevalent in low- and middle-income regions and is estimated to be four times higher than in high-income regions. Unaddressed near vision impairment exceeds 80% in western, eastern, and central sub-Saharan Africa. In high-income regions like North America, Australasia, Western Europe, and Asia-Pacific, rates are reported to be lower than 10%. Population growth and aging are anticipated to heighten the risk of more individuals acquiring vision impairment, necessitating ongoing efforts to enhance preventive measures and address unmet needs in eye care services globally.

STRATEGIES TO ADDRESS EYE CONDITIONS TO AVOID VISION IMPAIRMENT

Effective interventions encompassing promotion, prevention, treatment, and rehabilitation play a crucial role in addressing the diverse needs associated with eye conditions and preventing vision impairment. While numerous cases of vision loss are preventable (e.g., those stemming from infections, trauma, unsafe traditional medicines, perinatal diseases, and nutrition-related diseases), some conditions require targeted efforts for early detection and timely treatment to avert irreversible vision loss.

Prevention

- **Targeting infections:** Emphasizing hygiene and preventive measures to curb infections.
- **Trauma prevention:** Promoting safety measures to prevent eye injuries.
- **Safe medication practices:** Educating on the safe use of medications to avoid adverse effects.
- **Perinatal care:** Ensuring proper perinatal care to reduce the risk of associated vision issues.
- **Nutritional education:** Addressing nutrition-related diseases impacting eye health.

Timely Treatment

- **Diabetic retinopathy:** Emphasizing early detection and prompt treatment to prevent irreversible vision loss.
- **Refractive error:** Facilitating widespread access to spectacles for refractive error correction.
- **Cataract:** Promoting accessibility to quality cataract surgery, a highly cost-effective intervention.

Global Disparities

Only 36% of individuals with distance vision impairment due to refractive error have received appropriate spectacles, and only 17% with vision impairment or blindness due to cataract have received quality surgery.

Treatment for Comfort and Pain Management

Addressing non-vision-impairing conditions such as dry eye, conjunctivitis, and blepharitis to alleviate discomfort and pain.

Vision Rehabilitation

Offering effective rehabilitation services for those with irreversible vision loss, including conditions like diabetic retinopathy, glaucoma, trauma-related consequences, and age-related macular degeneration.

As population growth and aging increase the risk of vision impairment, these comprehensive strategies underscore the importance of global collaboration to enhance awareness, accessibility to care, and the effectiveness of interventions across the spectrum of eye health.

NATIONAL IMMUNIZATION PROGRAMME

INTRODUCTION

Immunization is the process of making an individual immune or resistant to an infectious disease, typically by administering a vaccine. It is a crucial aspect of public health and preventive medicine aimed at protecting individuals and populations from potentially serious or life-threatening infections. Immunization works in three stages as shown in **Flowchart 5.6**.

Vaccination

Immunization typically begins with the administration of vaccines, which contain antigens derived from specific pathogens, such as viruses or bacteria. These antigens stimulate the immune system to recognize the pathogen as foreign and mount a defence response.

Immune Response

After vaccination, the immune system produces antibodies and memory cells specific to the antigen introduced by the vaccine. Antibodies are proteins that can recognize and neutralize the pathogen, while memory cells "remember" the pathogen and can mount a rapid and robust immune response upon re-exposure in the future.

Protection

Through the process of immunization, the individual develops immunity to the targeted disease, which can prevent infection altogether or reduce the severity of illness if the individual

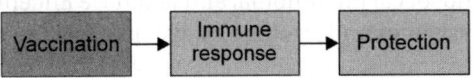

Flowchart 5.6: How immunization works?

is exposed to the pathogen. Immunization not only protects vaccinated individuals but also contributes to the concept of herd immunity, wherein a significant portion of the population becomes immune, making it difficult for the disease to spread within the community.

IMMUNIZATION

Immunization is considered one of the most effective and cost-effective public health interventions available. It has played a significant role in reducing the burden of infectious diseases worldwide, preventing millions of deaths and disabilities each year.

Immunization programs involve various components, including vaccine development and production, vaccination schedules and campaigns, monitoring vaccine safety and efficacy, and public education and advocacy. These programs are implemented at local, national, and global levels by governments, public health agencies, healthcare providers, and international organizations to ensure widespread coverage and protection against a range of infectious diseases.

According to World Health Organization, immunization stands as a triumph in global health and development, annually saving millions of lives. Vaccines reduce risks of getting a disease by working with your body's natural defences to build protection. When you get a vaccine, your immune system responds. With over 20 vaccines available, people of all ages enjoy extended, healthier lives. Immunization presently averts 3.5–5 million deaths annually, combating diseases such as diphtheria, tetanus, pertussis, influenza, and measles. Immunization is a key component of primary health care and an indisputable human right. The COVID-19 pandemic, associated disruptions, and COVID-19 vaccination efforts strained health systems in 2020 and 2021, resulting in dramatic setbacks. However, from a global perspective recovery is on the horizon.

Expanded Programme on Immunization

In India, the Expanded Programme on Immunization (EPI) was inaugurated in 1978 and later renamed the Universal Immunization Programme in 1985, extending its coverage beyond urban areas. In 1992, it became a part of the Child Survival and Safe Motherhood Programme, and in 1997, it was integrated into the National Reproductive and Child Health Programme. Since the inception of the National Rural Health Mission in 2005, the Universal Immunization Programme has remained an integral component.

Universal Immunization Programme

Universal Immunization Programme (UIP) in India targets approximately 2.67 crore newborns and 2.9 crore pregnant women annually, making it one of the largest public health initiatives in the country. It is widely acknowledged as one of the most cost-effective public health interventions, significantly contributing to the reduction of vaccine-preventable under-5 mortality rates.

Under the UIP, immunization is provided free of charge against 12 vaccine-preventable diseases nationwide, including diphtheria, pertussis, tetanus, polio, measles, rubella, severe forms of childhood tuberculosis, hepatitis B, and meningitis and pneumonia caused by hemophilus influenza type B. Additionally, sub-nationally, vaccination is offered against Rotavirus diarrhea, Pneumococcal pneumonia, and Japanese Encephalitis, with rotavirus and pneumococcal conjugate vaccines undergoing expansion, while the JE vaccine is administered only in endemic districts.

A child is considered fully immunized if they receive all due vaccines as per the national immunization schedule within the first year of their life. The UIP achieved significant milestones with the elimination of polio in 2014 and the eradication of maternal and neonatal tetanus in 2015.

Several vaccines have been introduced into the UIP in India to address various health concerns and improve public health outcomes:

Inactivated Polio Vaccine

Inactivated polio vaccine (IPV) was integrated into the UIP as part of the global polio end-game strategy to mitigate risks associated with the transition from trivalent Oral Polio Vaccine (tOPV) to bivalent Oral Polio Vaccine (bOPV). Introduced in November 2015 initially in 6 states, IPV coverage expanded nationwide by April 2016.

Rotavirus Vaccine

Rotavirus vaccine (RVV) was introduced in March 2016 to reduce mortality and morbidity caused by rotavirus diarrhea.

Measles Rubella Vaccine

India is committed to eliminating measles and controlling rubella. The measles rubella (MR) vaccine was introduced through phased campaigns in 2017. The campaign targeted around 41 crore children aged 9 months to 15 years, covering a significant portion of the country's population. Routine immunization now includes two doses at 9–12 months and 16–24 months, with the rubella component now part of routine immunization as MR vaccine.

Pneumococcal Conjugate Vaccine

Launched in May 2017, pneumococcal conjugate vaccine (PCV) aims to reduce infant mortality and morbidity caused by pneumococcal pneumonia.

Tetanus and Adult Diphtheria (Td) Vaccine

Td vaccine has replaced the tetanus toxoid (TT) vaccine in the UIP to address waning immunity against diphtheria in older age groups. Td vaccine is now administered to adolescents at 10 and 16 years of age, as well as to pregnant women.

Mission Indradhanush

Mission Indradhanush (MI) was inaugurated in December 2014 with the objective of elevating full immunization coverage among children to 90%. The initiative specifically targets regions with low immunization rates and areas that are difficult to reach, where the proportion of unvaccinated and partially vaccinated children is notably high.

As a pivotal component of public health efforts, MI was identified as a flagship scheme under both the Gram Swaraj Abhiyan and Extended Gram Swaraj Abhiyan. The Gram Swaraj Abhiyan encompassed 16,850 villages across 541 districts, while the Extended Gram Swaraj Abhiyan extended its coverage to 48,929 villages across 117 aspirational districts. Through MI, India aims to bolster immunization coverage, thereby fortifying the health and well-being of its population, particularly children who are most vulnerable to vaccine-preventable diseases.

New Initiatives

The initiatives in vaccine logistics and cold chain management in India encompass various aspects aimed at enhancing capacity, strengthening systems, and improving immunization programs. Here's a summary of these initiatives:

Capacity Building

National Cold Chain Training Center (NCCTE) in Pune and National Cold Chain & Vaccine Management Resource Center (NCCVMRC) in New Delhi have been established to provide technical training to cold chain technicians. Their focus is on repair and maintenance of cold chain equipment.

System Strengthening

The Government of India has implemented the Electronic Vaccine Intelligence Network (eVIN) system, which digitizes vaccine stock management, logistics, and temperature tracking at all levels of vaccine storage, from national to sub-district levels.

The eVIN system provides real-time visibility of vaccine stock positions and storage temperatures across all cold chain points, offering a comprehensive overview of the vaccine cold chain logistics system nationwide.

The eVIN system rollout has been completed in 12 states in the first phase and is ongoing in 9 states in the second phase. Eventually, eVIN is planned to be scaled up to cover the entire country.

National Cold Chain Management Information System

National Cold Chain Management Information System (NCCMIS) has been introduced to track cold chain equipment inventory, availability, and functionality, ensuring effective management of cold chain systems.

Immunization

- Programs include pulse polio immunization and routine immunization, which aim to vaccinate children against preventable diseases.
- Guidelines, reports, manuals, and formats are provided to support immunization efforts.
- Contacts for immunization are made available for coordination and information dissemination.
- These initiatives underscore India's commitment to ensuring the availability, proper storage, and efficient distribution of vaccines across the country, ultimately contributing to the success of immunization programs and improving public health outcomes.

CHAPTER 6

Drugs used in Optometry

Ajay Kumar Bhootra, Sumitra Agarwal

VASCULAR ENDOTHELIAL GROWTH FACTOR

Vascular endothelial growth factor (VEGF) is a signaling protein produced by cells throughout the body, including endothelial cells, which line the interior surface of blood vessels. It plays a pivotal role in angiogenesis, which is the formation of new blood vessels from pre-existing ones, and vasculogenesis, which is the formation of new blood vessels during embryonic development.

VEGF is crucial for various physiological processes, including:

Angiogenesis

VEGF promotes the growth of new blood vessels from pre-existing ones, a process essential for wound healing, tissue repair, and the female reproductive cycle.

Vasculogenesis

During embryonic development, VEGF plays a key role in the formation of the circulatory system by promoting the differentiation and proliferation of endothelial cells to form new blood vessels.

Vascular Permeability

VEGF increases the permeability of blood vessels, allowing fluids, nutrients, and oxygen to pass through vessel walls and reach surrounding tissues.

Inflammation

VEGF is involved in the regulation of inflammatory responses, including recruitment of immune cells to sites of injury or infection.

While VEGF is essential for normal physiological processes, dysregulation of VEGF expression and signaling can contribute to various pathological conditions, including:

Cancer

VEGF is overexpressed in many types of solid tumors, where it promotes the growth of new blood vessels to supply nutrients and oxygen to the tumor, a process known as tumor angiogenesis. Increased VEGF expression is associated with tumor progression, metastasis, and resistance to therapy.

Eye Diseases

In conditions such as age-related macular degeneration (AMD), diabetic retinopathy, and retinal vein occlusion, abnormal VEGF expression can lead to the growth of abnormal blood vessels in the retina, causing vision loss and other complications.

Cardiovascular Diseases

Dysregulated VEGF signaling is implicated in the pathogenesis of cardiovascular diseases such as coronary artery disease, peripheral artery disease and stroke.

Inflammatory Disorders

Aberrant VEGF expression contributes to the pathogenesis of inflammatory disorders such as rheumatoid arthritis and inflammatory bowel disease.

Due to its pivotal role in angiogenesis and vascular permeability, VEGF has become an important target for therapeutic intervention in various diseases, including cancer and eye disorders. Drugs that inhibit VEGF signaling, known as anti-VEGF therapies, have been developed and are widely used in the treatment of conditions such as cancer and certain eye diseases.

Anti-VEGF drugs are a class of medications designed to inhibit vascular endothelial growth factor (VEGF), a protein that plays a crucial role in angiogenesis (the formation of new blood vessels) and vascular permeability (the leakiness of blood vessels). These drugs are primarily used in the treatment of various eye conditions and certain types of cancer.

In ophthalmology, anti-VEGF drugs are primarily employed to treat conditions affecting the retina, particularly diseases associated with abnormal blood vessel growth and leakage, such as:

Age-related Macular Degeneration (AMD)

AMD is a leading cause of vision loss in older adults. Anti-VEGF drugs are used to treat the wet form of AMD, which involves abnormal blood vessel growth under the retina.

Diabetic Retinopathy

Diabetic retinopathy is a complication of diabetes characterized by damage to the blood vessels in the retina. Anti-VEGF drugs can help reduce abnormal blood vessel growth and leakage in diabetic retinopathy.

Macular Edema

Macular edema is the accumulation of fluid in the macula, the central part of the retina responsible for sharp, central vision. Anti-VEGF drugs can help reduce macular edema and improve vision.

Some commonly used anti-VEGF drugs in ophthalmology include:

Bevacizumab (Avastin)

Although not specifically approved for ophthalmic use, bevacizumab is frequently used off-label to treat various retinal conditions due to its anti-VEGF properties.

Ranibizumab (Lucentis)

Ranibizumab is approved for the treatment of wet AMD and other retinal diseases.

Aflibercept (Eylea)

Aflibercept is approved for the treatment of wet AMD, diabetic retinopathy, macular edema, and other retinal conditions.

Index

Page numbers followed by *f* refer to figure, *fc* refer to flowchart, and *t* refer to table.

A

Abbe number 98, 108, 109*t*
Abrasives 103
Absorption 111
    rate 82, 84
Accidental physical injuries 141
Accommodative dysfunction 185
Acoustic monitoring 80
Acrylic lenses 92
Adaptation time 211
Adaptive lenses 94
Adjustable strap pads 148
Administration technique 86
Adoption 268
Advocacy, effectiveness of 270
Aesthiometry 248
Aflibercept 284
Age-related macular degeneration 139, 140, 277, 278, 283, 284
Airway management 89
All India Ophthalmological Society 270
Allyl diglycol carbonate 92, 123
Alternative color vision tests 252
Aluminum 157, 159
Amblyopia 74
    treatment of 74
Amblyoscopes 259
American National Standards Institute 114, 115
Ametropia 215
Amplitude scan 255
Anatomical interpupillary distance 172*f*
Angiogenesis 283
Angle kappa, measurement of 259
Angle-closure glaucoma 52
Aniseikonia 185
Anisometropia 204
Anterior chamber
    angle 52, 244*f*, 246
        optimal examination of 246
    depth, assessment of 53
Antibiotic eye drops 69
Anti-reflective coatings 171
Anti-vascular endothelial growth factor drugs 62
Aperture 222
Aphakia 203
Applanation system, limitations of 217
Applanation tonometry 247
    semi-circles 217*f*
Aqueous deficient 13*t*
    dry eyes 13
Aqueous flare 234*f*
Artificial eye makers 196
A-scan 255
Aspheric lens 130, 131, 133, 133*t*
    profile 131*f*
Aspheric surface 133*f*
Asphericity, amount of 132*f*
Asthenopia 2

Asthenopic symptoms 193
Astigmatism 9, 10, 130, 203
    intensification of 10
    management of 10
    total 203
Atopic dermatitis 42
Atoric lens 130, 132
Atoric surface 132*f*
Atropine eye drops 8
    low dose 8
Audiobooks and voice-controlled devices 206
Auto refractometer 213, 214*f*, 215
    advent of 213
    clinical use of 214
    range of 215
Automated perimetry 253
Avastin 284
Aviator frames 153
Axial chromatic aberration 127*f*
Axis 99
    meridian 99
    specifies 99

B

Bagolini striated glasses 260
Base curve 100, 174, 212
Bausch and Lomb keratometer 261
Bell's palsy 25
Belt frame 143
Benjamin franklin 93
Best focus principle 214
Best form lens 129
Better vision 197
Bevacizumab 284
Bifocal lens 130, 132, 134
Bifocal spectacle lenses 134
Billiard's spectacle 188, 189*f*
Binocular vision 224
    estimation for state of 67
    grades of 259
Biocompatibility 201
Biomicroscope 228, 229
Bisphenol A 123
Bi-weekly disposable lenses 197
Black eye 73
Bladder care 90
Bleeding 55
Blepharitis 21, 21*f*
    anterior 22
    causes 22
    management of 23
    posterior 22
    types of 22, 22*t*
Blepharospasm 28, 28*f*
    diagnosis of 29
    exact cause of 28
    treatment of 29

Blind spot 61
Blindness 68, 71, 271, 276
    causes of 276, 277fc, 278
    childhood 272
    curable 265
    prevention of 265, 276
    total 276
Blood
    pressure 79
        control 58
        monitoring 78, 79
        range, normal 79
    sugar levels, tight control of 58
    vessels, growth of abnormal 283
Blue light exposure 140
Blue-yellow color blindness 75
Blurred vision 1, 10, 11, 17, 40, 49, 52, 58, 61
Blurriness, different types of 1
Body temperature, normal 76, 76t
Bonnet frame 142f
Bow frame 142f, 143f
Bowel care 90
Braille devices 72, 206
Branch retinal
    artery occlusion 63
    vein occlusion 63
Breathing
    difficulty 77
    support 89
Brightness scan 256
British Standard Classification of Refractive
        Index 108t
Broad beam 235, 235f, 236
    application 235
    procedure 236
    set-up 235
B-scan 255, 256
    ultrasonography 55
Bulbar conjunctival redness, severe 38
Burns 73
    chemical 73

C

Cancer 283
Capnography 80
Carbon fiber 156
    frames 157
Cardiac arrest 88
Cardiovascular diseases 284
    pathogenesis of 284
Cataract 48, 49f, 51, 271, 277, 278
    blindness control project 266
    causes of 49
    cortical 50
    family history of 49
    nuclear 49
    posterior subcapsular 50
    surgery 50
        campaigns 69
        improved quality of 271
        increased quantity of 271
    symptoms of 49
    types of 49, 50f
Cat-eye frames 153, 170

Catheter 83
Cells, identification of 235
Celluloid
    acetate 155
        material 144
    nitrate 155
    propionate 156
Central Coordination Committee 276
Central retinal
    artery occlusion 62
    vein occlusion 63
Central serous retinopathy 61
Central vision 284
Chalazion 20, 20f
    causes 20
    diagnosis of 21
    management of 21
    signs 20
    symptoms 20
Chemical stability 106, 116
Chinrest 258
Chromatic aberration 110f, 127, 134f
Ciliary congestion 37
Circular polarized lenses 137
Circulatory system, formation of 283
Clear vision, wider field of 131
Clinical ophthalmology, primary goal of 264
Clinical refraction 5
Clip-on spectacle 186
Closed-circuit television 72, 206
    systems 72
Cloudiness 129f
Cobalt blue filter 242, 243
Colmascope 104
Color blindness 74, 75
    cure for 75
    total 75
    types of 75
Color cosmetic contact lenses 198
Color perception 49, 137
    loss of 205
Color vision
    deficiency 75, 252
    testing 5
Commercial plastic photochromatic lens 94
Community
    engagement strategies 269
    ophthalmic practice 268
    ophthalmology 68, 263
        components of 263fc
        serves 264
        stands 263
        transcends 264
Community-based rehabilitation 264
    services 69
Comprehensive conjunctival examination 246
Comprehensive eye
    care facilities 265
    examination 7, 57
Concave lens 8, 210
    prismatic effect of 192f
Concomitant squint, types of 66
Conical beam 234
    examination 235
Conical cornea, optical treatment of 196

Conjunctiva 31
  diseases of 31
  examination 246
  palpebral 236
Conjunctival staining 13
Conjunctivitis 31, 32f
  allergic 32, 33
  bacterial 33
  causes of 33
  infectious 32
  non-infectious 32
  potential causes of 32
  types of 32t
Connective tissue disorders 51
Contact lens 10, 12, 195, 197, 198, 200-202, 239, 260
  clinical use of 202
  development of 196
  different types of 197
  fitting 243
  idea of 195
  manufacturing methods of 199
  material, general properties of 200
  surface 201f
    quality assessment 247
    wettability assessment 247
Contact tonometer 216
Continuous wear lenses 199
Contrast
  management 207
  sensitivity 205
  test 5
Convex lens 209
  prismatic effect of 192f
Cornea 36, 236, 246
  diseases of 37
  endothelial cells of 241
  inflammation of 37
  observe 239
Corneal abrasions 27
Corneal astigmatism, estimation of 262
Corneal blindness 271, 274
Corneal epithelium 233
  defect of 39
Corneal examination 234
Corneal health 71
Corneal infection 36
Corneal microcysts 239
Corneal opacity 40, 41
  causes of 40
Corneal radius, anterior 262
Corneal scarring 40, 233
  signs of 40
  symptoms of 40
Corneal surface 41
Corneal thickness mapping 251
Corneal topography 6, 8
Corneal transplantation 41
Corneal ulcer 39, 39f
  intensification of 39
  symptoms of 39
  treatment of 39
Coronary artery disease 284
Corrective lenses 8
  prescription of 9
  types of 116

Corridor length 101, 175
Corticosteroids 47
Cosmetic aspect spectacle dispensing 166
Cross curve 100
Crown 98, 118
    composition of 118
    glass 112
Cryotherapy 56
Crystalline lens 240, 247
    examination 247
    opacities 239
Curve variation factor 111
Cyclosporine 14
Cylinder 98, 115
    meridians 132f
    power 221
Cylindrical surface 99
Cystoid macular edema 62

D

Dacryocystitis 17, 17f
    causes of 17
    mild cases of 18
Dacryoscintigraphy 15
Daily disposable lenses 197
Dairy products 71
Debris left 106
Delivery systems 85
Demodex mites 22
Density 122
Depression curve 103
Descemet's membrane endothelial keratoplasty 44
Descemet's stripping automated endothelial keratoplasty 44
Destructive surgery, types of 64
Deuteranopia 252
Deviation
    angle of 67
    measurement of angle of 259
Diabetes 49
Diabetic retinopathy 55, 57, 58, 271, 273, 277, 278, 283, 284
Diamond face 161, 161f
Dichroic coating method 138
Difficulty seeing 10, 11, 49, 58
Diffuse illumination 236
    set up 237f
Digital device 173
    usage 180
Dilated eye exam 8
Dilated fundus examination 6
Dimensional stability 106, 116
Direct illumination 233, 236, 237, 238f
Direct ophthalmoscope 223, 223f
Direct retro-illumination 240
Dispersion
    high 109
    low 109
    medium 109
Disposable soft contact lens 196
Distance vision impairment, causes of 278
Distorted vision 2, 10, 58, 61
District Blindness Control Societies, strengthen functioning of 271
Diverse eye care delivery systems 70

Dominant eye 179
Double refraction 120
Double vision 2, 16, 49, 193
Drainage implant devices 54
Drooping eyelid 23, 24
Drop ball test 113f
Dry eye 2, 12, 13, 36, 185
    development of 13
    syndrome 24
    treatment options of 14
Dynamic adjustment plays 230

E

Eale's disease 63
Eccentric fixation 259
Ectropion 30, 30f, 31
    causes of 31
    treatment of 31
Eczema 42
Edema 239
Edger vomit 105
Elasticity, modulus of 202
Electronic devices 72
Electrooculogram 60, 257
Elevated body temperature 77
Elevated intraocular pressure 52
Embryonic development 283
Endophthalmitis 48, 58
    diagnosis of 48
    treatment of 48
Endoscopic dacryocystorhinostomy 18
Endothelial dysfunction 44
Engage voluntary organizations 265
ENT surgery 225
Entropion 29, 29f
    causes 30
    symptoms of 30
    treatment of 30
Enucleation 64
Epiphora 16, 17
    causes of 15
Epiretinal membrane 58
Episcleritis 44
    diagnosis of 45
Epithelial defect 38
Epithelial erosions 239
Epithelium 234
Erbium 118
Ergonomics 225
Esotropia 67
    accommodative 259
Establish comprehensive eye care
    facilities 265
Etching 101
Evaporative dry eyes 13t
Evisceration 64, 65
Excellence, center of 275
Exercise 78
Exophthalmometer 254, 254f
Exophthalmometry techniques 254
Exotropia 67
Extended wear lenses 199
Extraocular muscles 65
Eye Bank Association of India 270

Eye 26, 68
    alignment issues 194
    anterior 236
    camps 267, 273
    care 89
        infrastructure development 275
        institutions 273
        professionals 191
        services 265, 267
    contusions 73
    crossing of 67
    discomfort 10
    diseases 1, 283
        advanced centers for 70
        diagnosis of 223
    donation 274
    drops 26, 54
    examination of 1, 4, 10
    health education
        activities 269
        intensification of 268
    injuries 49, 55
    irritation 12, 27
    lid involvement 36
    movement 68
    pain 52
        severe 48
    redness 30
    removal of 16
    screening programs 69
        regular organizing of 69
    simple visual inspection of 41
    socket 68
    squeezing 3
    strain 11
    surgery 225
    watering of 14, 16
    wear 95f
Eyeball, destructive surgeries of 64
Eyeglasses 10
Eyelid 18
    abnormalities 16
    diseases of 18
    hygiene 23
    involuntary closure of 29
    oil glands, infection of 18
    surgery, clip on 25
    taping 31
Eyestrain 10
Eyewear technology 146
Eylea 284

F

Face description 167
Facial complexion 167
    study of 166
Facial nerve paralysis 26
    signs of 26
Facial shape 166, 167
    study of 166
Fatigue 36
Feedback mechanism, incorporation of 269
Femtosecond laser-assisted cataract surgery 51
Ferric oxide 118

Index

Fever 17, 68, 76
    causes of 77
    consideration for 76
    management of 77
Film lamination method 138
Filters, use of 242
Final checking completes process 165
Fine focus control 225
Flare, identification of 235
Fleischer's ring 23
Flexi wear 198
Flip-up spectacles 186
Floaters 4, 58
Flow rate 85
Fluorescein
    angiography 6, 55, 57, 60
    dye 15
    staining 38
Folding frame 144, 145f, 187, 187f
Forehead
    rest 258
    thermometers 76
Foreign body sensation 3, 26, 27, 30, 36, 38
Foster collaboration 270
Four mirror gonio lens 250
Fracture, orbital 68
Frame 144
    bridge of 147, 147f
    choice of 159
    ergonomics 167
        study of 166
    front 146, 147f
    material 170
        study of 166
        types of 154
    measurement of 176f
    pantoscopic angle of 186
    selection 162
    shape 169fc, 177
        study of 166
    specific measurements 175, 176fc
        position of 177, 177fc
    styles 169, 169fc
        study of 166
Free-form technology 101
Front curve 212
Fuchs' dystrophy 44
Full-rim frames 152, 183
Fundamental elements 116
Fundus fluorescein angiography 274
Fused bifocal design 135f
Fused multifocal lenses 136
Fusional amplitudes, measurement of 259

G

Galilean type biomicroscope 228, 229f
Gaze, cardinal directions of 259
Gender-wise classification 154
Glare 164
    and light sensitivity 40
    protection 140
Glass
    components selection 117
    distribution 120

lens 106
    blank manufacturing 116
    single magic pair of 207
    types of 120
Glaucoma 52, 271, 273, 277, 278
    acute 36
    exact cause of 52
    management of 54
    monitoring 253
    treatment of 54
    types of 52, 54
Goldmann applanation tonometer 216, 216f
Goldmann prism 217f
Goldmann type gonioscope 250
Goldmann visual field test 254
Gonioscope 249
    lens 249
    parts of 249
    types of 249
Gonioscopy 53, 248
Gradual vision loss 58
Graves' disease 25, 68
Gravity, specific 112
Grenough type biomicroscope 228, 228f
Groover 105

H

Haag-Streit type
    illumination system 226
    slit lamp 227f
Haidinger brushes 259
Hair color 167
    study of 166
Half-eye
    frame 187f
    spectacles 187
Halos around lights 52
Hand edging 165
Handheld magnifiers 205
Haploscopes 259
Hardness 106, 116
Harmful ultraviolet radiation 139
Hazy vision 49
Head injuries 88
Headaches 10, 193
Headband frame 143
Healthcare, important aspects of 76
Health-program development 264
Hearing aid frame 187, 187f
Heart rate
    monitors 78
    normal resting 78
Hemianopia spectacles 187, 187f
Hemorrhage
    subconjunctival 36
    vitreous 54, 55
Hertel exophthalmometer 255
Heterophoria 66, 259
Heterotropia 66
High index 108, 133
    glass 112, 118
Highly sophisticated proprietary software 126
High-power lenses 72
Home oxygen therapy 85

Homogeneity 116
Horner's syndrome 24
Hospital retrieval programs 271
Hruby lens 248, 250
Human faces, types of 159
Human resource development 275
Humphrey visual field test 253
Hydration 90
Hydrophilic polymers 201
Hydroxyethyl methacrylate 196
Hyperdeviation 67
Hypermetropia 9, 202, 215
    symptoms of 9
Hyperopia 130
Hypertropia 67
Hypo-deviation 67
Hypoglycemia 89
Hypotropia 67

I

Illnesses, heat-related 77
Illuminating techniques, types of 236
Illumination
    control 207
    Köhler's principle of 226f
    system 229, 258
Immune
    cells, recruitment of 283
    reactions 36
    response 279
Immunization 280, 282
    primary 272
    process of 279
    programs 280
Impaired conjunctival function 71
Impaired tear production 71
Implantable lenses 12
Inactivated polio vaccine 281
Indian Council of Medical Research 276
Indian Medical Association 270
Indian National Trachoma Control Programme 69
Indirect illumination 226, 236, 238, 238f
Indirect ophthalmoscope 223, 223f
Indirect retro-illumination 240
Industrial protection glasses 116
Infections 18
    bacterial 77
    fungal 77
    prevention 90
    severe 88
    viral 77
Inflammation 38, 283
Inflammatory disorders 284
Information dissemination 270
Infrared radiation protection 139
Infrared thermometers 76
Infusion 83
    pump 87
Inhibit vascular endothelial growth factor 284
Injection 124
    location of 82-84
    routes, types of 81
Injury, sites of 283
Insufficient tear production 13

Intermittent heterophorias 259
International Organization for Standardization 113, 14
Interpupillary distance 171
    measurement determines 191
Intraocular lenses, advanced 51
Intraocular pressure 215, 216
Intraocular structure, inflammation of 36
Intravenous push 82
Ionic charge 202
Iris 236, 240, 247
    examination 247
    sphincter details 239
Iron
    oxide 125
    pigment, enhanced contrast for 243
Irritation 30
Ishihara chart 251
Ishihara plates book 252
Itching 36

J

Javal-Schiotz keratometer 261
Johannes Gutenberg's invention 96
Joints 149, 150f

K

Keratectomy
    photorefractive 10
    phototherapeutic 41
Keratitis 37, 38f
    primary 234
Keratoconus 41, 41f, 204
    diagnosis of 243
    progression of 42
    treatment of 43
Keratometer 260, 262
    general principle of 260
    types of 260
    uses of 260
Keratoplasty 41, 43, 274
    penetrating 44
    types of 43fc
Keyhole bridge 148, 148f
Knife-edge principle 214
Koeppe gonio lens 250
Krause's glands 12

L

Lacrimal apparatus, diseases of 12
Lacrimal canaliculi 12
Lacrimal puncta 12
Lacrimal sac 12
Lacrimal tumor 15, 16, 16f
Lagophthalmos 25, 25f, 26
    causes 25
    degree of 26
    primary symptom of 26
    treatment of 26
Large print materials 72
Laser
    peripheral iridotomy 54
    photocoagulation 56
    therapy 57, 58

Index

trabeculoplasty 54
treatment 248
Laser-assisted in situ keratomileusis 10
Lashes 236
    examination 246
Laufer's assertion 95
Lazy eye 74
Lens 91, 128, 129f, 130f, 200f, 210f, 221, 223
    actual fitting of 165
    base curve of 212
    blank 97
    center of 190, 191f
    clock 105
    defects 126, 128
        types of 126fc
    design 127, 129, 130, 130fc, 171
    diameter 97
    diseases of 48, 51
    edging 162
    fitting 181
        special types of 174
    focal power of 130
    form 104, 212
    geometric center of 191f
    grooving 103
    insertion 181, 182, 182f-184f
    magnification of 208, 210f
    marking 104
    material, types of 106fc
    mounting of 183
    optical performance of 130f
    polishing 102
    power 99, 193, 195, 212
    prescription 91, 97
    prismatic effect of 189
    producers 93
    selection 162
    size 127
    specific measurements 174, 175fc
    standards 113
    subluxation of 51
    surface 97, 102, 125
        sequential process for 125fc
    thickness 212
    visual performance of 191
    washer 106
Lensmeter 221f
    adjusting eye piece of 221f
    types of 218
Library frame 145f
Lids 236, 246
    diseases 36
    swelling 38
Light
    changes, speed of 213
    flashes of 4, 55
    height 227
    influence of reflection of 165
    intensity 227
    loss of 110t
    reflection, phenomenon of 110
    sensitive lenses 136
    sensitivity 27, 36, 38, 141
    source 222, 249
    width 227

Lime 118
Linear polarized lenses 137
Lipid deposits 248f
Liver 71
Low vision 271, 272
    aids 71, 205
        benefits of 205
        types of 205
    care 207
    practice, basic principle of 207
    service centers, establishment of 273
Lucentis 284

M

Macular edema 284
Macular hole 58
Maddox rod 260
Magnesia 118
Magnification 208, 224, 237-242
    high 228
    index 209
    low 228
    med-high 233
    medium 228
Magnifiers 72, 205
Manokel 142f
Manual lensmeter 219, 219f
Manual pulse measurement 78
Manual refractometer 213
Mask
    non-rebreather 85
    use of 86
Mass 16
Measles rubella vaccine 281
Mechanical optics 91
Mechanical system 227f, 228
Medication administration 90
Meibomian gland 18
    evaluation 13
Melting 119
    point 116
Meridian 99, 115
Metal alloys 157, 158
Metal frames 151, 157
Metallic oxide coatings 139
Microcysts 239
Microincision cataract surgery 51
Minus lens
    prescription 186
    thinner edge profile of 109f
Mirror 223, 258
Mismatch lens 184
Mission Indradhanush 281
Mitsui chemicals 92
Mobile eye units 267
Modern slit lamps 230
Monel alloys 157, 158
Monitoring eye health 224
Monochromatic aberrations 127
Monocular diplopia 49
Monocular interpupillary distance 98
Monocular telescopes 72
Monomer, preparation of 123
Monovision 12

Index

Motion sickness 211
Mould assembly 123
Mucopurulent discharge 17, 38
Multifocal glasses 12
Multifocal lens 130, 132, 134
Multipurpose district mobile ophthalmic units 267
Muscle pulling sensation 193
Myasthenia gravis 24
Mydriasis 67
Myopia 7, 130, 202
    control lenses 8
    severe 8
    signs of 7
    symptoms of 7

N

Narrow beam 231
Nasal cannula 85
Nasolacrimal duct 12
National Blindness and Visual Impairment Survey 273
National Cold Chain Management Information System 282
National Cold Chain Training Center 282
National Health Policy of India 266
National Immunization Programme 279
National Patent Development Corporation 196
National Programme for Control of Blindness 69, 265, 266, 270
    and Vision Impairment 269
Near vision impairment, causes of 278
Nebulization 76, 86
Nebulizer device 86
Neoplasm 36
Neovascularization 239
Nerves, dysfunction of 65
Neurological disorder 24
Neurological monitoring 90
Neuromuscular disorder 24
Neurosurgery 225
Neutral density 242, 243
Newton's ring 103
Nickel
    alloys 157
    silver 158
Night blindness 70
Niobium 118
Non-contact tonometer 216, 217, 218f
Non-invasive techniques 251
Nutrition 90
Nutritional education 278
Nyctalopia 70
Nylon 156
    monofilament cord 182

O

Objective auto refractometer, limitations of 215
Observation 57
Occlusion treatment 67
Octopus perimetry 253
Ocular curve 100, 175
Ocular discharge 30
Ocular injuries, first-aid in 73
Ocular motility test 24
Ocular movement, examination of 67
Ocular surface integrity 243
Omega-3 fatty acids 14
One-position keratometer 261, 261f
Open-angle glaucoma 52
Ophthalmic lens 91, 114
    blank 117fc
        manufacture 116
    designs 130
    development of plastic material for 123
    evolution of 93
    material 106
    types of 133
Ophthalmic prescription lens making 124
Ophthalmology 1
Ophthalmoscopes 222
Ophthalmoscopy 6, 53
Opportunistic screening 273
Optic atrophy 64
Optic nerve 36
    assessment of 224
    diseases of 63
Optic neuritis 63
Optical aberrations 126
    types of 126fc
Optical coherence tomography 6, 53, 55, 60, 251
Optical lenses 126
Optical section 232, 232f
Optician uses prism prescription 194
Optometry, drugs used in 283
Optyl 145, 157
Oral thermometers 76
Orbit 68
    diseases of 68
Orbital cellulitis 68
Orbital exenteration 16, 64, 65
Orthokeratology 8
Orthoptic exercise 67
Orthoptic instruments 259
Oval face 159, 160f
Over-the-counter artificial tear drops 14
Oxygen
    masks 85
    permeability 200
    tent 85
    therapy 76, 84
    titration of 85
    transmission 200f

P

Pachymetry 53, 247, 250
Pad 148
    arms 149, 149f
    different types of 148f
Pain 44
    management 83, 84, 279
    severe 38
Panophthalmitis 48
Pantoscopic tilt 177, 178f
Papillary reaction, examination of 67
Papilledema 64
Pebble lenses 91
Perimeters, types of 253
Perimetry 53
Perinatal care 278

Periodic check-ups, establish routine of 272
Peripheral artery disease 284
Peripheral corneal erosion 238f
Peripheral vision
    changes 211
    loss of 4, 52, 55
Permanent blur vision 1
Permanent infrastructure, establishment of 267
Phacoemulsification 50
Photochromatic lens 118, 136, 136t
    benefits of 136
Photochromatic tints 93
Photochromic polarized lenses 137
Photography 53, 248
Photophobia 30, 39, 48
Physical trauma protection 141
Pince-nez frame 144, 145f
Pince-nez style 96
Pinguecula 35, 35f
Pinhole spectacle 188, 188f
Plano cylinder 99
Plastic
    frames 151, 155
    lens 94, 122
        blank manufacturing 122
        material, types of 98
    materials 144
    polymer 92
    spectacle lenses 107
    surgery 225
Plates, types of 252
Pneumococcal conjugate vaccine 281
Poisoning 88
Polarized lenses 136
    advantages of 137
    principle of 137
Polished lens surface 125
Polyhydroxyethyl methacrylate 196, 198
Polycarbonate 112, 124
Polymer 122
Polymerization 123
Polymerized methyl methacrylate 92
Polymethyl methacrylate 196
Posterior segment abnormalities 215
Potassium 118
Power meridian 99
Power reading scale 221f
Precious metals gold 157
Prentice rule states 193
Presbyopia 11, 204, 278
    correction of 94
    management of 11
    onset of 11
Prescription
    eyeglasses 8, 10
    frames 153
Pressure
    diastolic 79
    systolic 79
Previous eye surgery, complications of 58
Primary deviation, measurement of 259
Primary eye care 267
Prism 100, 192f, 194, 223
    amount of 193
    correction 194

    dispensing of 189, 193
    power 193
Prismatic power 116
Progressive lenses 12
Proptosis 68
    measurement 254
Protanopia 252
Protective lenses 139
Protein 248f
Pseudomyopia 215
Pterygium 34, 34f
    causes 34
    mild cases of 35
Ptosis 23, 23f
    acquired 24
    causes 23
    degree of 24
    evaluation of 24
    frames 188
    mild 25
    permanent 24
    spectacle 188f
    treatment of 25
Public health
    ophthalmology 263
    sciences 264
Puffy eyes 36
Pulse
    monitoring 78
        methods of 78
    oximetry 78, 80
Punctal plugs 14
Pupil 36, 236
Pupillary distance, incorrect measurement of 186
Pupillary response, absent 48
Pus 68

Q

Quality control 121, 162

R

Ranibizumab 284
Ray-Ban shape 145f
Ray-deflection principle 214
Reading
    frames 154
    glasses 11, 72
Rectal thermometers 76
Recumbent spectacles 188, 188f
Red eyes 3, 36
    causes 36
    management of 37
    treatment of 37
Red free filter 243
Red-green color blindness 75
Redness 27, 44
    around eye 68
Reflectance 110
Reflex epiphora 30
Refraction 9, 10
    error of 6, 6fc
    index 98
    test 8

Refractive error 50, 74, 271, 276, 278
    calculation of 214
    correction of 66, 67
Refractive index 107, 108, 110, 112
Refractive surgery 9, 10, 12
Refractometer 213
    operates 213
Regular monitoring 54, 90
Resin lens 106, 139
Respiration monitoring 79
Respiratory depth 80
Respiratory rate 80
Respiratory rhythm 80
Retina 240, 283
    diseases of 58
Retinal correspondence
    estimation of 259
    treatment of abnormal 259
Retinal detachment 57, 59
Retinal examination 9, 10, 57, 60, 223
Retinal vein occlusion 63, 283
Retinoblastoma 62
Retinopathy, hypertensive 58, 59
Retinoscopic principle 214
Retinoscopy 5
Retro-illumination 236, 239, 240, 240*f*
Rhegmatogenous retinal detachment 60
Rigid gas permeable contact lenses 198
Rimless frame 145*f*, 152, 183
Rivet frame 142, 142*f*
Rocking pads 148
Rolled gold 157, 158
Rotate power wheel 221
Rotavirus vaccine 281
Round face 153, 160, 160*f*

S

Saddle bridge 148
    ideal fitting of 148*f*
Safe medication practices 278
Scales 258
Scatter light 128
Scheiner disc principle 214
Schirmer's test 13, 14
School Eye Health Programs 69
Sclera 236
    diseases of 44
Scleritis 45
    causes of 45
    symptoms of 45
    treatment of 46
Sclerotic illumination 236
Sclerotic scatter 226
Screen magnification software 206
Seborrheic dermatitis 22
Secondary deviation, measurement of 259
Secondary eye care 267
Segment inset 105, 175
Seizures 77, 89
Semi-finished lens 124
Semi-rimless frame 146*f*, 152
Sensitivity 48, 51, 185
Service delivery, enhance quality of 265
Set up low vision service centers 273

Sexually transmitted infections 32
Silica 118
Silicone hydrogel lenses 198
Silver 157
Simpler lens care 197
Single control element 229
Skin care 89
Sleep, lack of 36
Sleep-wake cycle 140
Slit illumination
    system 227
    unit 227*f*
Slit lamp 227*f*, 229, 230, 233
    additional use of 247
    base of 229*f*
    basic parts of 227
    beam reaches 247
    biomicroscope 15, 27, 225
    clinical use of 230
    examination 5, 38, 60, 231*fc*, 245
    illumination 226*f*
    principles of 225
    types of 226
    user experience of 230
Sodium 118
Soft contact lenses 198, 248*f*
Soft hydrogel lenses 198
Soft lens manufacturing methods 200
Soft metal alloy 125
Solid tumors, types of 283
Special dispensing measurements 174, 174*fc*
Specific surgical technique 31
Spectacles 91, 95, 166
    dispensing 161
        steps of 162*fc*
    evolution of 97
    frame 141, 151
        classification of 152*fc*
        clip on 187*f*
        parts of 146c
        selection, laws of 159*fc*
        temple of 143, 149*f*
    functional dispensing of 161
    glass blanks 117*f*
    intolerance 184
    lenses 92, 138, 211
        effectiveness of 93
    mounted magnifiers 206
    special types of 186
Spectrum, infra-red end of 118
Specular illumination 236, 241, 241*f*
Sphere 131*f*
Spheric surface 133*f*
Spherical lens 130, 131
    surface 131*f*
Sphero-cylinder 99
Spirometry 80
Sports
    frames 153, 188
    sunglass 189*f*
Spring loaded joints 150, 150*f*
Square face 161, 161*f*
Square frames 153
Squint 74
    latent 66
    manifest 66

non-paralytic 66
paralytic 65
Standard visual acuity test 42
Staphylococcus aureus 32
Staphyloma 46
   anterior 46
   causes 46
   management of 46
   posterior 46
   types of 46*t*
Stereomicroscope system 227*f*, 228
Stereopsis, presence of 259
Stones 128
Strabismus 65, 65*f*, 67
   intensification of 67
   types of 65
Strategies Under Vision 2020: Right to Sight Program 270*fc*
Streptococcus pneumoniae 32
Stress 128, 129*f*
Striae 128, 129*f*
Stroke 88, 284
Stroma 234
Stromal infiltrates 38
Strontium 118
Stye 18, 19*f*, 20, 20*t*, 151
   diagnosis of 19
   types of 19*t*
Superficial keratopathy 30
Suppression, treatment of 259
Supra frames 182
Surface power 101, 104
Surgery 51, 57
Sussman gonio lens 250
Swan-Jacobs gonio lens 250
Sweating 77
Swelling around eye 16, 68
Swimming sunglass 189, 189*f*
Synoptophore 258
   uses of 258

T

Tangential illumination 236, 242
   lies, primary significance of 242
Task specific spectacles 186
Tear 17, 36, 57
   artificial 13, 31
   duct blockage 15
   excessive 14, 48
   film
      debris 241
      evaluation 14
      examination 246
      lipid layer 241
Tele-ophthalmology Network Units 267
Telescopic lenses 206
Temperature, monitoring 76
Temple frame 144*f*
Tetanus
   and adult diphtheria vaccine 281
   toxoid 281
Thermal expansion 122
Thermoplastics 123
   manufacturing of 124
Thermosetting, manufacturing of 123

Thread frame 142*f*
Tinted lenses 138
Titanium 157
Tolerance 115, 116
Tonometry 5, 53
Top joint frames 168*f*
Total corneal power, estimation of 262
Trabeculectomy 54
Trachoma 277
Traditional lenses 197
Transparency 106
Transverse test 104
Trauma 36, 51, 68, 88
   prevention 278
   signs of 24
Triangular face 161, 161*f*
Trichiasis 15, 26, 27, 27*f*, 28
   causes of 27
   symptoms of 27
   treatment options of 28
Trifocal lens 134, 135*f*
Tritanopia 252
Tumor
   angiogenesis 283
   orbital 68
Tunnel vision 52
Two-position keratometer 261, 261*f*
Tyndall's phenomenon 234*f*

U

Ulcers 27
Ultrasound
   imaging 6, 57, 60
   pachymetry 251
Ultraviolet light 35
Ultraviolet radiation 49
   protection 139
Uncut lens 165, 190
Unisex frames 154
Universal Immunization Programme 280
Upswept shape frame 146*f*
Uvea, diseases of 47
Uveitis 36, 47
   intensification of 47

V

Vaccinations 77, 279
Vacuoles 239
van Herrick technique 244, 244*f*
Varnish 102
Vascular abnormalities 68
Vascular endothelial growth factor 283
Vascular permeability 283
Vasculogenesis 283
Venturi mask 85
Vertex 104
   distance 174*f*, 178, 212
   distance measurement 173
Vertical beam 233
Vertical phoria 185
Vertical strabismus 67
Very high index 108
Vesicles, epithelial 239

Vision 16, 48, 140, 164
    changes 68
    disturbances 38
    field of 58
    impairment 278
    loss 283
    rehabilitation 279
    therapy 9, 66
Visual acuity 40, 165, 205
    examination of 67
    normal 44
    test 5, 9, 10, 24, 38, 60
Visual axis 191f
Visual distortion 211
Visual disturbances 51
Visual evoked
    potential 6, 257
    response 257
Visual field
    defect 205, 254
    examination 60
    test 6
        types of 253
Visual habits and biometric data 179, 179fc
Visual impairment 276
Visual inspection 80
Visual satisfaction
    stages of 164
    triad 164fc
Vitamin A
    deficiency 70
    supplementation 69
    sources of 71t
Vitrectomy 56, 57
    indications for 57
    procedure 58
Vitreous hemorrhage 54, 55
    symptoms of 55

Vitreous humor, evaluation of 224
Vitreous opacities 56, 57
    causes of 56
    intensification of 57
Volk lens 248
Vomiting, persistent 77

W

Wandering eye 67
Warm compresses 13, 19
Watering eyes, treatment of 15
Wayfarer frames 153
Wide beam 233, 233f
Widespread refraction services 272
Wolfring's glands 12
Worth 4-dot test 260
Wounds, puncture 73

X

X chromosome 74
Xerophthalmia 71

Y

Y chromosome 74
Yellow filter 242, 243

Z

Zeis, gland 18
Zeiss type
    gonioscope 250
    illumination system 226
    slit lamp 227f
Zero curvature, line of 99
Zirconium 118
Zyl frames 181